INDUSTRIAL MICROBIOLOGY

INDUSTRIAL MICROBIOLOGY

THIRD EDITION

(In two colours)

L E Casida J R

Pennsylvania State University

NEW AGE TECHNO PRESS

An Imprint of

NEW AGE INTERNATIONAL (P) LIMITED, PUBLISHERS

LONDON • NEW DELHI

Bangalore • Chennai • Cochin • Guwahati • Hyderabad • Kolkata • Mumbai

Visit us at www.newagepublishers.com

Published by New Age International (P) Ltd., Publishers
First Edition: 1968
Third Edition (*In two colours*): **2026**

GLOBAL OFFICES

- **New Delhi** — **NEW AGE INTERNATIONAL (P) LIMITED, PUBLISHERS**
  7/30 A, Daryaganj, New Delhi-110002, (INDIA), **Tel.:** (011) 23253472, 23253771
  E-mail: contactus@newagepublishers.com • Visit us at www.newagepublishers.com
- **London** — **NEW AGE INTERNATIONAL (UK) LTD.**
  27 Old Gloucester Street, London, WC1N 3AX, UK
  E-mail: info@newacademicscience.co.uk • Visit us at www.newacademicscience.co.uk

BRANCHES

- **Bangalore** — 37/10, 8th Cross (Near Hanuman Temple), Azad Nagar, Chamarajpet, Bangalore- 560 018
  Tel.: (080) 26756823, **E-mail: bangalore@newagepublishers.com**
- **Chennai** — 26, Damodaran Street, T. Nagar, Chennai-600 017, **Tel.:** (044) 24353401
  E-mail: chennai@newagepublishers.com
- **Cochin** — CC-39/1016, Carrier Station Road, Ernakulam South, Cochin-682 016
  Tel.: (0484) 4051304, **E-mail: cochin@newagepublishers.com**
- **Guwahati** — Hemsen Complex, Mohd. Shah Road, Paltan Bazar, Near Starline Hotel
  Guwahati-781 008, **Tel.:** (0361) 2513881, **E-mail: guwahati@newagepublishers.com**
- **Hyderabad** — 105, 1st Floor, Madhiray Kaveri Tower, 3-2-19, Azam Jahi Road, Near Kumar Theater
  Nimboliadda Kachiguda, Hyderabad-500 027, **Tel.:** (040) 24652456
  E-mail: hyderabad@newagepublishers.com
- **Kolkata** — RDB Chambers (Formerly Lotus Cinema) 106A, 1st Floor, S N Banerjee Road
  Kolkata-700 014, **Tel.:** (033) 22273773, **E-mail: kolkata@newagepublishers.com**
- **Mumbai** — 142C, Victor House, Ground Floor, N.M. Joshi Marg, Lower Parel, Mumbai-400 013
  Tel.: (022) 24927869, 24915415, **E-mail: mumbai@newagepublishers.com**
- **New Delhi** — 22, Golden House, Daryaganj, New Delhi-110 002, **Tel.:** (011) 23262368, 23262370
  E-mail: sales@newagepublishers.com

C-25-02-14586

Printed in India at Parmanand Offset, Delhi.
Typeset at In-house, Delhi.

NEW AGE INTERNATIONAL (P) LIMITED, PUBLISHERS
7/30 A, Daryaganj, New Delhi - 110002
Visit us at **www.newagepublishers.com**
(CIN: U74899DL1966PTC004618)

Preface to the Third Edition

After the good response of the earlier editions it is a pleasure for us to present the third edition. In this edition some Reagents and Buffers are added for the benefit of the students. Necessary corrections are incorporated in response to the suggestions made by many teachers and students and all attempts are made to make the book error free.

We would like to acknowledge the valuable advice and suggestions of many instructors and students who used the earlier editions. We would be grateful to our esteem readers for suggestions in the interest of the subject.

Publisher

Preface to the First Edition

Industrial microbiology encompasses a broad and complex area of study. It includes the many uses of microorganisms to produce products of economic value and to decompose the wastes of municipalities and industry. In addition, it includes the prevention of unwanted growth of microorganisms and the resultant deterioration of natural and man-made materials. Various disciplines, in addition to microbiology *per se*, also must be considered as part of industrial microbiology. Among these disciplines are engineering, economics, and patent law—subjects not normally considered to be within the realm of study for a course in microbiology.

This book was written as an introductory text to provide the college junior or senior student, or the industrial technician needing to gain an insight into this area, with a working knowledge of the theory and practice of various aspects of industrial microbiology. Since the entire field of industrial microbiology could not be covered in a single book, some readers may find what they consider to be glaring omissions. Also, extensive presentations of the physiology and genetics of microoranisms are not included in this book, nor are extensive descriptions of individual groups of microorganisms. While these considerations are of distinct importance to industrial microbiology, I feel that the student either will have already studied these areas or can consult text and reference books for pertinent or additional information.

Individual subjects within the boundaries of industrial microbiology cannot be penetrated in depth in an introductory textbook. In fact, it is considered that penetration in depth is not desirable in an introductory text on this subject, since information should be presented in a form usable in the learning process and not in the form of a reference manual. Therefore, I have written this book in terms of the most commonly practiced industrial uses of microorganisms, with emphasis on industrial fermentations. I have assumed that most of the students reading this text will find employment in the fermentation industries, and that a knowledge of this area will allow the student to think and work in other areas not specifically covered by the material presented.

The style and sequence of presentation of material in this book departs somewhat from that employed in other books on the subject. Since many industrial fermentation processes are basically similar, with similar underlying concepts, a knowledge of the concepts and workings of one process allows an understanding of other processes that differ only in the microorganisms used, or in variables such as aeration, agitation, temperature, and incubation period. Thus, in this book, certain fermentation processes are considered as "type" fermentations, and are described at greater length than are similar fermentations that differ only by the above parameters. While this approach does not tell the student precisely how to carry out each of the known fermentation processes, it does allow him to grasp more easily the basic concepts underlying the various fermentations without having to contend with a vast array of process variables that may or may not be important. Information on these process variables may be found in reference books, patents, review articles, and published symposia, assuming, of course, that the actual process details are not industrial secrets.

Some of the industrial fermentation processes presented are not actually practiced at the present time. In most instances, this is because the economics favor nonmicrobial processes for producing the same or similar products. However, the concepts on which these fermentation processes are based are valid and, with an improvement in the process or a change in its economic picture, the process might become commercially practical.

Various concepts of industrial microbiology research also are considered in this book, as are some of the techniques employed in the handling of industrial cultures, and in the detection, assay, and purification of fermentation products. A consideration of research is included, not only because the student may find employment in an industrial research laboratory but also because the concepts of an industrial process will be more clearly understood if the research approaches required for the discovery and development of the process are understood. An understanding of the handling of industrial culture and of the detection, assay, and purification of industrial fermentation products is of considerable importance because, without these procedures, an industrial fermentation process could not exist. Obviously, new techniques are continuously being developed, but they usually are somewhat similar to present techniques, or their use will be better understood when based on a knowledge of presently available techniques.

This book also explores areas of industrial microbiology not normally included in texts on the subject. Thus, the economics associated with industrial microbiology industries are considered, and salient points of patent law are outlined. The purpose of this is to enable the student to think in these terms when considering the applications and possibilities of industrial microbiology.

Thus, overall, I hope that, through the use of this book, the student will gain insight into many of the aspects of industrial microbiology. He should understand how to isolate and grow microorganisms of industrial importance, how physical and chemical factors of the microorganisms' environment affect growth, and how to dissociate growth from biochemical synthesis. He should understand the known metabolic pathways of microorganisms and how they can be controlled. He should know the morphological and physiological growth patterns of microorganisms of industrial importance. He should understand the economics of the production of microbial products of industrial importance, and of competition on the open market. He should be familiar with at least certain points of patent law, and with the competitive position afforded by patents. He should have a working knowledge of the genetics and physiology of microorganisms, and should understand the problems associated with and the methods for control of culture stability. He should be familiar with the types, operations and limitations of fermentation equipment, and should understand the procedures for growing microorganisms on a large scale and for providing, for example, sufficient aeration, temperature control, and antifoam control. Finally, he should be familiar with how new industrial fermentation processes are discovered and developed to an economically feasible state. Knowledge in these areas combined with an understanding of the concepts of various presently practiced industrial fermentation processes should allow the student to work with confidence in industry.

I thank the following individuals for reading and commenting on various portions of this manuscript : F. W. Tanner of Charles Pfizer and Co., Inc. ; I. L. Wolk of Merck and Co., Inc. ; J. S. Isherwood of the Pittsburgh Brewing Co.; R. G. Beaman of Yeomans Brothers Co.; and E. S. Lindstrom, L. N. Zimmerman, C. F. Pootjes, and W. A. Eberhartt of Pennsylvania State University.

L. E. Casida, Jr.

Contents

PART I

INTRODUCTION

CHAPTER 1

Definition and Scope of Industrial Microbiology

Industrial microbiology deals with all forms of microbiology which have an economic aspect. It deals with those areas of microbiology on which, in some manner, a monetary value can be placed, regardless of whether the microbiology involves a fermentation product or some form of deterioration, disease, or waste disposal. In most instances, the economic criterion applies to a desire either to cause or to allow some specific type of growth or metabolic activity or to prevent microbial growth. These considerations make it apparent that industrial microbiology is a very broad area for study. In fact, many nonindustrial areas of microbiology are important to industrial microbiology, and should be taken into consideration in understanding the concepts and practice of industrial microbiology. These areas include, among others, soil and agricultural microbiology, medical microbiology, microbial physiology, cytology and morphology, virology, genetics, marine microbiology, food and dairy microbiology, and immunology. Disciplines not normally considered to be included in microbiology also are important to industrial microbiology and include organic, inorganic, and physical chemistry, biochemistry, engineering, medicine, economics, sales, and law, particularly patent law. Governmental regulations on the use of certain substrates and the sale of certain products also are relevant to industrial microbiology, as are considerations of space and marine exploration. Furthermore, areas not presently considered to have any relationship to industrial microbiology, under the proper conditions, easily can become a matter for consideration.

Industries for which industrial microbiology has no apparent application sometimes become interested in or are forced to become interested in this subject. They may merely wish to diversify their overall product line, or they may wish to employ microorganisms to bring about some change in a raw material, by-product, or product normally associated with the company's production activities. At the other end of the scale, microorganisms may bring about deterioration or, in some other manner, modify a product in an unwanted manner so that an industrial concern is forced to consider the industrial aspects of microbial activity. As an example, an industrial concern producing fiberglass may have no apparent need for a knowledge of industrial microbiology. But, if a change or improvement in some processing step suddenly allows microbial growth on the sizing applied to the glass fibers, then industrial microbiology immediately assumes importance.

It should now be apparent that there are many facets to industrial microbiology. Examples of particular areas of application include the sterilizations, deterioration, and quality control associated with the production and handling of food and beverage products, as well as the deterioration of, for example, fabrics, metals, concrete, wood, jet fuels, paper, animal feeds, and medicinal preparations. Also included are the methods for and the problems associated with the disposal of wastes from municipalities or industrial concerns. Microorganisms are industrially employed as a means for prospecting for new oil reserves, and for obtaining better oil recovery from present reserves. The industrial microbiologist is interested in ways of combating disease agents of plants, animals and man. He is concerned with the microbe's ability to modify a soil environment for the growing of green plants, particularly with the relationship of microorganisms to soil fertility, and with the ability of the soil microbe to degrade man-made pesticides and other chemicals that find their way into soil.

Industrial microbiology concerns itself with the isolation and description of microorganisms from natural environments, such as soil or water, and with the cultural conditions required for obtaining rapid and massive growth of these organisms in the laboratory and in large-scale cultural vessels commonly known as fermentors. Obviously, the design, sterilization, and use of these fermentors is of importance.

The means for the detection and assay of chemical products of microbial activity is a part of industrial microbiology, as are the recovery, chemical purification, packaging, and marketing of fermentation products. Thus, the ability of microorganisms to convert inexpensive raw materials, or substrates, to economically valuable organic compounds obviously is of considerable concern to the industrial microbiologist. Also of great interest is the economic value of the microbial cells themselves, and of the intracellular and extracellular enzymes elaborated by the organisms. The activities of these enzymes are important to the success of an industrial fermentation process, because they are associated with the microorganism's ability to attack, degrade, and utilize components of the medium, and to accumulate fermentation products. Microbial enzymes in themselves can be economic products; for example, microbially produced invertases, anylases, and proteases. On the other end of the scale, however, microbial enzymes also mediate the deterioration and spoilage caused by microorganisms.

Thus, fermentation products may be components of the microbial cells, the cells themselves, intracellular or extracellular enzymes, or chemicals which are produced or altered by the cells. Examples of various of the commercially important products of microbial activity are listed in Table 1.1. This list necessarily is not complete, since newly discovered products are continually coming to the forefront.

Table 1.1 Products of microbial activity having present or potential commercial importance

1.	Antibiotics: streptomycin, penicillin, the tetracyclines, erythromycin, polymyxin, bacitracin, etc.
2.	Organic solvents: acetone, butanol, ethanol, amyl alcohol, etc.
3.	Gases: carbon dioxide and hydrogen
4.	Beverages: wine, beer and distilled
5.	Foods: cheeses, fermented milks, pickles, sauerkraut, soy sauce, yeast bread, vinegar, mushrooms, and acidulants such as citric acid
6.	Flavoring agents: monosodium glutamate and nucleotides
7.	Organic acids: lactic, acetic, citric, gluconic, butyric, fumaric, itaconic, kojic, etc.
8.	Glycerol
9.	Amino acids: L-glutamic acid and L-lysine
10.	Steroids
11.	Wide range of compounds used as chemical intermediates for further chemical synthesis of economically valuable products
12.	Bakers' yeast
13.	Food and feed yeast
14.	Legume inoculant
15.	Bacterial insecticides: for example, *Bacillus thuringiensis*
16.	Vitamins and other growth stimulants: B_{12}, riboflavin, vitamin A and the gibberellins
17.	Enzymes: anylases, proteases, pectinases, invertase, etc.
18.	Fats

Patents are of importance to industrial microbiology in that they provide a certain degree of economic protection to an inventor (and to his employer) for a new fermentation process or product. Thus, patents provide the impetus for the expenditure of the huge sums of money ofter required for the research and development associated with new fermentation processes.

Industrial microbiology is often considered to be purely an area of applied microbiology, Thus, purely theoretical aspects should provide little interest to the industrial microbiologist. However, this frequently is not a true statement. Purely theoretical research being carried out at a university or governmental laboratory can well have applicability for industrial microbiology. For example, a study of keto-acid intermediates in the metabolism of a microorganism may yield the information that the addition to the growth medium of high levels of an ammonium salt or of urea causes amino acids to accumulate in the medium. This observation may be of value in explaining a metabolic pathway or pathways for the theoretical study of the microorganism, but at the same time, if further explored from the industrial microbiology standpoint, it could yield a process for the commercial production of amino acids. Thus, academic observations can yield practical possibilities, and industrial fermentation industries often keep a close watch on theoretical studies being carried out in universities and in other laboratories. In fact, industrial concerns may have research personnel of their own carrying out studies of a purely theoretical nature which have no initially apparent economic possibilities.

This consideration also works in reverse. Discoveries of new industrial microbial processes for producing fermentation products or for combating deterioration often raise questions of an academic nature. These questions relate to the physiology, morphology, and genetic make-up of microorganisms, and to the medical implications, mode of action, and the like, of chemical compounds. For instance, newly discovered antibiotics may be in commercial production and actually be employed for some time in combating disease before the chemical structure of the antibiotic has been deciphered or its mode of action has been elucidated.

Thus, in studying industrial microbiology, the student should concentrate on the economic aspects of how man makes use of or combats the activities of microorganisms. But, at the same time, the student must not lose sight of the basic concepts of microbiology which have no immediately apparent money-making possibilities.

Chapter 2

Historical Development of Industrial Microbiology Concepts

Industrial microbiology is a relatively new science, as is all of microbiology. As a science, it is a little more than 100 years old; as an art, it dates back into antiquity. However, a few of the present-day practices of industrial microbiology are more of an art than a science. The basic concepts of industrial microbiology and the academic undertones associated with it will be better understood if we first consider some of its historical aspects. Only major historical findings are considered, and the reader is referred to the collection of outstanding scientific publications by early scientists as assembled by Brock (1961). Additional information of historical interest is included with the pertinent chapters, and it is of interest in certain instances to compare the findings of the early investigators with the present concepts and practices as described in the chapters of the individual fermentations.

Before proceeding further, it is necessary to define the term "fermentation," especially since this term is used extensively in this and later chapters. Through the years, this word has gained new meanings, while retaining the old. Originally, fermentation referred to the bubbling observed when sugar and starchy materials underwent a transformation to yield alcoholic beverages. Later, this term was applied to the process in which alcohol was formed from sugar, regardless of whether the causative agent was or was not biological. Pasteur then entered the picture. He considered fermentation to apply to those anaerobic reactions through which microorganisms obtained energy for growth in the absence of oxygen. Today, fermentation has a much broader meaning. It applies to both the aerobic and the anaerobic metabolic activities of microorganisms in which specific chemical changes are brought about in an organic substrate. In fact, from an industrial microbiology standpoint the meaning is yet broader, and includes almost any process mediated by or involving microorganisms in which a product of economic value accrues.

Before the time of Leeuwenhoek, who lived and worked in the 17th century, individual microbial cells had not been observed. In fact, no one had done more than to postulate that possibly forms of life might exist smaller than could be seen with the unaided eye. However, industrial microbiology was practiced before the time of Leeuwenhoek, but the practice was purely an art. Thus, certain processes involving microorganisms were repeatable, after a fashion, if one followed the proper steps in carrying out the process. Man practiced these processes back into antiquity, and the first usage of most of the processes is, in large part, unknown. However, once man became agrarian and began to raise his own crops, he had access to the substrate materials for microbial fermentation activity, and at least theoretically, was in a position to carry out certain of the known fermentation processes. Thus, to a certain extent, we can predict for any group of people in antiquity the possible types of microbial fermentations which they might have practiced merely by considering the particular crops produced in their agriculture. Honey probably was available even to the earliest civilizations without requiring specific effort for its production and, therefore, fermented honey, or mead, may have provided one of the earliest alcoholic beverage fermentations for man. Manna also was easily obtainable, and it underwent fermentation in a manner analogous to that of honey to yield a fermented drink. Other early fermentation processes practiced by man included the leavening of bread, the retting of flax, the production of various alcoholic beverages (including beer, wine and mead), the production of vinegar by allowing wine to sour, and the production of various fermented foods and milks. The decomposition of various organic materials, particularly foods, was well known and, as man's knowledge progressed, he realized that the incorporation in foods of spices and high concentrations of salt helped to retard food spoilage. Obviously, the diseased states of plants, animals, and man were well known and, of course, empirical cures of one type or another were developed for these diseases. Although outstanding scientific discoveries were being made in other fields of learning throughout this period, the causes of the above phenomena could only be hypothesized, because the microscope had not been invented and, hence, was not available for observation of the causative agents. Also, the analytical chemical methods, which were available, were meager and in themselves were poorly understood.

In the 17th century, Antony van Leeuwenhoek of Delft, Holland, ground lenses as a hobby. With these lenses he was able to build a microscope with just enough magnification to allow observation of some of the larger microbial forms. This microscope had only a single lens and, obviously, his skill at grinding must have been rather extraordinary. He did not pass on this skill to others, but maintained strict secrecy on his methods of grinding. Of more importance, however, was the fact that Leeuwenhoek employed his own powers of observation in conjunction with his microscope to examine materials at hand so as to determine what they might consist of or contain. His observations were carefully recorded (as should be those for any scientific investigation) and transmitted to the august Royal Society of London where they were read before the Society and then published. Leeuwenhoek's letters of 1677 and 1684 to the Royal Society described several microorganisms that he had observed in water containing ground pepper, tartar from the teeth, and saliva. In addition, in his letter of 1684, he described his experiments on the inhibitory effect of acetic acid on microorganisms. He rinsed his mouth with vinegar and also suspended some of the tartar in vinegar. The mouth rinse reduced the number of microorganisms on the surface of the tartar, and the suspension of the tartar in vinegar killed the organisms. He further noted that one particular type of microorganism seemed to be more sensitive to the vinegar than the others. Thus, not only did he observe the bactericidal effect of acidity, but he also noted that certain microorganisms were more resistant to acidity than were others. A further publication by Leeuwenhoek in 1680 is of particular importance in relation to industrial microbiology. In this letter, he described beer yeast as being very small spherical or oval granules. Many people had observed beer yeast in mass before this time, because it tended to settle from the brew in the later stages of the fermentation. Leeuwenhoek's observation was important, because it revealed that this yeast mass actually was composed of many minute spherical forms. However, his observations did not experimentally establish that these minutes forms were living entities.

Leeuwenhoek's "wee beasties" remained a scientific curiosity for many years, although other research workers postulated that possibly they might be associated with disease and putrefaction. The resolving power of the available microscopes was not great enough to allow exacting studies of these microorganisms, nor were there techniques available for the isolation and maintenance of pure cultures or for the sterilization of growth media.

Although the further development of the microscope tended to parallel or slightly precede further discoveries concerning microorganisms. It is of distinct interest that these further discoveries and their relationship to industrial microbiology came about not because of any great interest in the morphology or activities of microorganisms, or because of an interest in improving specific fermentation processes, but because of a theoretical problem that had been bothering learned men for a considerable period of time. This theoretical problem concerned spontaneous generation; that is, could life spring forth from dead or inanimate materials. Redi's experiments in the 17th century demonstrated that the macro concepts of spontaneous generation were fallacious; mice did not spring forth de novo from old rags, nor did maggots from meat. These experiments, however, did not explain the apparent spontaneous generation at the micro-level, such as the spontaneous appearance of microscopically observable microorganisms in solutions of organic materials, particularly in sugar solutions undergoing alcoholic fermentation. Scientific controversy over this micro-level spontaneous generation challenged the best minds of the time, and from this controversy came the beginnings of modern microbiology and industrial microbiology, as well as the techniques for their study. Some of these techniques are still in use today, and several of the basic concepts derived from these studies are still valid.

In his paper of 1799, Lazaro Spallanzani attempted to disprove spontaneous generation by hermetically sealing infusions of seeds in flasks, followed by heating of the flasks for varying periods of time in a boiling water bath. In these experiments, he observed that a short period of heating killed one group of microorganisms, probably the protozoa, and that the smaller organisms, probably the bacteria, were more resistant to heating. Thus, his experiments first demonstrated the difference in heat resistance of various types of organisms and that prolonged heating may be necessary for sterilization. Microbial growth occurred when Spallanzani's flasks were opened and exposed to the atmosphere. Questions were raised by other investigators as to whether this growth reflected introduction into the medium from the air of new viable organism, or whether the organisms originally present in the flasks were not killed by the heat, and were just waiting for the introduction of air to resume growth. These investigators also proposed an alternate hypothesis that supported the spontaneous generation theory—that the heat had, in fact, killed the microorganisms, but that the reentry of atmosphere into the media in the flasks had caused the spontaneous transformation of inert medium components into living microorganisms.

Theodore Schwann, in his publication of 1837, attempted to answer the criticism of Spallanzani's experiments that air reintroduced into the sterilized medium could cause the spontaneous formation of life from the medium components. Using an approach somewhat similar to that of spallanzani's, he demonstrated that a sterilized meat broth did not undergo putrefaction; that is, microbial growth did not occur if fresh heated air was introduced into the medium. Thus, Schwann managed to sterilize air, a technique of great importance for modern-day forced-aeration submerged fermentations.

In the same paper, Schwann presented his studies on the association of microbial activity with the beer yeast alcoholic sugar fermentation. He transferred beer yeast to flasks of sucrose solution, then stoppered and heated all of the flasks. After cooling, air was allowed to reenter part of the flasks through heated tubes, a procedure that did not remove the oxygen of the air. Unheated air was allowed to enter other flasks, and all of the flasks were then stoppered and incubated. After a prolonged period, fermentation (that is, the evolution of carbon dioxide) was not evident in the flasks that had received heated air, while fermentations occurred within four to six weeks in those flasks receiving unheated air. In regard to the spontaneous generation theory, he concluded that "Thus, in alcoholic fermentation as in putrefaction, it is not the oxygen of the air which causes this to occur, but a substance in the air which is destroyed by heat." This statement nicely outlined the concept of airborne contamination.

In this paper, Schwann also considered that the alcoholic fermentation might possibly be caused by living organisms that destroyed the sugar, in the process producing alcohol and carbon dioxide. He wished to determine what types of microorganism might be involved, particularly whether they were infusoria, which consisted primarily of protozoa and bacteria, or molds (yeasts). His experimental approach was to employ selective metabolic poisons. Strychnine solution was used as a specific poison for the infusoria, and potassium arsenate as a general Poison for both forms. His results demonstrated that strychnine had no effect on the alcoholic fermentation, while several drops of arsenate completely abolished it. Therefore, he concluded that he should look for a "plant" (a mold or yeast) as the responsible agent.

Microscopes by this time had developed to the point that schwann was able to observe the yeast and, in fact, was the first to observe and descibe a yeast in the process of growing. He observed budding, and concluded that the organism was fungal-like. He inoculated fresh grape juice with beer yeast, and noted an increase in the numbers of micro-organisms with a morphology resembling that for yeast as observed in the beer fermentation. He further noted correlations between the time of appearance of the yeast in the grape juice, the rate of yeast growth, and the initiation of the carbon dioxide evolution of sugar fermentation. He also noted that inoculation of the grape juice brought about a quicker alcoholic fermentation than did merely relying on natural inoculation, obviously a concept aplied in most modern industrial microbiology processes. He further stated that, "It is highly probable that the development of the fungus (sugar fungus) causes the fermentation."

It was previously known that the presence of nitrogen-containing substances was necessary for an alcoholic fermentation to proceed. Schwann correctly deduced that this observation was important from the microbial standpoint, and offered his opinion that "...it appears that nitrogen is necessary for the life of the plant (yeast) as it is probable that every fungus contains nitrogen." Thus, he stated the basis for the compounding of nutrient media for microbial growth. In fact, the amounts and types of nitrogen sources often are of critical importance for the media employed in present-day industrial fermentation processes.

Schwann further proposed a simple explanation for the alcohol fermentation that defined the relationship of carbohydrate substrate to both growth and alcohol production. He stated that "The alcoholic fermentation must be considered to be that decomposition which occurs when the sugar fungus (yeast) utilizes sugar and nitrogen containing substances for its growth, in the process of which the elements of these substances which do not go into the plant (yeast) are preferentially converted into alcohol."

Charles Cagniard-Latour (1838) confirmed and extended Schwann's descriptions of the growth and morphology of yeast cells. Microscopes allowing 300-to 400-power magnification were available by this time, and Cagniard-Latour utilized a microscope of this type, in conjunction with an ocular micrometer, to study the beer yeast. By studying samples removed hourly form a beer fermentation, he observed that the cells varied in size, but that all were 10 microns or less in diameter. He observed budding of the yeast, and demonstrated that the buds actually were attached to the mother cells and not merely a fortuitous positioning of small yeast cells. He also observed bud scars on the yeast cells.

By utilizing microscopic counts during the progress of the alcoholic fermentation, he was able to demostrate that the increase in both the numbers and the weight of the cells during the fermentation corresponded with a seven-fold increase over that initially introduced. He therefore concluded that this represented multiplication of the yeast on a complete nutrient medium. Cagniard-Latour also observed that, although yeast would ferment a simple sugar solution without a nitrogen source being present, the cells did not grow. In other words, they did not increase in weight. Under these conditions, the cells also demonstrated a progressive loss of fermenting ability.

M. Gay-Lussac had previously demostrated that oxygen was required for initiation of the alcoholic fermentation, but that it was not required for the further progress of the fermentation. Cagniard-Latour explained this observation by showing that yeasts were able to grow anaerobically. However, he concluded that oxygen was required for the "germination" of the yeast.

Based on his studies, Cagniard-Latour stated that the erratic variations in fermentations commonly encountered by brewers and distillers, even with great care in their operations, agreed with the hypothesis "...that the alcoholic fermentation is caused by bodies endowed with life, because who knows in how many different ways such similar bodies can be affected..." He also concluded, as did Schwann, that the alcohol fermentation was the result of the living growth of yeast on sugar to form carbon dioxide and ethanol from the sugar. In addition, however, he noted that yeast cells did not die when frozen or when maintained in the absence of water. These observations are still valid today.

At the time that Schwann and Cagniard-Latour were presenting their studies to the scientific public, the well-known and influential chemist, Justis Liebig (1839), used his influence and scholarly status to proclaim that all of the reported apparently living activity observed by these and other workers was really the result of chemical and physical reactions going on in the medium. He reasoned, without much in the way of experimental proof, that beer yeast and all other organic materials undergoing decomposition really were merely unstable chemical substances which could transmit their instability to fermentable substrates such as sugar, and that the latter also were somewhat unstable, because their elements were held together only weakly. Thus, it remained for Louis Pasteur to finally discredit, presumably for all time, the theory of spontaneous generation. In a sense, we owe a debt of gratitude to Liebig for keeping alive the spontaneous generation theory because, without his influence, Pasteur probably would not have been induced to study microbial fermentations and to establish the bases for modern-day microbiology.

According to Brock (1961), Pasteur's paper published in 1857 represented the beginning of the science of microbiology. This was Pasteur's first reported study of a fermentation, and it was concerned not with the alcohol fermentation but with the lactic acid fermentation. In this paper, Pasteur stated that the lactic acid fermentation was caused by living microorganisms, and he described their microscopic appearance. He also described a medium for lactic acid production. Furthermore, he separated the bacteria from the fermentation medium by washing the cells, but was not able to get the cells into pure culture. In fact, at this time, the concept of pure culture micorbiology did not exist, and this lack of pure cultures caused some difficulty for Pasteur in accurately studying this fermentation.

Pasteur's report of 1860 provided the first example of the use of a synthetic medium for microbiological studies. This medium contained only trace elements, ammonium salt and sugar, with no complex organic materials (such as protein) being added. With this medium, he was able to quantitatively study the alcoholic fermentation in such a manner as to be able to show that, during the fermentation, the yeast increased in weight with a consequent increase in the carbon and nitrogen contents of the overall cell batch. Also, he observed that the increase in yeast protein in this synthetic medium was accompanied by a related decrease in the ammoniacal nitrogen of the medium, demonstrating that substrate nitrogen was being incorporated into the yeast cells. Finally, in this paper Pasteur demonstrated that fermentation of the sugar required the multiplication of the yeast cells; in other words, in this medium spontaneous generation did not explain the presence of fermentation. It should be noted that others, including Liebig, had difficulty in reproducing these experiments, apparently because Pasteur used a rather large inoculum of yeast cells while the other workers used a comparatively lesser inoculum. As will be noted later, Pasteur was fortunate that he did use a large inoculum, because it tended to carry over growth factors required for initiation of the growth of the yeast.

Pasteur's studies were often hampered by the fact that he was not using pure cultures. In one of his publications of 1861 (1861a), he reasoned deductively that some of the products of the lactic acid fermentation described in his previous studies possibly could be attributed to the presence of more than one organism in the culture. Specifically, he reasoned that the butyric acid present as a fermentation product must have resulted from a different fermentation being carried out by a different organism simultaneously with that of the lactic acid fermentation. Previously, he had microscopically observed that other bacteria were present, but had concluded that they were growing on the butyric acid as a carbon source, not producing it as a fermentation product. In the 1861 a publication, Pasteur described the morphology of a fairly large bacterium and showed that it multiplied and produced butyric acid when transferred to fresh medium (including synthetic medium). However, possibly of more importance as a result of this study was the fact that he was able to set forth the concept of the strictly anaerobic microorganism. He passed a stream of air through some of the cultures and a stream of carbon dioxide through others. The latter provided anaerobic growth conditions. By this experimental approach, he was able to show that the microorganism associated with the butyric acid fermentation was actually killed by air, and that air caused cessation of the fermentation. In addition, he showed that this bacterium could live indefinitely and multiply in the complete absence of air or free oxygen. Today these qualities are known characteristics of strict anaerobes.

Another of Pasteur's 1861 studies (1861b), as well as later studies, revealed what has since become known as the "Pasteur effect"–a phenomenon in which the growth and physiology of a yeast (or other microorganism) differs depending on whether it is grown under aerobic or anaerobic conditions. Pasteur observed that under anaerobic conditions relatively less growth occurred, and that a large amount of sugar was converted to alcohol. He reasoned that the yeast was obtaining its required oxygen from the sugar molecule. Under aerobic incubation conditions less sugar was decomposed, and a greater portion of the sugar was converted to yeast cellular materials. Also, in the presence of air, little if any alcohol was produced and, in fact, air actually inhibited the fermentative decomposition of the sugar, that is, alcohol formation. It should be noted that, since pasteur's time, the Pasteur effect has been demonstrated in other microorganisms and in higher forms of life. Pasteur also noted that the yeast could grow aerobically on certain carbon sources such as amino acids or organic acids, but not anaerobically. These happen to be the carbon sources which cannot be anaerobically fermented to yield oxygen to the organism for its metabolism.

The famous death knell to spontaneous generation came in pasteur's publication of 1861c. He first showed that microrganisms could occur as airborne contaminants by collecting organisms with an air sampler onto a special cotton, and then dissolving the cotton and transferring the organisms to glass microscope slides. Since his air sampler actually filtered the organisms from the air onto the cotton, this may be the first if not one of the early uses of cotton plugs to filter organisms from the air. Microscopic observations of the slides prepared in this manner revealed that a "large number" of microorganisms occurred in air. Pasteur then proceeded to sterilize media in his famous "swan-necked flasks" (Figure 2.1), so as to show that growth could not occur in sterile media unless airborne contamination had occurred. These flasks did not utilize cotton plugs, but the necks of the flasks were drawn out and curved in such a fashion that microorganisms that entered along with the free passage of air into the flasks were trapped on the walls of

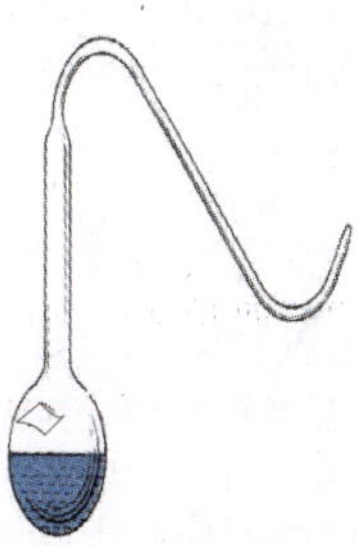

Figure 2.1 Pasteur's swan-necked flask used in experiments disproving spontaneous generation.

the curved drawn-out neck. Thus, this study also demonstrated the sterilization and maintenance of asepsis of fermentation media; the partial sterilization of media, or pasteurization, came at a later date.

None of Pasteur's studies, as described, utilized pure cultures of microorganisms. Thus, we must marvel at his ability to obtain scientifically valid results with mixed cultures of microorganisms, although obviously in several instances his cultures contained only a low level of growth of unwanted organisms. It remained for Lister in 1878 to demonstrate the first technique for obtaining pure cultures of microorganisms. Lister was attempting to study the bacterium associated with the lactic acid fermentation, but realized that a contaminating microorganism also was present in low numbers. He reasoned that, if sequential dilutions of the culture were prepared, the contaminating microorganism probably would not be present in some of the greater dilutions which would still contain the microorganism of interest. Therefore, he used a microscope counting technique to determine the extent of dilution required for disappearance of the contaminant and to determine how much dilution the principal organism of the mixed culture could withstand and still be observable in microscopic preparations. Using these end-point determinations, he then devised the dilution to extinction procedure (most probable number) to evaluate the actual numbers of the principal organism in his cultures, and to isolate this organism in pure culture. Actually, Lister encountered considerable difficulty in explaining to others the theoretical basis of this procedure. Today, however, this procedure is the basis for determinations of numbers of microorganisms by the most probable number technique, and it still is sometimes used for the isolation of microorganisms. While Lister's experimental approach, in fact, did yield the first pure cultures of microorganisms, his use of microscope counting to determine the approximate end points for his dilution scheme was somewhat fallacious. Thus, later workers realized that approximately 100,000 microorganisms per milliliter are required before an average of one microorganism per field can be observed with the compound microscope at 1000-fold magnification.

As is apparent by this time, several workers had developed procedures for the sterilization of nutrient media. As a result, a food preservation industry rapidly developed which used hermetically sealed tin cans and heating temperatures of boiling water. However, several workers, including Pasteur and Schwann, at times had noted, in their sterilization experiments, that temperatures greater than that of boiling water were required to obtain sterilization of aqueous solutions or suspensions of organic materials. In this regard, the food preservation industry also encountered some difficulty with certain foods, particularly peas, in that spoilage sometimes occurred even though the cans had been heated in boiling water. It was assumed that this was due largely to the protection against heat afforded to the microoorganisms by the solid character of the food being preserved. However, Ferdinand Cohn reasoned in a different manner. He felt that perhaps certain microorganisms might exist which possessed a considerably greater heat resistance than did the organisms previously studied. In his publication of 1876, Cohn described an alternation of heating at 100°C and incubation of a hay infusion such that an enrichment culture developed that contained a spore forming bacillus. He described this bacillus and its process of sporeforming bacillus. He described this bacillus and its process of spore formation, and then demonstrated its high level of heat resistance. Obviously, this discovery was of great importance to the canning industry, as well as to other areas of industrial microbiology and to microbiology in general. His technique of "intermittent sterilization" still finds some use today in instances in which the material to be sterilized is somewhat heat sensitive, or in which there are bacterial spores present with exceptional heat resistance. The initial heat treatment causes "heat-shocking." with consequent germination of the spores during incubation, to yield the less resistant vegetative forms which are then killed by the next heat treatment.

Lister's technique for obtaining pure cultures of microorganisms could be successfully employed only if one of the various microorganisms of a mixture was present in considerably greater numbers than were the other organisms. Also, his technique was complicated and rather laborious to carry out. Robert Koch had been studying the relationship of microorganisms to disease, but was encountering difficulty in not being able to work with pure cultures of the disease-producing microorganisms, especially since Lister's technique was not feasible for his studies. Koch's observation that boiled potato slices on incubation allowed development of colonies of microorganisms and that these colonies could be transferred to fresh potato slices prompted him to search for a solidifying agent which could be added to liquid medium so as to provide a similar type of colonial growth. Potato slices could not be used for his animal pathogens, since these organisms did not grow on this substrate. He therefore employed gelatin as a solidifying agent (Koch, 1881), and, as a result, was able to obtain individual colonies well separated from each other on the surface of the gelatin medium. He assumed, correctly, that most of these colonies had arisen from a single cell. Furthermore, he realized that colony morphology, as developed on his gelatin plates, could be utilized for the description and identification of microorganisms, and that this technique also could be used for the purification of cultures. The benefits accruing to industrial microbiology and to microbiology, in general, from this technique obviously cannot be overestimated. A paper by koch in 1882 described the use of solidified blood serum as slopes in cotton-plugged test tubes instead of gelatin to allow the use of the elevated incubation temperatures at which gelatin assumes a liquid state. Later, Frau Hesse, the wife of one of Koch's students, realized that agar provided a solidifying agent that demonstrated none of the faults of gelatin or of solidified blood serum.

While Koch's plating procedures provided tremendous advantages for the study of microorganisms, there was still the problem of a suitable culture vessel. In 1887, Petri solved this proplem by describing what is now known as the Petri plate, a culture dish that is still used extensively today.

Studies on the alcoholic fermentation by various workers over a period of years had conclusively shown that living yeast cells were the causative agents. However, with further studies on this fermentation, various individuals postulated that, possibly, it was mediated by an enzyme associated with the yeast. Hydrolytic enzymes of various types were already known. To determine whether a yeast enzyme might actually mediate the alcoholic fermentation, Eduard Buchner (1897) ground up yeast cells and expressed the juice from the broken cells. He then filtered the juice to obtain a clear solution, and mixed the solution with a concentrated sugar solution. On incubation, carbon dioxide was evolved, and he identified and quantitated the ethyl alcohol that was formed. In other words, the cell-free yeast juice carried out the alcoholic fermentation. He considered that the active agent was a soluble proteinatious enzyme, because filtration that removed all the yeast cell fragments had no effect, and because the activity was not susceptible to chloroform treatment. Furthermore, the activity was sensitive to elevated temperatures and to drying. He called this enzyme "zymase" and considered it probable that zymase, under natural conditions, was extracellular and operated in the medium outside the yeast cells. Thus, Buchner was the first to demonstrate enzymatically mediated fermentation reactions (other than hydrolytic reactions). However, because of the state of the art at that time, he was in error on two points. It is now known that zymase is not a single enzyme, but a series of enzymes making up the Meyerhof-Embden scheme for sugar catabolism, and that these enzymes are not normally extracellular but function within the yeast cell.

As previously stated, Pasteur was successful in obtaining yeast growth in a synthetic medium, while certain of his colleagues could not reproduce his experiments. Apparently, this was because his colleagues employed lower inoculation levels than did Pasteur. In succeeding years, other instances were recorded in which more than a minimal inoculum level was required to obtain growth of microorganisms in synthetic media. Wildiers (1901) solved this problem, at least in part, by demonstrating that yeast has a vitamin requirement for growth. He applied the name "bios" to this growth factor, or vitamin, and this was the first demonstration of a growth factor, requirement for microorganisms. Wildiers obtained the bios factor by extracting boiled yeast and, when this extract was utilized in conjunction with a low-level yeast inoculum, growth ensured in synthetic media. Wildiers hypothesized that animals might also require this growth factor. Also, he felt that this growth factor actually might be a mixture of several vitamins, a point experimentally proven by others at a later date. Since Wildiers' time, vitamins obviously have assumed great importance in animal and human nutrition as well as in the nutrition of microorganisms. Today, not only are vitamins important in industrial microbiology, since they affect the growth and fermentative capability of industrial microorganisms, but also at least some of the vitamins have become commercially valuable products of the fermentation industry.

Bacteriophage present a constant threat to modern-day fermentation processes employing bacteria and actinomycetes. F. d' Herelle (1917) coined the name "bacteriophge" for the filterable parasite of the dysentery bacillus that he was studying. He mixed feces with cells of this bacterium and, after enrichment culture and bacteriological filtration, obtained a broth filtrate capable of causing complete lysis when mixed with a culture of the bacillus. Furthermore, this activity occurred repeatedly on successive transfers of bacteriologically filtered culture broths containing the agent to fresh cultures of the bacillus.

He observed that plaque formation occurred on agar plates seeded with the host organism, and that the formation of plaques could be used to determine the numbers of bacteriophage occurring in a lysed culture of the bacillus. He determined that the bacteriophage did not multiply in the absence of its living host. He also determined the host specificity range for this phage, and predicted that phages might exist for other microorganisms. While his discoveries have proved to be of great importance in industrial microbiology, microbial genetics, and other areas of microbiology, his primary hope for bacteriophage-that they could be used medicinally to treat disease or to confer immunity–has not been realized.

A concept with broad implications for industrial microbiology was outlined by Kluyver in 1924. His publication entitled "Unity and Diversity in the Metabolism of Microorganisms" discussed the striking diversity and yet basic similarities of metabolic pathways and of thermodynamic considerations among microorganisms as well as higher forms of life. Previous researchers had concentrated on demonstrating the diversity of end products of microbial metabolism and the diversity of nutritional requirements for the growth of both aerobic and anaerobic microorganisms. Kluyver pointed out, however, that regardless of all this diversity, there was an underlying unity among microorganisms (and higher forms of life) in both the metabolic pathways utilized and the associated energy release and utilization. He based these conclusions, in part, on observations that, by adjusting the growth medium or cultural conditions, one could change the type of metabolic intermediates (or end products) which accumulated during the growth of various microorganisms. Usually, relatively few of these compounds accumulated, because the product of one enzyme of a metabolic pathway was immediately acted on by the next enzyme of the metabolic sequence. By utilizing this approach, it was apparent that certain intermediate compounds actually were common to apparently diverse metabolic pathways. Thus, although many products of microbial metabolism were possible, their formation was associated with relatively fewer metabolic pathways for the dissimilation of organic molecules. These studies and conclusions allowed a more rational approach to the study of microbial Physiology and, hence, to the development of our understanding of how to control the activities of microbial synthesis to yield products of economic value.

By far the most widely known medicinal product of microbial fermentation today is penicillin. However, the discovery of penicillin by Alexander Fleming in 1929 was based solely on a chance observation in the laboratory of a contaminated Petri dish, and on a considerable curiosity on the part of Fleming as to the cause and potential of the phenomenon observed. A Petri plate of *Staphylococcus aureus* which had been setting on a laboratory bench for a period of time became contaminated with a mold that caused the *Staphylococcus* colonies in its vicinity first to become transparent and then to lyse. Actually, other workers had observed similar phenomena on Petri plates, but had not followed up their observations. Fleming subcultured the mold and, on growing it in liquid medium, noted that a bactericidal and bacteriolytic principle had accumulated in the culture broth. It was found that the mold was a species of *Penicillum*, and that other fungal species did not produce this antibiotic principle. Therefore, he applied the name "penicillin" to the active agent occurring in the mold broth filtrates.

Fleming employed streak plates to determine the bacterial inhibition spectrum for penicillin. These plates were prepared by first cutting a trough along one side of the plate, and then filling the trough with a mixture of agar and penicillin. The test organisms were streaked at right angles to the penicillin trough and, on incubation, the relative degrees of inhibition were determined by measuring the distances over which the penicillin, as it diffused from the trough, had inhibited growth of the test organisms. Fleming also employed the dilution tube assay to determine the bacterial inhibition spectrum, as well as to assay the potencies of various penicillin preparations. He demonstrated that penicillin possessed a low toxicity level for man and animals and, as such, possibly might have therapeutic value in the treatment of bacterial infections. Other characteristics of penicillin reported by Fleming related to the effect of heat and pH on the antibiotic, its filterability through a Seitz filter, its water and solvent solubilities, its rate of formation and disappearance with time in culture flasks, and its comparative production on various culture media. Finally, Fleming pointed out that penicillin could be used as a selective inhibitor to allow the isolation of microorganisms insensitive to or only slightly sensitive to penicillin from large populations of organisms sensitive to the antibiotic.

The further history of penicillin development and of the penicillin industry appears elsewhere in this book. The discovery of penicillin alerted research works to the possibility that other microorganisms right synthesize antibiotics. Thus, with intensive research effort during the Second World War and thereafter, streptomycin, chloramphenicol, the tetracyclenes, and a series of other antibiotics of great commercial and medicinal value were discovered.

The use of metabolically blocked mutants of microorganisms is relatively recent, but of great importance. Many investigators were involved, and the reader is referred to a review by Adelberg (1953). The study of genetic blocks has contributed greatly to our knowledge of microbial genetics and, at the same time, has provided a means for irecting microorganisms to accumulate large amounts of metabolic intermediates that normally, because of their transient existence in metabolic pathways, would not accumulate to any extent in cultures. Nevertheless, the relationship between the point in metabolic pathway a which a genetic block occurs and the particular organic compound that accumulates has not always been clear. It is only recently that the mechanisms associated with certain of these metabolic blocks are becoming understood.

It should now be obvious, from this brief history that many of the earlier researchers did not set out to solve a problem or to interpret their results in terms of industrial microbiology applications. However, it is apparent that many of these studies do have a strong bearing on the technology and thinking of modern-day industrial microbiology, as well as on the technology of the times in which the studies were carried out. Also, we see that many of the techniques and the concepts developed are still valid today. A discussion of possible directions that industrial microbiology might take in the future is presented in the last chapter of this book.

References

Adelberg, E.A. 1953. The use of metabolically blocked organisms for the analysis of biosynthetic pathways. *Bacteriol. Rev.,* **17**,253-267.

Brock, T. 1961. *Milestones in microbiology.* Prentice-Hall, Inc., Englewood Cliffs, N.J.

Buchner, E. 1897. Alkoholische Gahrung ohne Hefezellen. *Berichte der Deutschen Chemischen Gesellschaft,* **30,** 117–124.

Cagniard-Latour, C. 1838. Memoire sur la fermentation vineuse. *Annales de Chimie et de Physique,* **68,** 206–222.

Cohn, F. 1876. Untersuchungen Bacterien. IV. Beitrage zur Biologie der Bacillen. *Beitrage zur Biologie der Pflanzen* **2**, 249–276.

Fleming, A. 1929. On the antibacterial action of cultures of a Pencillium, with special reference to their use in the isolation of *B. influenzae. British. J. Exp. pathol.,* **10,** 226–236.

d'Herelle, F. 1917. Sur un microbe invisible antagoniste des bacilles

dysenteriques. *Comptes rendus de l'Academie des sciences,* **165,** 373–375.

Kluyver, A.J. 1924. Eenheid en versheidenheid in de stofwisseling der microben. *Chemisch Weekblad,* **21,** 266.

Koch, R. 1881. Zur Untersuchung von pathogenen Organismen. *Mittheilungen aus dem kaiserlichen Gesundheitsamte,* **1**,1–48.

Koch, R. 1882. Die Atiologie der Tuberkulose. Berliner Klinischen Wochenschrift, No. 15, April 10, 1882, pp. 221–230.

van Leeuwenhoek, A .1677. Concerning little animals observed in rain-, well-, sea-, and snow-water; as also in water wherein pepper had lain infused.

Philosophical Trans. of the Royal Soc. of London, **11(133),** 821–831.

van Leeuwenhoek, A 1680. See Brock, T. 1961, p.23.

van Leeuwenhoek, A. 1684. Some microscopical observations about animals in the scurf of the teeth. *Philosophical Trans. of the Royal Soc. of London,* **14 (159),** 568–574.

Liebig, J. 1839. Ueber die Erscheinungen der Gahrung, Faulniss and Verwesung, and ihre Ursachen. *Annalen der Physik and chemie*, **48,** 106–150

Lister, J. 1878. On the lactic fermentation and its bearings on pathology.

Trans. Pathol. Soc. London, **29,** 425–467.

Pasteur, L. 1857. Memoire sur la fermentation appelee lactique. *Comptes rendus de l' Academie des sciences*, **45,** 913–916.

Pasteur, L. 1860. Memoire sur la fermentation alcoolique. *Annales de Chimie et de Physique,* 3rd series **58,** 323–426.

Pasteur, L. 1861a. Animalcues infusoires vivant sans gaz oxygene libre et determinant des fermentations. *Comptes rendus de l' Academie des sciences*, **52,** 344–347.

Pasteur, L. 1861b. Influence de l'oxygene sur le developement de la levure et la fermentation alcoolique. *Bulletin de la Societe chimique de Paris*, June 28,

1861, pp. 79–80 (Resume).

Pasteur, L. 1861c. Memoire sur les corpuscles organises qui existent dans l'atmosphere. Examen de la doctrine des generations spontanees. *Annales des sciences naturelles,* 4th series, **16,** 5–98.

Petri, R. J. 1887. Eine kleine Modification des Koch's schen Plattenverfahrens. *Centralblatt fur Bacteriologie and Parasitenkunde*, **1,** 279–280.

Schwann, T. 1837. Vorlaufige Mittheilung, betreffend Versuche uber die Weingahrung and Faulnis. *Annolen der Physik and Chemie,* **41,** 184–193.

Spallanzani, L. 1799. Observations and experiments upon the animalcula of infusions. See Brock, T. 1961, pp. 13–16.

Wildiers, E. 1901. Nouvelle substance indispensable au development de la levure. *La Cellule*, **18,** 313–332.

Chapter 3

Fermentation Equipment and Its Use

The industrial usage of microorganisms often requires that they be grown in large vessels containing considerable quantities of nutritive media. These vessels are commonly called fermentors, and they can be quite complicated in design, since frequently they must provide for the control and observation of many facets of microbial growth and biosynthesis. Therefore, before we can consider the development of a fermentation process or the mechanics of existing fermentations, we must know something of the design and operation of those fermentors and their auxiliary equipment, and of the limitations imposed by these fermentors on the ways in which microorganisms can be cultivated on an industrial scale.

Industrial fermentors are designed to provide the best possible growth and biosynthesis conditions for industrially important microbial cultures, and to allow ease of manipulation for all operations associated with the use of the fermentors. These vessels must be strong enough to withstand the pressures of large volumes of aqueous medium, but at the same time, the materials from which they are fabricated must not be corroded by the fermentation product nor contribute toxic ions to the growth medium. Since most industrial fermentations utilize pure cultures, the fermentors must make some provision for the control of or prevention of the growth of contaminating microorganisms. If the growth of the fermentation microorganism is to occur aerobically, then provision must be made for rapid incorporation of sterile air into the medium in such a manner that the oxygen of this air is dissolved in the medium and, therefore, readily available to the microorganism, and that the carbon dioxide resulting from microbial metabolism is largely flushed from the medium. Some form of stirring should be available, if not accomplished by gas evolution during `microbial growth, to both mix the organisms through the medium and to make nutrients and oxygen more available to the individual microbe. The fermentor should provide for the intermittent addition of antifoam agents as demanded by the foaming status of the medium. Some form of temperature control should be available so as to maintain a constant predetermined temperature in the fermentor during growth of the organism. The fermentor should provide aseptic means for the withdrawal of culture samples during the fermentation as well as for the introduction of inoculum at the initiation of the fermentation. A mechanism for detecting pH values of the culture medium and for adjusting these values during growth is often required, even if this consists only in withdrawing a sample from the fermentor for pH determination followed by addition of alkali or acid to the fermentation medium. Ancillary to the fermentor there should be additional inoculum or seed tanks, actually smaller-sized fermentors, in which inoculum is produced and then added directly to the fermentor without employing extensive piping, which can magnify contamination problems. Other vessels may be required for mixing medium constituents and water in the preparation of large batches of medium for addition to production scale fermentors. Some means also must be provided for the sterilization of this medium and of antifoam. For many fermentations, air filters or some means

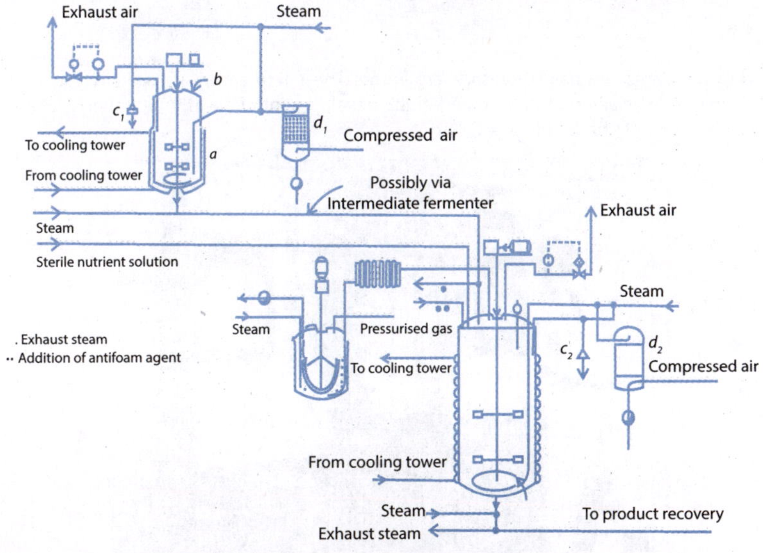

Figure 3.1 Flow sheet showing layout of fermentation plant. a, Seed tank. b, Inoculation port. c_1, c_2, Sampling devices. d_1, d_2, Filters. e, Substrate container. f, Sterile filter. g, Reaction tank. h, Electrode for foam control. i, Cooling coils. (Muller and Kieslich, 1966, *Angew Chem. Internat*. Edit., 5, 653–662.)

of sterilization must be present between the source of high pressure air and its entry into the fermentor. Lastly, there must be a drain in the bottom of the fermentor or some mechanism provided for removing the completed fermentation broth from the tank, and access must be had to the inside of the fermentor so that it can be thoroughly cleaned between fermentation runs. An example of the manner in which these various components of a fermentation plant are operated in conjunction with each other is presented as a fermentation plant flow sheet, Figure 3.1.

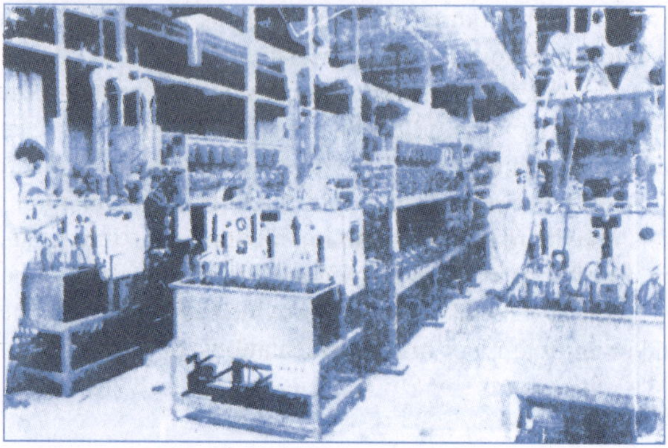

Figure 3.2 Banks of small laboratory fermentors. These fermentors are used in research on existing commercial fermentations and in the development of new fermentation processes. Photo courtesy of Charles Pfizer & C., Inc.

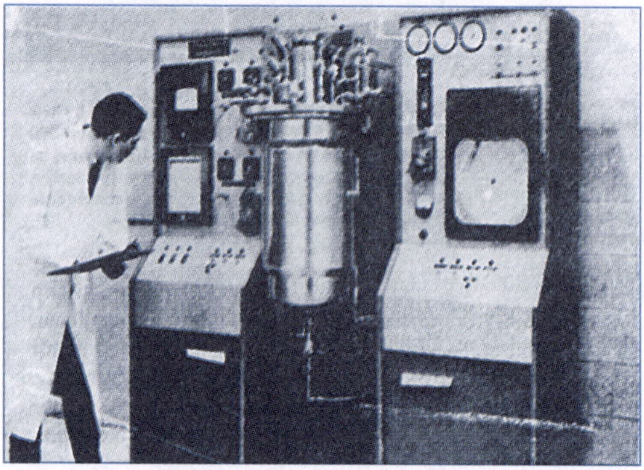

Figure 3.3 Fermacell fermentor for pilot-plant studies. This fermentor is available in three sizes providing working volumes of up to 40 (as pictured), 100, or 200 liters, and it can be used for either batch or continuous culture and provides automatic pH and foam control. Photo courtesy of New Brunswick Scientific Co., Inc.

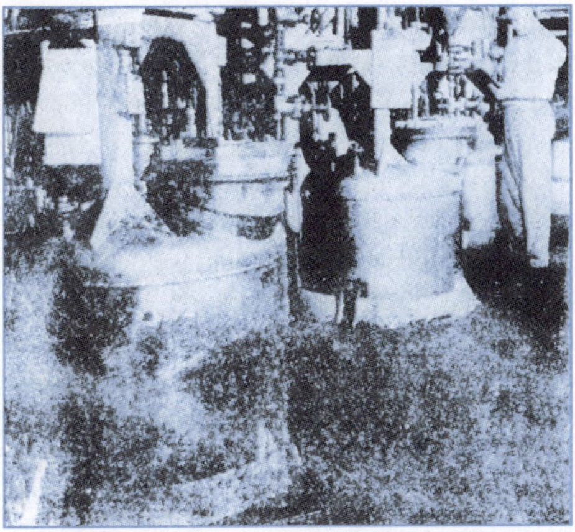

Figure 3.4 Larger pilot-plant fermentors used in the study of process variables for new fermentations. Similar fermentors range in size from 25 through 50, 100 and 500 gallon total volume capacities, and they duplicate the size, shape, and accessories of large production fermentors. As a result, the techniques of fermentation production for new processes can be perfected in these fermentors before the fermentation goes into actual production. Photo courtesy of Charles Pfizer and Co., Inc.

Fermentors are available in varying sizes. These sizes are usually stated based on the total volume capacity of the fermentor. However, the actual

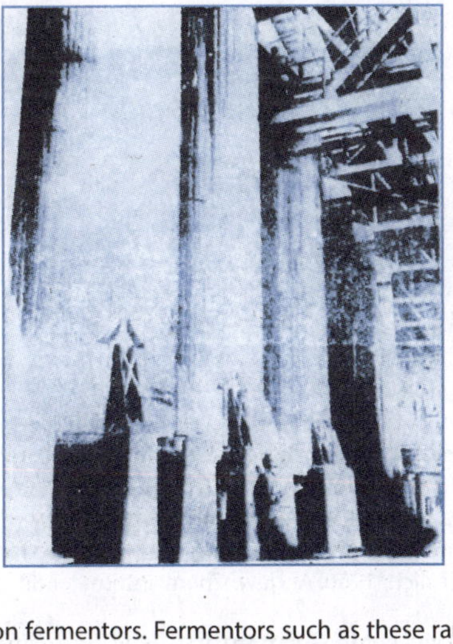

Figure 3.5 Large production fermentors. Fermentors such as these range in size from 5000 or 10,000 gallons total capacity to approximately 100,000 gallons. Photo courtesy of Charles Pfizer and Co., Inc.

operating volume in a fermentor is always less than that of the total volume, because a "head space" must be left at the top of the fermentor above the liquid medium to allow for splashing, foaming, and aeration of the liquid. This head space usually occupies a fifth to a quarter or more of the volume of the fermentor. Small laboratory fermentors (Figures 3.2 and 3.14) have a total volume of one to two liters of medium with a maximum of about 12 to 15 liters. Pilot plant fermentors, which are used in larger-scale studies of fermentations, often are in the size range of 25 to 100 gallons and up to 2000 gallons total volume (see Figures 3.3 and 3.4). Larger fermentors for industrial production of fermentation products or microbial cells (Figures 3.5 to 3.7) range from 5000 or 10,000 gallons total capacity to approximately 100,000 gallons. Fermentors of a size larger than this are rare but, when used, are often in the shape of spheres (Horton spheres) and are of 250,000 to 500,000 gallon total capacity.

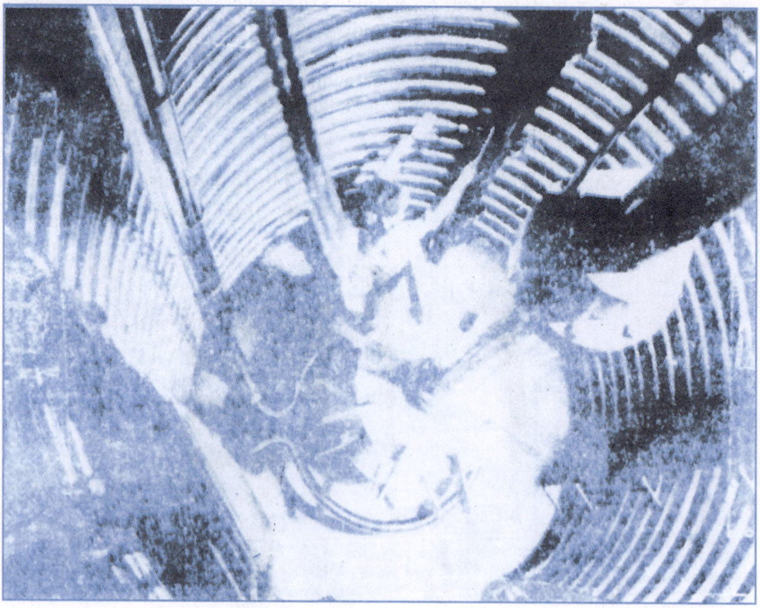

Figure 3.6 Interior view of large production fermentor of conventional design. Notice the cooling coils along the wall, the two impellers mounted one above the other on a shaft through the top of the fermentor, the circular sparger below the impellers, and the baffles on the wall of the fermentor. This view is from the top of the fermentor looking towards its bottom. (Muller and Kieslich, 1966. Angew. Chem. internat. Edit., 5,653–662.)

Small laboratory-scale fermentors used in groups of two to three or more allow great flexibility in research for the development of fermentation processes. Thus, several experimental variables with adequate controls can be tested side by side in these small fermentors. In addition, the optimum fermentation conditions, as determined in these fermentors, often are applicable in "scale-up" to fermentations in much larger fermentation tanks. The small tanks also may be used to produce inoculum for inoculating larger tanks and these tanks as inoculum for yet larger tanks. If we assume that about one to five percent by volume of inoculum is required for most fermentations, we can then decide the sizes of fermentation vessels required to build up enough inoculum to inoculate a very large tank, such as a 100,000 gallon tank. However, we must remember that there is a difference between fermentor capacity and working volume of the fermentor.

The small laboratory scale fermentors are designed so that they possess great flexibility in providing varying conditions for the growth of microorganisms. At the same time, they can be adjusted to provide microbial growth conditions similar to those found in the largest of industrial production tanks. Thus, fermentors, large or small, are somewhat similar in

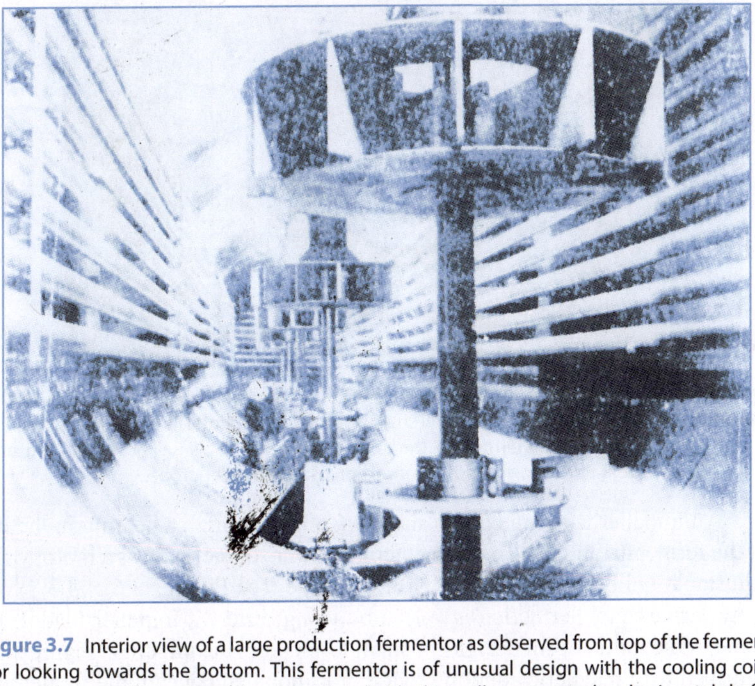

Figure 3.7 Interior view of a large production fermentor as observed from top of the fermentor looking towards the bottom. This fermentor is of unusual design with the cooling coils mounted vertically on the walls, and with individual impellers mounted on horizontal shafts at various heights in the fermentor. Photo courtesy of Merck and Co., Inc.

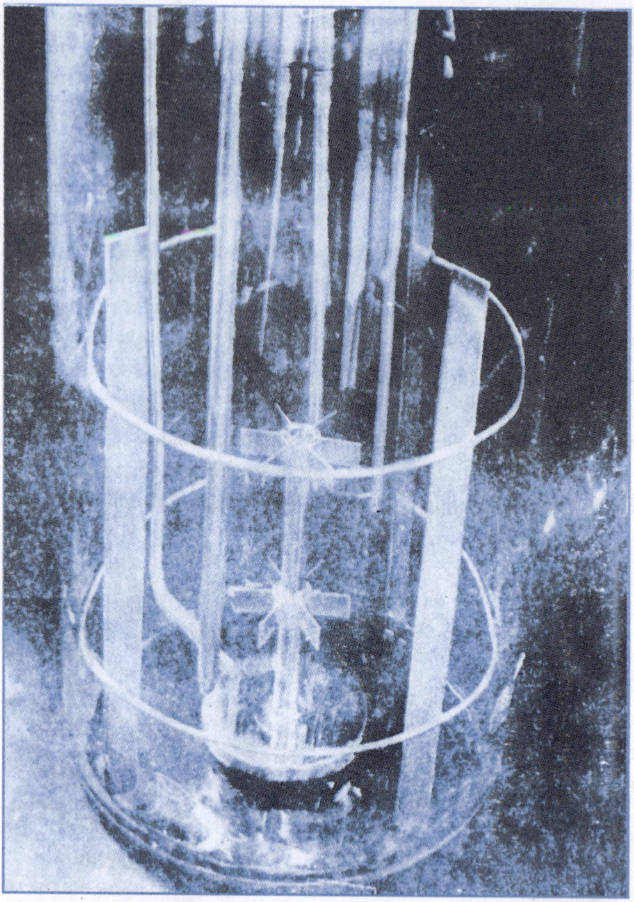

Figure 3.8 Interior view of a 12-liter total capacity VirTis magnetic drive fermentor. Notice the double impeller mounted on a small shaft attached to the bottom of the fermentor, the baffles along the wall of the fermentor, the tubular sparger with a small hole in its end, and the metal tube next to the sparger for the insertion of a thermistor probe.

An impeller is mounted to a shaft extending through a bearing in the lid of the fermentor and driven by an external power source, such as a motor with adjustable pulleys and belts, or by direct drive (see Figures 3.6 and 3.7). In direct drive, impeller action is varied by using different impeller blades. In some of the more recent designs of small fermentors the impeller (Figure 3.8) is driven by a magnetic coupling to a motor mounted beneath the fermentor. The height of the impeller blade or blades above the bottom of the fermentor is adjusted so that, when rotated at a relatively high speed, vigorous stirring and agitation of the medium is accomplished. At very high rotation speeds, the medium is thrown up against the sides of the fermentor so that a marked vortex occurs with the impeller at the bottom of the vortex (see Figures 3.9 and 3.10).

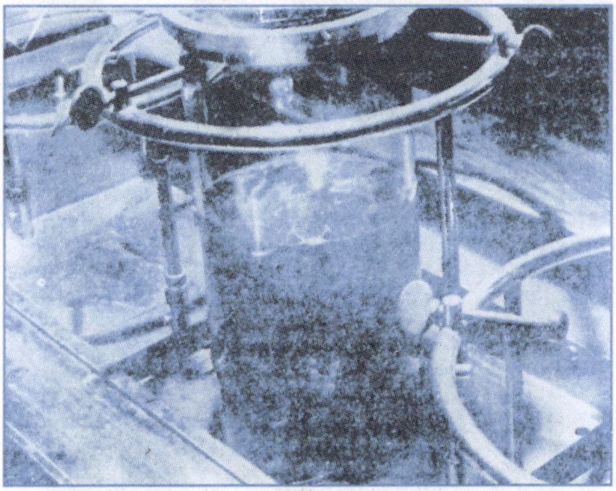

Figure 3.9 Vortex created by rapidly rotating impellers in a fermentor with baffles removed. The liquid has been thrown to the walls of the fermentor in such a manner that both of the impeller blades are virtually free of liquid. With the power supply turned off, the top impeller blade in this fermentor was submerged approximately one inch below the surface of the liquid.

In fermentations such as that for producing baker's yeast, contamination is not a serious problem. The low pH of the medium and the inclusion of lactic acid prevent growth of most bacterial contaminants. If, as in this fermentation, the fermentation economics preclude the cost of air sterilization, then the

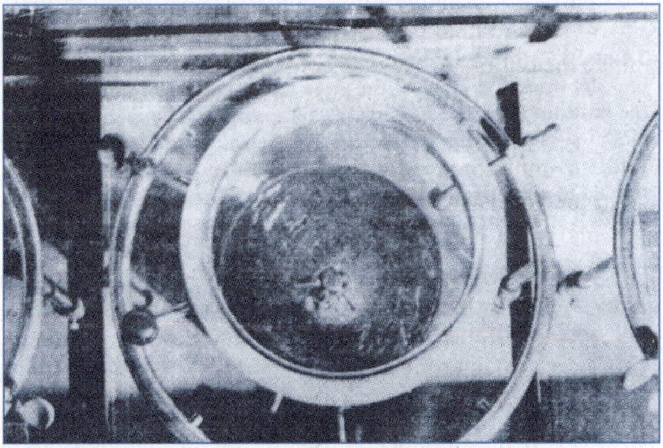

Figure 3.10 As for Figure 3.9 but vortex observed from above the fermentor. Again, notice that even the bottom impeller blades are partially free of liquid.

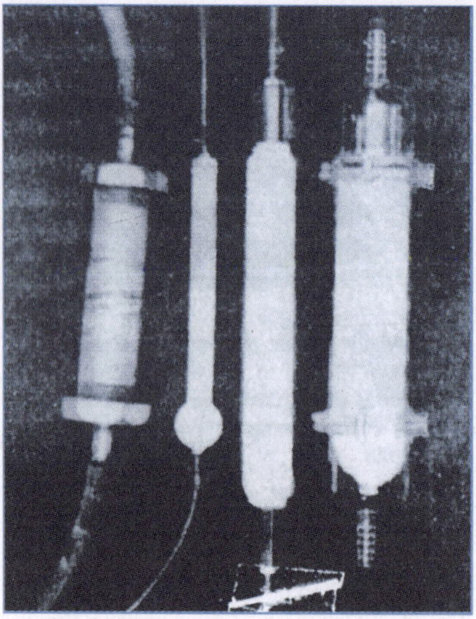

Figure 3.11 Air filters packed with glass wool as used in conjunction with various laboratory fermentors. The filters are fabricated of metal, plastic, or glass and the larger filters measure approximately 1 foot in length by 1.5 to 2 inches in diameter.

air may be merely cleaned by passage through a liquid such as glycerol or oil. However, most aerobic fermentations require that sterile air under pressure be introduced into the fermentation vessel. The cheapest means for sterilization of air is to pass it through a sterile filter (Figure 3.11) composed of glass wool, carbon particles, or some other finely divided material that will trap microorganisms present in the air. Beyond this filter, the air is carried through sterile piping to the bottom of the fermentor beneath the impeller blades. Here the air passes into a sparger which may be designed in various ways but which often consists of a pipe with minute holes (1/64 to 1/32 inch or larger in size) that allow the air under pressure to escape as tiny air bubbles into the liquid medium. Sparger holes smaller than this require too great an air pressure for economical bubble formation. Spargers in fermentors for growth of mycelium-forming organisms often utilize 1/4-inch holes to prevent plugging of the holes by hyphal growth. Pipes crimped at the end or with a single small hole (Figure 3.8) to produce a stream of air bubbles also are employed in some instances. The air bubbles from the sparger are picked up and dispersed through the medium by the action of the impeller blades mounted above the sparger. However, if the impeller is rotating rapidly enough that a marked vortex of the medium occurs, the air bubbles may escape directly through the shallow layer of medium above the impeller into the atmosphere of the head space (Figure 3.10). Thus, the rotation rate of the impeller blade should be great enough to allow through mixing of the medium but not so great that air from the sparger escapes without being dissolved in the medium for use by the microorganism. The smaller the bubbles of air produced by the sparger, the greater is the bubble surface area and the more likely is the oxygen of that air to pass across the bubble boundary and dissolve in the liquid of the medium. However, small air bubbles require greater air pressure for their formation through the fine holes of the sparger. Since sterile air is a costly item for an industrial fermentation, the size of the air bubbles, therefore, must be adjusted to give the greatest possible aeration without greatly increasing the overall cost of the fermentation.

In some very large fermentation tanks, an impeller is not utilized. The medium is stirred by the directed rush of air bubbles from a sparger at the bottom of the tank. These tanks are specially designed and usually do not contain baffles.

Fermentation tanks are never tightly sealed; there must be some place for escape of the air that has been introduced into the fermentor or for escape of the fermentation gases evolved during the growth of anaerobic microorganisms. We might assume that a fermentation vessel with openings in it large enough to allow the escape of considerable volumes of air would be prone to contamination problems. However, this is not the case, because the air entering the tank or the anaerobic fermentation gases produced in the tank create a positive pressure so that air or gas rush out through the air leaks in the tank. Dust carrying contaminating microorganisms cannot, therefore, enter the tank. Aeration and agitation of the aqueous medium in the tank creates an aerosol in the head space, and some of this aerosol escapes with the air from the tank. The aerosol fouls the packing around the impeller shaft where it enters the fermentor and allows possible entry of contamination at this point. A steam seal helps to prevent this contamination, although it causes some deterioration of the packing material. Fermentation microorganisms which are plant or animal pathogens require specially designed fermentors to handle the aerosol. All air escaping from the tank is collected and incinerated or treated in some other manner to destroy the escaping microorganisms.

For any given fermentor, the size of the sparger air bubbles is usually fixed, and the air flow rate during the fermentation cannot be changed by altering the size of the sparger holes. However, the air flow rate can be changed by changing the pressure on the air line. The ability to change air flow rates, which are usually measured in volumes of air per volume of medium per minute (Figure 3.12), may be of importance in fermentations where an initial high rate of aeration is required, to build up a large cell population, after which more anaerobic fermentation conditions are called for.

Impeller action in a fermentation tank tends to spin the liquid in a circular motion and, as previously stated, can create a vortex above the impeller. Under these conditions, it is possible for the liquid to spin in such a manner that suspended solids or microbial cells tend to remain in the same relative position in relation to the moving liquid without actually being mixed through it. Also, segments of the medium may remain adjacent to other segments of the medium, because the liquid is spinning as a mass. This results in relatively little splashing at the liquid surface so that a relatively small amount of medium surface is exposed to the atmosphere in the head space of the tank. This condition causes decreased aeration, since the medium

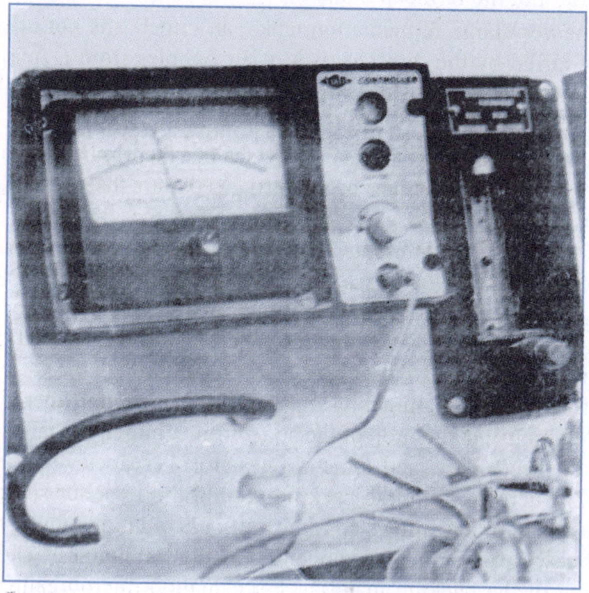

Figure 3.12 Temperature and aeration flow-rate controls for laboratory fermentors. As regards the air–flow meter at the right, notice the small ball suspended in the stream of incoming air. The height at which this ball becomes suspended in the air stream provides a relative measure of the air–flow rate, but does not measure air–flow in terms of volume of air per volume of medium per minute. The latter determination must be made on the air as it enters or escapes from the fermentor.

is aerated both by air from the sparger and by air incorporated at the surface of the medium. To correct this situation, verticle baffles (Figures 3.6 and 3.8) are often attached to the inside wall of the fermentor. These baffles disrupts the flow pattern of the liquid so that much greater mixing and turbulence of the liquid will occur.

Aeration and agitation of a liquid medium can cause the production of foam. This is particularly true of media containing high levels of proteins or peptides. In contrast, media composed largely of inorganic components and relatively pure sugars are much less likely to cause foaming problems. Proteolytic bacteria (that is, bacteria that degrade proteins to peptides and further) cause particularly serious foam problems, because the foam due to peptides can be quite stable. In fact, in fermentations utilizing organisms that do not usually cause foam problems on high protein media, the occurrence of a stable foam may be an indication that contamination by these organisms has occurred. In any event, foam must be controlled if a fermentation is to be carried out in a proper manner. If the foam is not controlled, it will rise in the head space of the tank (Figure 3.13) and be forced from the tank along with the spent air. This condition often causes contamination of the fermentation from organisms picked up by the breaking of some of the foam which then drains back into the tank. Excessive foaming also causes other problems for a fermentation. In extreme cases, a considerable volume of the medium may be forced from the tank as foam. Also, the presence of excessive foam in a tank impedes aeration by limiting gas exchange between the medium and the atmosphere of the head space.

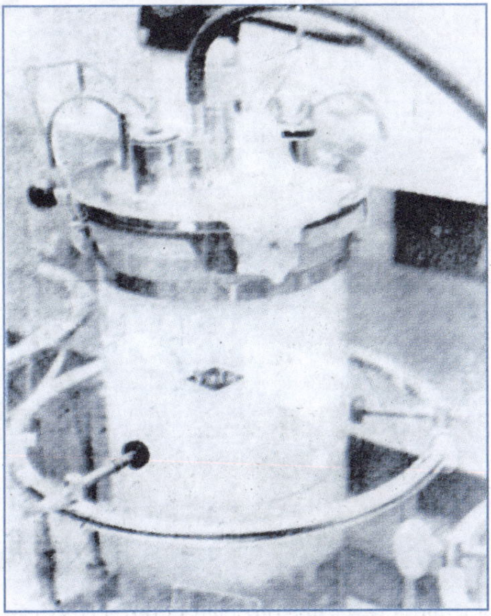

Figure 3.13 Small fermentor foaming over. The occurrence of excessive foam, as in this picture, can cause contamination of the fermentation if not already contaminated.

The usual procedure for controlling foam is to add an antifoam agent (Figure 3.14), although a supplementary impeller blade mounted high in the tank may at times be effective. An antifoam agent lowers surface tention and, in the process, decreases the stability of the foam bubbles so that they burst. The antifoam may be added at media make-up (before sterilization), or it may be added after sterilization or as called for during the fermentation. There are two types of antifoam agents: inert antifoams and antifoams made from crude organic materials. The latter antifoam agents usually are not effective as foam control agents if added to the medium before sterilization. They must be sterilized separately and then added to the fermentation as needed. When foaming occurs, only enough antifoam is added to break the foam, since excess antifoam may be toxic to the microorganism and, generally, is not effective in holding down foam in a succeeding foam build-up. Thus, the correct amount of antifoam must be added each time foaming becomes a problem.

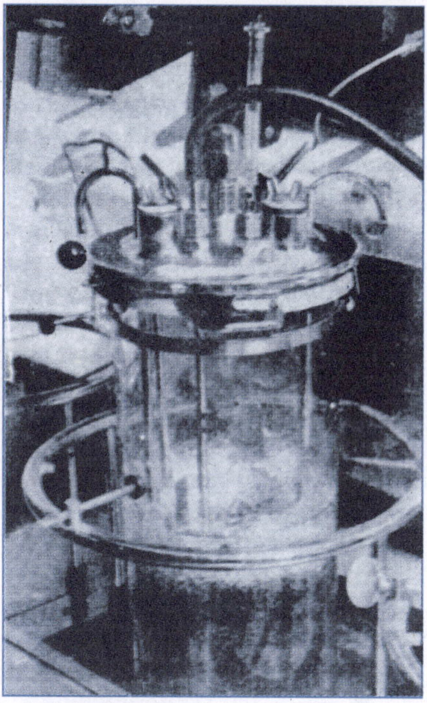

Figure 3.14 Small fermentor as pictured in Figure 3.13 except that a small amount of silicone antifoam agent was added from the small syringe mounted in the head of the fermentor. The foam broke almost immediately on the antifoam agent.

Antifoam agents are often difficult to sterilize, particularly if they are of an oily nature, because of poor heat penetration and transport through the oil. Thus, we must first be certain that the sterilizing procedure being used renders the antifoam free of microbial life.

The antifoam agents comprised of crude organic materials are of several types. Animal and vegetable oils are often used, for example, lard oil, corn oil, and soybean oil. Long-chain alcohols such as octadecanol also are of value. In addition, mixtures of oils and alcohols are effective in controlling foam, for example, lard oil mixed with octadecanol for penicillin fermentations. These antifoam agents are not inert; as previously mentioned, an excess of the antifoam may be toxic. Also, the antifoam may provide nutrients such as fatty acids for the organism, which occurs in certain antibiotic fermentations by organisms of the Streptomyces genus. The fatty acids also may lower the pH of the medium and this must be considered in the pH control of the fermentation.

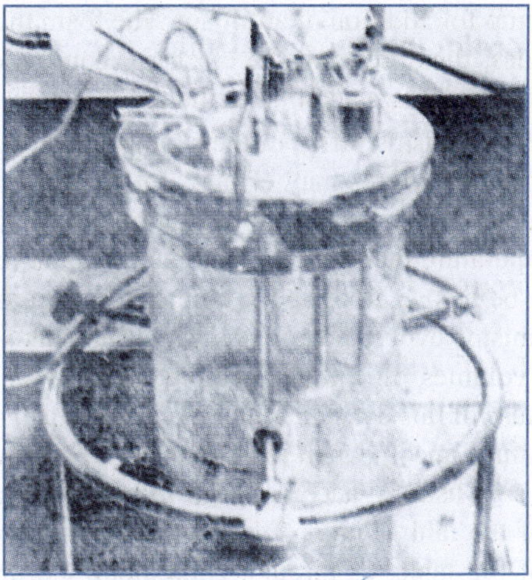

Figure 3.15 Small fermentor being cooled by water sprayed onto its outer surface. Notice the thermistor probe inserted in a metal tube projecting through the head of the fermentor for control of the spray-water temperature.

The use of inert antifoam agents, such as various silicone compounds, is the ideal way to control foam, but these agents, generally, are too expensive for use in large-scale industrial fermentations. The only effect of these compounds on the fermentation appears to be that of controlling foam; they are not utilized by the microorganism nor are they toxic. They may be added to the fermentation medium at make-up before sterilization, and they are still somewhat effective after sterilization, although build-up of a stable foam during the fermentation may require further additions of the antifoam agent. The inert antifoam agents are of particular value in initial research on a new fermentation, since they allow study of the fermentation in the absence of the toxic or nutritional factors contributed by the more crude agents.

When antifoam is required in a tank, it is added either manually or electrically. Obviously, manual addition requires that someone continuously observe the tank so that the antifoam can be added as required. Electrical addition of antifoam is usually preferred, therefore, because, being automatic, it requires little attention. To accomplish this automatic addition, a sensing mechanism is employed to determine when the foam has risen into the head space of the fermentor. Such a devise is provided by two electrodes mounted in the top of the fermentor and which project part way into the head space of the fermentor. These electrodes are connected to a pump associated with a reservoir of sterile antifoam and, as the foam rises in the fermentor, it touches the two electrodes, in the process allowing current to flow between them so as to activate the pump for addition of antifoam. The foam then collapses away from the electrodes, thus breaking the electrical connection between them and stopping further antifoam addition to the fermentor.

Various microorganisms differ in their temperature optima for growth, and these growth temperatures may or may not coincide with the optimum temperature as determined for the fermentation itself. It is the optimum fermentation temperature that must be maintained in the fermentor, and this temperature may be below, at, or above ambient temperature. Metabolically active microorganisms evolve heat which can accumulate to a considerable degree in large volumes of culture medium, such as in large production fermentors. Because of this consideration, more often than not, the fermentor must be cooled in some manner to maintain the optimum fermentation temperature. This is usually accomplished either by spraying cold water on the outside of the tank (Figure 3.15) or by passing cold water through jacketed walls of the tanks or through coils along the inside walls of the tank (Figures 3.6 and 3.7). For most fermentations, it is not economically feasible to cool the water used for this purpose and, hence, a source of naturally cold water is essential. Should a fermentation require temperatures above ambient, heat may be applied by passing steam through the coils or jacket of the fermentor. Also, when sterilized medium is initially added to a fermentor before inoculation, it is cooled only to that temperature at which the fermentation is to be conducted.

Pure culture fermentations usually require that the medium be srerilized. In small laboratory fermentors, the medium is placed directly in the fermentor, and the fermentor is then autoclaved. However, for larger tanks, this usually is not feasible. For these tanks, the medium constituents at double to triple strength are mixed with water in a separate mixing tank or tanks, and the resulting medium is then pumped through retention tubes and heat exchangers before passing into the large empty fermentation tank that has been previously sterilized by live steam. A mechanical vacuum breaker (a butterfly valve) on the tank prevents a vacuum build-up and consequent collapse of the tank during the period in which the freshly steamed fermentor is cooling before receiving the sterilized medium. The retention tubes contain steam jet heaters that inject high-pressure steam into the medium to sterilize it as it passes through the pipes, and the rate of passage (two to ten minutes per unit of medium) is adjusted to provide complete media sterilization without overcooking. The heat exchangers (a pipe containing the medium within a second pipe containing cool water moving in the opposite direction) cool the medium before delivery to the fermentor. After entry into the fermentor, the medium is then diluted to volume by sterile water that also has passed through the retention tubes and heat exchangers.

The medium must receive sufficient heat treatment to be sterile, but not enough so that it becomes overcooked. The later media often demonstrate poor growth or low yields in comparison to properly sterilized media, and this can be attributed to the action of heat on various components of the medium, as for example, phosphates reacting with sugars. Also, the decreases in pH commonly associated with medium sterilization may be magnified in overcooked media.

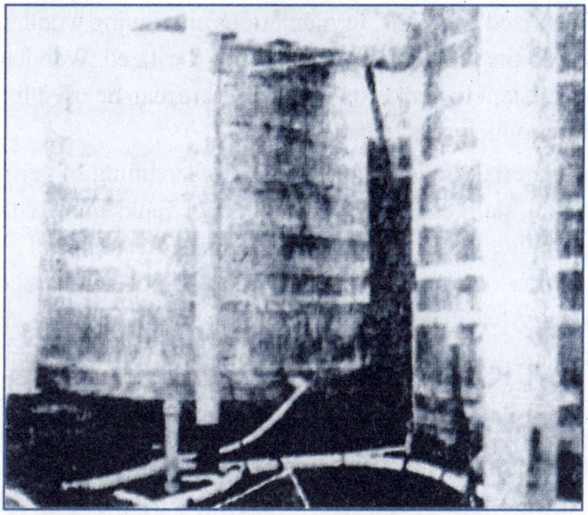

Figure 3.16 Cypress tanks formerly used in the brewing of beer. Courtesy of the Pittsburgh Brewing Co.

Sterilization of the medium is not required for some fermentations, however. Usually, these are the fermentations that utilize some built-in means for control of contamination. Also, they often are the fermentations for which the overall economics do not allow the expense of media sterilization. Examples are certain yeast fermentations that are conducted at relatively low pH values, fermentations utilizing as carbon substrate compounds that are toxic to most microorganisms (as, for example, certain hydrocarbons or ethanol), fermentation utilizing carbon substrates that are not attacked by most microorganisms (such as methane gas), fermentations using massive inoculum, and fermentations with poorly available nutrients present in dilute form and with other toxic agents present (such as with *Torula* yeast growing on sulfite waste liquor).

Various fermentation products, such as lactic acid, or medium components, such as the high salt content in the medium for chlorotetracycline production, are corrosive and may attack the inside lining of the fermentation tank (and also the linings of retention tubes, holding tanks, and product work-up tanks). This consideration dictates that tanks for these fermentations be constructed of materials resistant to corrosion. Certain other fermentations are quite sensitive to metallic ions that may dissolve from the liner of the tank. Thus, the construction material for a fermentation tank must be considered in regard to the particular fermentation that is to be conducted in the tank. In this case, California redwood or cypress wood (Figure 3.16). However, wood cannot easily be sterilized and, thus, fermentations employing wooden tanks must be those in which the medium normally is not sterilized. Wooden tanks also are somewhat resistant to corrosion and, therefore, can be used for fermentations such as that producing lactic acid.

Other materials for the construction of or lining of fermentation tanks include copper, stainless steel, iron, and glass. Tanks lined with stainless steel or glass are quite expensive, and these tanks are used only if necessitated by fermentation requirements and can be justified by the economics of the fermentation. Also, because of fabrication problems and susceptibility to mechanical and heat-shock breakage, the glass liners are limited to smaller tanks. Copper-lined tanks find use in certain steps in the brewing of beer. Thus, the filtered mash is boiled with hops in copper-lined tanks, although the actual fermentation may be carried out in tanks lined with glass. Tanks constructed of cast iron were used extensively in the early days of penicillin production. Later, when this fermentation was conducted in other tanks, such as those with stainless steel liners, it was found that the yields of penicillin decreased instead of the expected increase. The reason for this became obvious when the inside surfaces of these tanks were inspected. The stainless steel surface was smooth. In contrast, the cast iron surface had become markedly pitted and rough, factors that contributed to the baffling and shearing components of the fermentor design.

Tanks for anaerobic fermentations present different requirements. In most instances, provision for the introduction of air into the fermentation is not required, with the exception being those fermentations that require an initial aeration to build up a high cell yield before anaerobic conditions are imposed. In addition, an anaerobic fermentation may not utilize an impeller or other mixing device. However, some anaerobic fermentations require initial mixing of the inoculum through the fermentation medium, but may not need further mixing, because the rising of evolved fermentation gases tends to provide sufficient mixing.

The fact that air is not introduced into the fermentation tank does not automatically provide anaerobic conditions for the fermentation. There is still a head space above the fermentation medium which is filled with atmosphere containing oxygen. Some microorganisms, such as certain of the lactic acid-producing bacteria, are microaerophilic and can withstand small amounts of oxygen, even though the fermentation is essentially anaerobic. Other microorganisms, such as members of the genus *Clostridium*, are obligate anaerobes and cannot withstand the presence of oxygen. This type of organism can be successfully grown in a fermentation tank without extensive changes in design or use of expensive apparatus to remove oxygen from the atmosphere if the proper precautions are taken. A thick gelatinous medium is used which impedes the penetration of oxygen. The medium is sterilized immediately prior to inoculation, which drives out dissolved oxygen, and the inoculum is introduced into the bottom of the tank immediately on cooling of the medium to the proper temperature for the fermentation and before oxygen has had a chance to penetrate into the medium. In a fermentation such as this, carbon dioxide and hydrogen are evolved, so that as soon as the fermentation is progressing vigorously, the oxygen in the atmosphere of the head space is flushed from the tank. These fermentation gases are economically valuable, and provision often is made to collect the gases as they emanate from the production fermentors. The carbon dioxide has been utilized in the past for production of dry ice and the synthesis of methanol. The hydrogen is valuable for use as a catalyst in chemical reductions. This gas mixture also can be used to flush the atmosphere from freshly inoculated tanks of *Clostridium* organisms, with the gas evolved from a vigorous fermentation being piped directly to newly inoculated tanks.

The fermentation equipment discussed thus far is that which is most often employed in the industrial growth of cells and for the production of their biosynthetic products. However, other types of equipment are employed in specific instances, particularly for aerobic fermentations. Drum fermentors have been described but only rarely used commercially. The fermentation medium is placed in an internally baffled, metal (often aluminum) drum with a spindle at either end to allow rotation of the drum. The revolving of the drum causes splashing of the medium, mixing, and aeration, although additional air may be piped into one end of the fermentor and exhausted at the other end.

The treatment of municipal and industrial waste waters (see Chapter 14) utilizes two types of fermentation apparatus which, possible, might not be considered as fermentation equipment, although organic matter decomposition fermentations are carried out in them. The "activated sludge" treatment of municipal waste utilizes the aerated submerged fermentation approach. Aerobic microbial degradation of the organic components of the waste water occurs in a deep, elongated or round tank which is fully exposed to the atmosphere, and air under pressure is introduced from the walls of the tank into the lower reaches of the water volume so as to provide oxygen for the microorganisms and, at the same time, mixing of the water. The second waste-water treatment fermentation utilizes the "trickling filter" system, in which the incoming water are sprayed over a deep bed of rocks. Microorganisms able to oxidatively degrade the organic wastes cling to these rocks and, as the waste water trickles down through the rock bed, its organic components are decomposed.

The trickling filter concept is also applied in a more conventional fermentative approach, the "vinegar generator". In order to oxidize ethyl alcohol to the acetic acid of vinegar, a high column packed with some material such as beech wood shavings is employed. Alcohol is introduced at the top of the column and, as it percolates through the column, it is oxidized by *Acetobacter* species of bacteria to acetic acid.

Fermentations utilizing fungi, more often than not, are conducted as aerated submerged fermentations. The penicillin fermentation is an example (see Chapter 17). However, in the early days of penicillin production before the advent of aerated deep tanks, the *Penicillium* mold was grown as a mycelial mat on the surface of stationary liquid medium. The medium was contained in flat bottles, and the bottles were incubated on their sides in temperature controlled rooms. Yields of penicillin were low, because of the inherent low-yielding capacity of the fungal strains used, and because of the poor fermentation design characteristics of these bottles. Thus, nutrients became exhausted in the liquid levels immediately beneath the mycelial mat, and fresh nutrients were available only by diffusion from the bottom of the bottle. Carbon dioxide was trapped under the mycelium, and the carbon dioxide evolved into the atmosphere above the mycelium tended to flush other gases, including oxygen, from the bottle. In other words, aeration and nutrient conditions were inadequate for good growth of the mold and production of penicillin. These problems were largely corrected when submerged, aerated fermentation conditions were applied.

The surface fungal mycelial mat approach to fermentations, however, is still utilized today in certain fermentations, such as that for the production of citric acid, although submerged aerated fermentations for this acid also are extensively employed today. The yields of the two fermentative approaches compare favorably. The surface mat culture of citric acid is accomplished by placing the fermentation medium in shallow, open pans in racks in a constant temperature room, and the medium is inoculated by spraying spores of *Aspergillus niger* across the surface of the medium. The open pans can be used, because contamination is not a particular problem, and because they allow good gas diffusion too and away from the surface of the mat.

"Continuous fermentations" are fermentations that are run continuously without emptying the fermentor at each harvest of microbial cells or biosynthetic products (see Chapter 13). Fresh medium is continuously or intermittently added to the fermentation to replace spent nutrients, and a portion of the fluid, which contains cells or biosynthetic products, from the fermentor is continuously or intermittently withdrawn for recovery of the product. By controlling the concentration of some limiting component of the nutrients, the organism is maintained in a specific phase of its growth cycle so that it will continue growth almost indefinitely in this phase. Aside from the inherent problems of contamination, genetic stability, and the like, associated with this type of fermentation, there is a requirement that the fermentation have special sensing devices for pH, rate of cell growth and product formation, and other factors of the fermentation, that it have metering facilities for introduction of fresh nutrients, and that there be valves and piping for the withdrawal of a portion of the culture during the fermentation for recovery of products. In some instances, such as in the growth of *Torula* yeast in sulfite waste liquor, little problem is encountered, and monitoring, metering, and product recovery requirements are at a minimum. Other continuous fermentations may require much more elaborate facilities and design, as for example, the Acetator and Cavitator fermentors described in Chapter 21 for vinegar production.

Gaseous carbon nutrients as components of fermentation media present special problems in fermentation equipment design. Methane and ethane are good examples of this point, and fermentors, such as the "bubble cap" fermentor, have been designed to allow utilization of such substrates. A bubble-cap fermentor is a tank containing a series of horizontal plates (Figure 3.17). Each plate supports nutrients medium without a carbon source, and the medium is inoculated with the required microorganism. Each plate also has short, vertical pipes connected to its upper surface and projecting just above the surface of the liquid medium. A hole in the bottom of this pipe allows contact with the atmosphere above the medium in the next lower plate. The top of each of these small pipes is covered with an inverted cuplike cap so

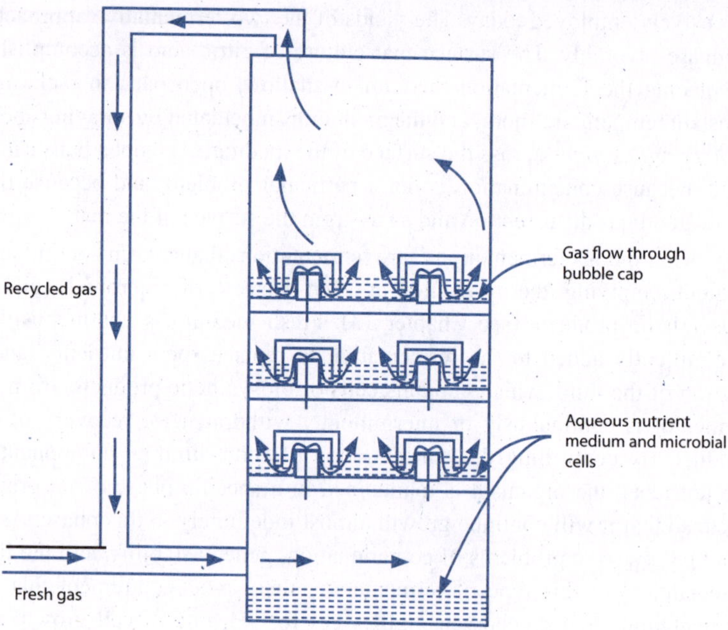

Figure 3.17 Bubble-cap fermentor design to allow microbial attack on gaseous substrates such as gaseous hydrocarbons. (M. S. Taggart Jr., March 19, 1946, U.S. 2,396,900).

that the lower rim of the inverted cap extends beneath the surface of the nutrient medium. Hydrocarbon gas is introduced at the bottom of the fermentor beneath the plates and rises through the pipes of each plate, escaping from each pipe beneath the surface of the liquid medium because of the inverted cap loosely covering the pipe. Thus, gas not oxidized at one plate level in the fermentor rises to the next plate to again be exposed to microbial oxidation.

Gas rising completely through the fermentor can be recycled to the bottom of the fermentor for another passage. Obviously, an alternate procedure for fermenting gaseous substrates is to introduce them with the air through the sparger in a submerged aerated fermentation. However, unless special precautions are taken, much of the gaseous substrate will be lost with the air exhausted from the fermentor.

Fermentations utilizing liquid carbon substrates immiscible with water, such as liquid hydrocarbons that float on the surface of the aqueous medium, can be handled in one three ways. Tanks for submerged aerated fermentations are most often used, with vigorous impeller agitation dispersing the hydrocarbon as small oil droplets throughout the aqueous medium. An emulsifying agent can also be added to aid in this dispersion. The second possibility, although rarely used, is to employ what might be described as a "lift" or "cyclic" fermentor. The hydrocarbon substrate is allowed to float on the surface of the aqueous medium, and aqueous medium containing microorganisms is withdrawn continuously from the bottom of the fermentor to a vertical small-bore lift pipe at the side of the fermentor. The column of medium in this pipe is raised, either by introduction of sterile air under pressure or by mechanical pumping, to the top of the fermentor where it is sprayed over the surface of the hydrocarbon. This spraying, and the introduction of sterile air into the lift pipe or into the head space of the fermentor, keeps the medium well aerated. In addition, the passage of the condensed aqueous spray down through the floating hydrocarbon layer brings microorganisms in the spray into continuous contact with the hydrocarbon and, if the spray is forceful, tends to break up the layering effect of the hydrocarbon on the liquid surface.

The third fermentor design for immiscible liquid substrates pumps a mixture of aqueous culture and immiscible substrate from the main reservoir of the fermentor, and then forces it through a nozzle against a baffle arrangement. The resulting well-mixed and aerated splash then falls back to the culture reservoir below.

PART II

BASIS AND DEVELOPMENT OF INDUSTRIAL FERMENTATION PROCESSES

Industrial fermentations are money-making ventures, and the competition is keen. More than one industrial concern may carry out the same fermentation and even use a similar microorganism. Also, the fermentation product may have to compete on the open market with a similar product that is produced by a nonmicrobial process. Therefore, to be competitive, an industrial fermentation must produce high yields of product at least possible expense, and the recovery of the product to salable form must be efficient and not add greatly to the cost of the fermentation.

How have such economically competitive fermentations arrived at their present states of excellence? These fermentations did not just suddenly appear in their present form : someone had to discover the possibility for such a fermentation and then develop a way to make it economically feasible on a large-scale production basis. Thus, research is required to discover the fermentation in the first place, and additional research is required to adapt the fermentation to existing types of fermentation equipment and to increase the yields of product. Studies also are required to find a means for recovery of the product from the culture broth in such a state that it can be offered on the open market. As industrial production continues over a period of time, it is necessary to maintain the competitive advantage of the process by further research designed to increase yields or, possible, to better the procedures for product recovery. Thus, a continuous research program is required both for the development of a new fermentation process and for the continuing production of products that utilize existing processes.

What, then, are the research and development approaches that are employed for the finding of a microorganism of economic value and for the developing of its potential as a fermentation process that can be carried out on a production scale? We must start with the microorganism itself. Where do we find such a microorganism? Stock culture collections are a possibility, but the organisms in these collections have only rarely proven to be of value. In most instances, these organisms were not originally deposited in the stock culture collection because of their ability to produce good yields of some product or, if they were, there probably already exists a patented process that utilizes the organism. Several microbial fermentations are known to occur in nature. For example, if we are interested in finding a microorganisms to convert lactose to lactic acid, we might investigate milk that has soured. In this instance, It would already be known that the desired product had been produced in the milk and that the respective bacteria would be present. Often, however, we find that the particular fermentation of interest does not occur in nature, although it will proceed in the laboratory if the conditions are right. While not helping in the search for industrial microorganisms, the latter observation is of value, since the concept of patents for microbial fermentation processes is based, at least in part, on the premise that, by providing the proper set of conditions, man directs a microorganism to produce a product in the laboratory of production fermentor which it does not produce in nature.

Microorganisms can be isolated at random from various natural sources and tested individually for their fermentation potential, but the chances of finding one of value by this means are not very great. Only a very few members of a natural microbial population will possess the characteristics being sought. Thus, to find a microorganism that can do what we want it to do is not a simple matter.

The most successful approach to finding such a microorganism is to utilize some technique that will allow the obtaining and testing of large numbers of microorganisms, but without requiring that extensive studies be carried out on each individual organism. Such a technique is available and is known as "screening". The screening technique is used in various forms, depending on the type of microorganism that is desired, on the particular product of interest, and on the source from which the microorganisms are to be obtained.

To make effective use of the screening approach, we first must have access to a natural microbial source that contains many different types of microorganisms whether most of these organisms are or not known to possess the biosynthetic abilities in which we are interested. The best source from which to obtain a wide variety of microorganisms is the soil. Another source, which has not yet been explored to any extent, is sea water or marine mud. Examples of other natural microbial sources are compost, rumen contents, domestic sewage undergoing treatment, manure, and spoiled foodstuffs or feedstuffs.

Why is soil the ideal source from which to obtain diverse types of microorganisms? The answer is evident if we consider that much of the debris of the world finds its way onto and into the soil and is there decomposed by one microorganism or another. Thus, we might consider soil as being a huge natural fermentation vat whose organisms are involved in the decomposition and resynthesis of simple to complex organic materials, and in the oxidation, reduction, and other chemical changes of inorganic materials. Usually, more than one type, and often many types, of soil microorganisms are able to carry out each of these individual biochemical or chemical transformations.

While it is known that many different types of microorganisms occur in the soil, it is not so evident just what portion of these organisms have, to date, been isolated to pure laboratory culture. Various workers have estimated that plate counting and isolation procedures for total numbers and types of soil microorganisms, even though utilizing the best known media and incubation conditions, probably allow less than one percent of the soil microorganisms to be grown in the laboratory. If this statement is reversed, we find that 99 percent or greater of the soil microorganisms may not yet have been cultivated in the laboratory. Apparently, these microorganisms are waiting for someone to devise a medium and cultural conditions that will allow their growth in the laboratory. Obviously, this is of interest to one who wishes to isolate organisms with new biosynthetic capabilities, because it means that, at least with soil, there are many microorganisms not previously described which are just waiting to be isolated and evaluated.

The soil also allows a certain degree of manipulation in the relative levels of the components of its microbial population before application of screening and isolation procedures. The level of available nutrients in soil usually is relatively low, and the microbial competition for these nutrients is keen. If a particular nutrient is added to moistened soil and the soil is incubated, a relatively greater growth response occurs among those soil microorganisms able to attack this nutrient, thus simplifying the isolation of these particular organisms. In other words, we can carry out an "enrichment" in soil for microorganisms of interest. Likewise, the soil may be incubated in liquid laboratory media to enrich for specific organisms before isolation is attempted. A natural enrichment occurs in soil in the region of plant roots, and the microorganisms in this area may be different from those in adjacent soil not penetrated by roots. This "rhizosphere effect" is caused by root secretions and dead or sloughed root debris which serve as microbial nutrients.

The choice of approach for isolating soil microorganisms depends on several factors. However, certain questions need to be answered before a decision is made.

1. Is it to be an aerobic, microaerophilic or anaerobic fermentation?
2. Is the product to be microbial cells or a chemical compound?
3. Is the interest only in a specific group of microorganisms, such as the Streptomyces genus for antibiotic production, or are all possible types of microorganisms to be considered?
4. Is there interest only in a specified product or group of products, or are all possible products produced by certain types of organisms to be considered?
5. Will the microorganism only be required to better the yield of an already existing fermentation?
6. Is there a specific carbon or nitrogen substrate is to be utilized in the nutrition of the organism and biosynthesis of product?
7. Are any of the potential fermentation substrates insoluble or immiscible with water?
8. Is the fermentation to be a one-or two-step enzymatic transformation of a substrate, or is it intended for the microorganism to totally degrade a substrate, such as a carbohydrate, to small organic molecules, such as acetate, and then resynthesize products of value from the small molecules?
9. Are the expected fermentation products either acidic or alkaline in nature?
10. Are mutants such as auxotrophs likely to be employed for the fermentation?
11. Will metabolic poisons or alternate electron acceptors be employed in the fermentation?
12. Is the product to be optically or biologically active ?
13. Is the product sensitive to autooxidation, hydrolysis, or other unwanted change?
14. Is any constituents of the medium volatile, or is the fermentation product volatile?
15. Are there flavor, color, or esthetic considerations associated with the product?
16. Is the microorganism likely to require unusual temperature, aeration, pH, or other conditions for growth?

17. Are any of the nutritional substrates at low concentration likely to be toxic to the organism, or will toxicity become apparent if high concentrations are employed?
18. Is the product of the fermentation in itself likely to be an inhibitor of the fermentations?
19. Is the fermentation process likely to employ more than one fermentative step, or is more than one microorganism likely to be required?
20. Will mating types of the organisms be required?
21. Is the microbial fermentative agent likely to be a plant or animal pathogen that will require special handling and disposal?
22. Will the microorganism require a prolonged period of incubation both during isolation and during later stages of growth in the laboratory and in production?
23. Will possible valuable by-products be produced during the fermentation?
24. Is the fermentation product closely related to some intermediate of the tricarboxylic acid or Meyerhof-Embden cycles or to intermediates of other well-known metabolic sequences?

The answers to all of these questions are important. However, only a relatively few of these factors will be considered as they apply to screening approaches.

Chapter 4

Screening

PRIMARY SCREENING

Screening may be defined as the use of highly selective procedures to allow the detection and isolation of only those microorganisms of interest from among a large microbial population. Thus, to be effective, screening must in one or a few steps allow the discarding of many valueless microorganisms, while at the same time allowing the easy detection of the small percentage of useful microorganisms that are present in the population. The concept of screening will be illustrated by citing specific examples of screening procedures that are or have been commonly employed in industrial research programs. In each instance, except for that of the crowded-plate technique, a natural microbial source such as soil is diluted to provide a cell concentration such that aliquots spread, sprayed, or applied in some manner to the surfaces of agar plates (Figure 4.1), will yield colonies not touching neighboring colonies.

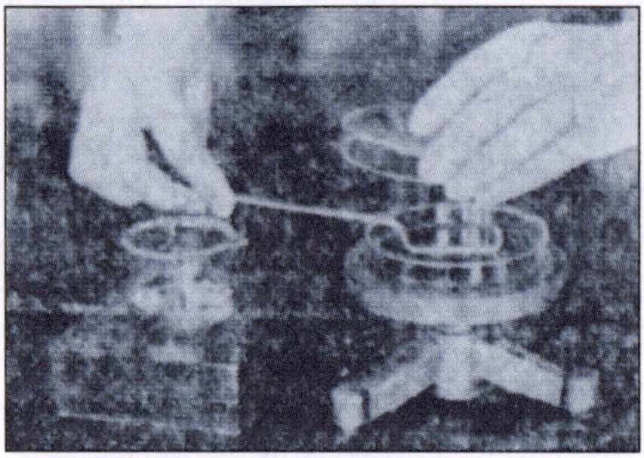

Figure 4.1 Spread plating of soil dilutions. An 0.1 to 0.2 ml portion of a soil dilution is applied to the agar surface by pipette, then spread across the surface with a sterile glass rod. The rod is sterilized by dipping it in alcohol and then burning off the residual alcohol. The plate is setting on a spreading wheel which is rotated to allow a more even spreading of the sample.

Microorganisms producing organic acid or amines from various carbon substrates often can be detected by the incorporation of a pH-indicating dye,

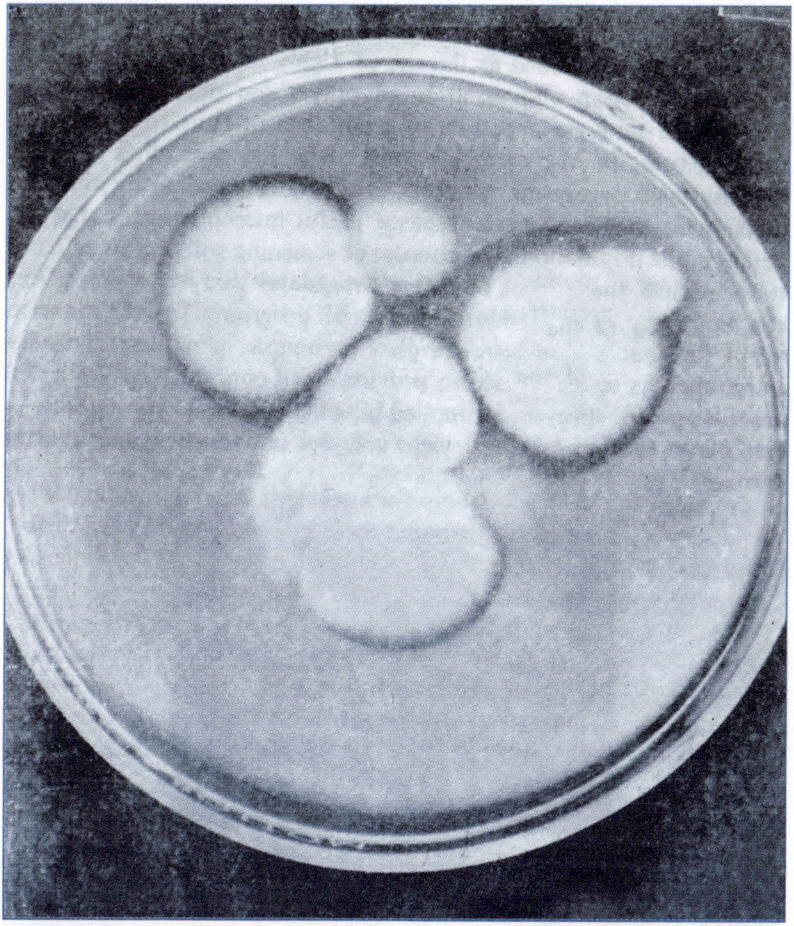

Figure 4.2 Detection of fungi capable of producing organic acids by incorporation of $CaCO_3$ into the agar medium. Notice the areas of dissolved $CaCO_3$ adjacent to several of the colonies.

such as neutral red or bromthymol blue, into a poorly buffered agar nutrient medium. The production of these compounds is indicated by a change in the color of the indicating dye in the vicinity of the colony to a color representing an acidic or alkaline reaction. The usefulness of this procedure is increased if media of greater buffer capacity are utilized so that only those microorganisms that produce considerable quantities of the acid or amine can induce changes in the color of the dye. An alternative procedure for detecting organic-acid production involves the incorporation of calcium carbonate in the medium so that organic-acid production is indicated by a cleared zone of dissolved calcium carbonate around the colony (Figure 4.2). These procedures are not foolproof, however, since inorganic acids or bases also are potential products of microbial growth. For instance, if the nitrogen source of the medium is the nitrogen of ammonium sulfate the organism may utilize the ammonium ion, leaving behind the sulfate ion as sulfuric acid, a condition indistinguishable from organic-acid production. Thus, cultures yielding positive reactions require further testing to be sure that an organic acid or base actually has been produced.

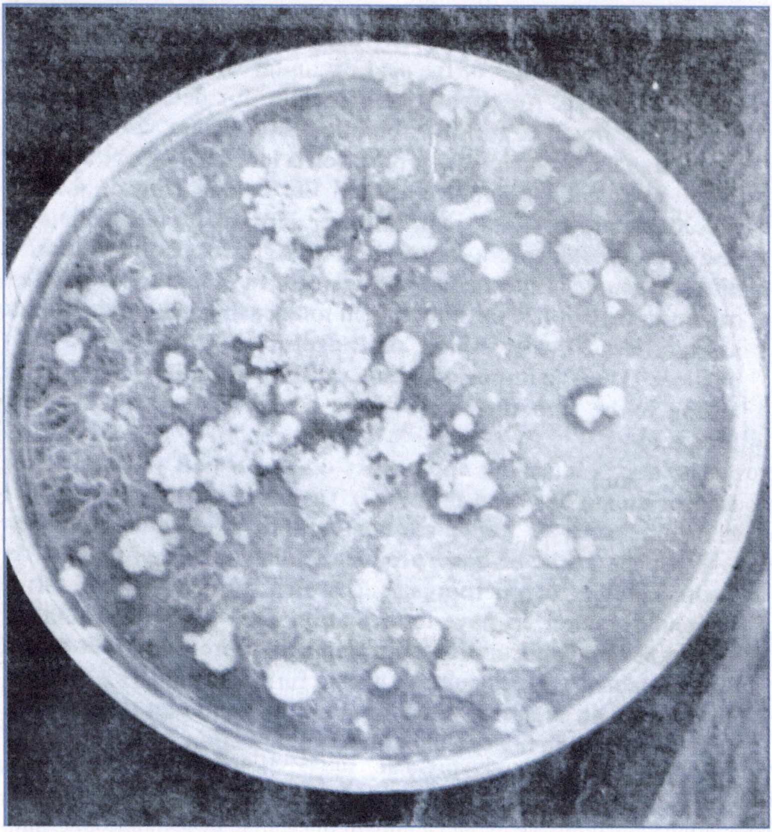

Figure 4.3 Crowded-plate screening for antibiotic-producing microorganisms. Notice the inhibition of growth adjacent to several of the colonies.

The above screening approaches do not tell us just which organic acid or amine has been produced. Therefore, further testing by some procedure such as paper chromatography is required to determine whether the acidic or basic product actually is one of interest. In any event, colonies of microorganisms which, through use of this initial screening, appear to have fermentation potential should immediately be purified and subcultured onto slants of appropriate agar medium to be maintained as stock cultures during further testing. It is discouraging to discover an organism showing good fermentation potential only to find that, through faulty technique, contamination, or for other reasons, the culture has been lost.

The screening approach also has been employed extensively in the search for microorganisms capable of producing useful antibiotics. The simplest screening technique for antibiotic producers is the "crowded-plate" procedure. This technique is used when we are interested only in finding microorganisms that produce an antibiotic without regard to what types of microorganisms may be sensitive to the antibiotic. The soil or other source of microorganisms is diluted only to a cell concentration such that agar plates prepared from these dilutions will be crowded with individual colonies on the surface of the agar; that is, 300 to 400 or more colonies per plate. Colonies producing antibiotic activity are indicated by an area of agar around the colony that is free of growth of other colonies (Figure 4.3). Such a colony is subcultured to a similar medium (Figure 4.4), and purified by streaking (Figure 4.5), before making stock cultures. The purified culture is then ready for testing to find what types of microorganisms are sensitive to the antibiotic, the "microbial inhibition spectrum".

As previously discussed for other primary screening techniques, the crowded-plate procedure also does not necessarily select an antibiotic-producing microorganism, because the inhibition area around the colony sometimes can be attributed to other causes. Notable among these are a marked change in the pH value of the medium resulting from the metabolism of the colony, or a rapid utilization of critical nutrients in the immediate vicinity of the colony. Thus, further testing again is required to prove that the inhibitory activity associated with a microorganism can really be attributed to the presence of an antibiotic.

The crowded-plate technique, as described has only limited application, since usually we are interested in finding a microorganism producing antibiotic activity against specific microorganisms and not against the unknown microorganisms that were by chance on the plate in the vicinity of an antibiotic-producing microorganism. Antibiotic screening is improved, therefore, by the incorporation into the procedure of a "test organism," that

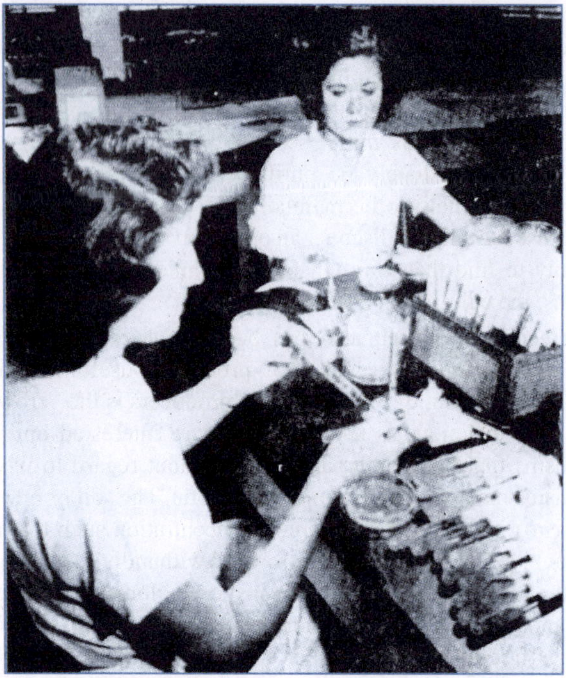

Figure 4.4 Subculture of microorganisms from primary screening plates. Photo courtesy of Charles Pfizer and Co., Inc.

is, an organism used as an indicator for the presence of specific antibiotic activity. Dilutions of soil or of other microbial sources are applied to the surfaces of agar plates so that well-isolated colonies will develope, roughly 30 to 200 colonies per plate. The plates are incubated until the colonies are a few millimeters in diameter, and so that antibiotic production will have occurred for those organisms having this potential. A suspension of the test organism is then sprayed or applied in some manner to the surface of the agar, and the plates are further incubated to allow growth of the test organism. Antibiotic activity is indicated by zones of inhibited growth of the organism around antibiotic-producing colonies (see Figure 4.6). In addition, a rough approximation of the relative amounts of antibiotic produced by various colonies can be gained by measuring in millimeters the diameters of the zones of inhibited test-organism growth. Antibiotic-producing colonies again must be isolated and purified before further testing.

A similar screening approach can be used to find microorganisms capable of synthesizing extracellular vitamins, amino acids, or other metabolities. However, the medium at make-up must be totally lacking in the metabolite

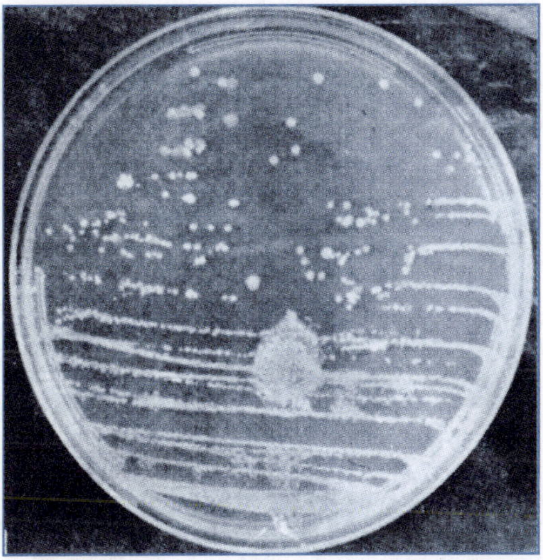

(a)

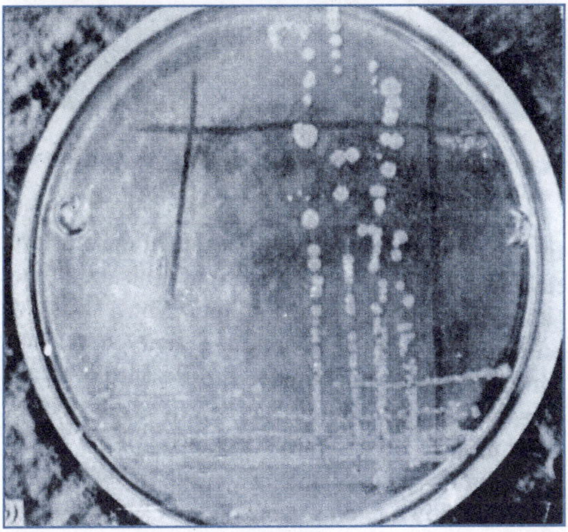

(b)

Figure 4.5 Streak plates prepared in two different ways for culture purification. For plate A, the organisms were largely cleaned from the inoculating loop by making close streaks of the loop near one side of the plate before separating the streaks by a greater distance across the surface of the agar. For plate B, four parallel streaks were made along one edge of the plate, then the loop was flamed, cooled, and drawn perpendicularly across the original streaks. This procedure was repeated twice more, as shown by the guide lines marked on the back of the plate.

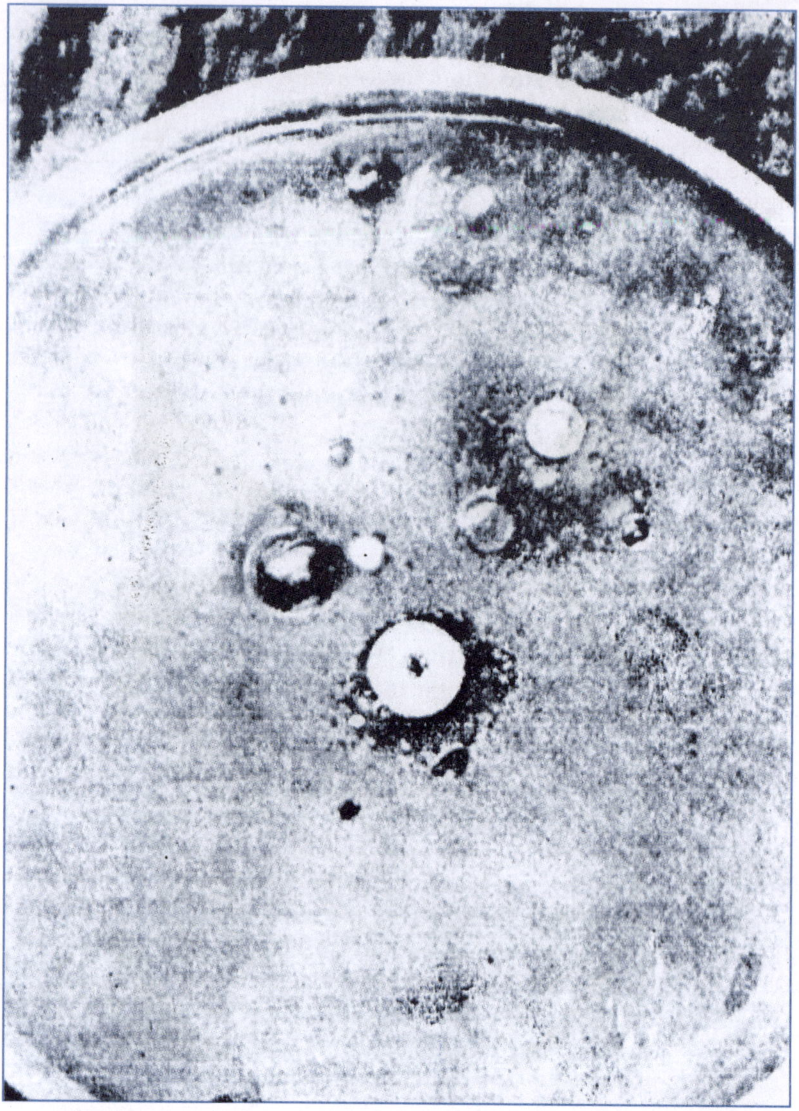

Figure 4.6 Use of a test organism in screening for antibiotic-producing microorganisms from soil. A Petri plate exhibiting many colonies of soil organisms was sprayed with a suspension of *Escherichia coli* cells (the test organism) before further incubation of the plate. The plate in this figure had many colonies on it before spraying, but only a few of the colonies are visible after growth of the test organism. Notice the zone of inhibited *E. coli* growth surrounding the large white *Streptomyces* colony.

under consideration. Again the microbial source is diluted and plated to provide well-isolated colonies, and the test organism is applied to the plates before further incubation. The choice of the particular test organism to be used is critical. It must possess a definite growth requirement for the particular metabolite, and for that metabolite only, so that production of this compound will be indicated by zones of growth, or at least increased growth, of the test organism adjacent to colonies that have produced the metabolite.

At times, we wish to screen a microbial source in order to find microorganisms capable of utilizing a specific carbon or nitrogen nutrient for growth and biosynthesis. To accomplish this objective, the plating medium is made up so as to contain the particular nutrient as its only source, respectively, of carbon or nitrogen. Dilutions of soil are applied to the plates, and the colonies appearing after incubation are assumed to possess the desired attribute. However, each organism must be tested further, since its growth under these conditions possibly could be attributed to nutrient sources other than those incorporated in the medium. Thus, if only low dilutions of soil are employed, there may be a carry-over of carbon and nitrogen nutrients from the soil which would allow at least limited growth of many microorganisms on the plating medium. Also, a microorganism on the plate which can utilize the specific carbon or nitrogen substrate may only partially degrade it or, in the process, may synthesize other carbon or nitrogen compounds that will allow growth of a few adjacent microorganisms that normally could not grow because of lack of the metabolite.

A modification of the latter technique is employed when volatile substrates such as hydrocarbons, low molecular weight alcohols, and similar carbon sources are being considered. With these substrates, often it is not necessary to incorporate the specific substrate into the agar medium. The dilutions from a microbial source are applied to plates of agar media containing all nutrients but the specific substrate, and the specific substrate is placed in the lid of the Petri plate after inversion of the plate. Enough vapors from the volatile substrate rise to the surface of the agar within this closed atmosphere to provide the specific nutrient for the microorganisms. Obviously, this procedure is of particular value when the volatile substrate is either immiscible or insoluble in water and, hence, difficult to disperse in an agar medium.

These are but a few examples of primary screening techniques. A good mental exercise is to pick several organic compounds and try to determine how we might screen for microorganisms capable of producing these compounds.

SECONDARY SCREENING

Primary screening allows the detection and isolation of microorganisms that possess potentially interesting industrial applications. This screening is usually followed by a secondary screening to further test the capabilities of and gain information about these organisms. The primary screening may have yielded only a few microorganisms, or many microorganisms may have been obtained. Probably, however, only a very small number of these organisms will have any real commercial value, because primary screening determines which microorganisms are able to produce a compound without providing much idea of the production or yield potential for the organisms. In contrast, secondary screening allows the further sorting out of those microorganisms that have real value for industrial processes, and the discarding of those lacking this potential. Organisms of the latter type must be discarded as soon as possible from research studies because of the high expense of such studies.

Secondary screening is conducted on agar plates, in flasks or small fermentors containing liquid media, or as a combination of these approaches. The use of agar plates, although not as sensitive as liquid culture, is of advantage for initial secondary screening, because more information is obtained with the expenditure of a similar amount of effort. Agar plates in an incubator take up relatively little space and do not require the amount of handling and work-up effort associated with liquid cultures. However, agar plate cultures provide only a limited indication of the actual product yield potentials among various isolates; to obtain this information, we must employ liquid culture, because liquid culture provides a much better picture of the nutritional, physical, and production responses of an organism to actual fermentation production conditions.

Secondary screening can be qualitative or quantitative in its approach. The qualitative approach, for example, tells us the spectrum or range of microorganisms which is sensitive to a newly discovered antibiotic. The quantitative approach tells us the yields of antibiotic which can be expected when the microorganism is grown in various differing media. However, there is not necessarily a distinct difference between qualitative and quantitative secondary screening. Thus, a qualitative screening for the "microbial inhibition spectrum" of an antibiotic determines which test organisms are sensitive to the antibiotic, but may, at the same time, yield information on the relative sensitivities of these organisms to the antibiotic.

Secondary screening should yield the types of information which are needed in order to evaluate the true potential of a microorganism for industrial usage. For example, secondary screening should determine what types of microorganisms are involved and whether they can be classified at least to families or genera. This information is of value, because it allows a comparison of the newly isolated organisms with those already described in the scientific and patent literatures as being able to produce fermentation products of commercial interest. Classification of the organisms also allows a prediction of whether they possess any pathogenicity for plants, animals, or man which would need to be considered in the handling of the organisms. In addition, to a certain extent, it allows a prediction of the growth characteristics and other requirements to be considered in studying these microorganisms. The classification of microorganisms often involves the expenditure of considerable time and effort, so that we may wish not to classify them except into broad groups until their distinct value as industrial prospects has been demonstrated. However, the organism should be classified as to species by the time a patent application is filed. We do not patent a microorganism as such, but the use of a newly described microorganism does help in obtaining a patent because it adds "novelty" or newness to the microbial process (see Chapter 15).

Secondary screening should determine whether the microorganisms are actually producing new chemical compounds not previously described or, alternatively, for fermentation processes that are already known, secondary screening should determine whether a more economical process is possible. Should the product be a newly discovered compound, it must be determined if it really has a use. Thus, patents are granted only for useful products. To determine whether a product actually is a newly discovered, compound, we can utilize paper, thin-layer, or other chromatographic procedures to compare the product with known compounds. These chromatographic approaches are of particular value in comparing new antibiotics with those previously described. Nevertheless, regardless of whether the fermentation product is or is not a new compound, secondary screening should detect real differences in product yield potentials among the various isolates. The organisms are grown for various periods of time and on various media in liquid culture so that quantitative assays may be performed. These studies involve much work and, if possible, they should not be made until agar-plate procedures have allowed the discarding of worthless cultures.

Secondary screening should reveal whether there are pH, aeration, or other critical requirements associated with particular microorganisms, both for the growth of the organism and for the formation of chemical products. The screening should also detect gross genetic instability in microbial cultures. Thus, a microorganism is of little value if it tends to mutate or change in some manner so that it loses its ability to accumulate high yields of product. Secondary screening should show whether certain medium constituents are missing or, possibly, are toxic to the growth of the organism or to its ability to accumulate fermentation products. It should show something of the chemical stability of the product, and of the product's solubility picture in various organic solvents. It should determine whether the product has a simple, complex, or even a macromolecular structure, if this information is not already available. It should show whether the product possesses physical properties, such as ultraviolet-light absorption or fluorescence, or chemical properties that can be employed to detect the compound during the use of paper chromatography or other analytical methods, and which also might be of value in predicting the structure of the compound.

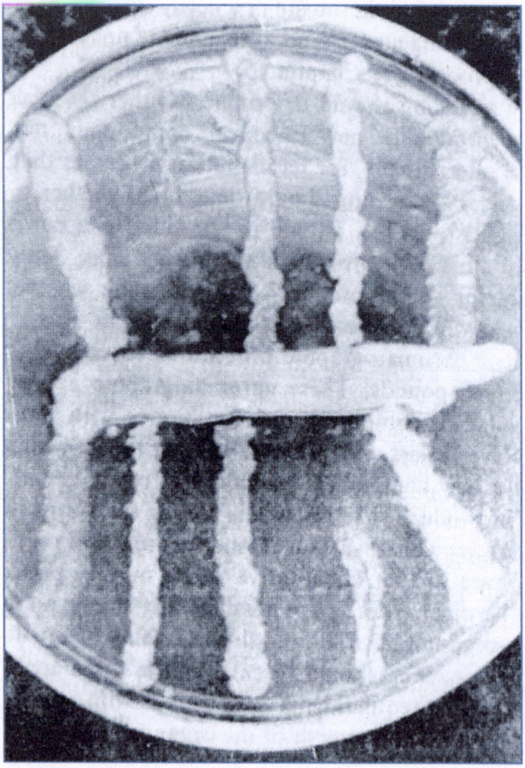

Figure 4.7 Giant colony inhibition spectrum. The growth along the central streak is that of a nonsporulated streptomycete. The lower group of test organisms (from left to right) and the upper group (from right to left) are, respectively, *Escherichia coli, Staphylococcus aureus, Pseudomonas aeruginosa, Saccharomyces cerevisiae*, and *Bacillus* cereus. As is apparent, the antibiotic produced by the streptomycete has demonstrated activity only against the yeast.

During the secondary screening associated with certain kinds of fermentation products, determinations should be made as to whether gross animal, plant or human toxicity can be attributed to the fermentation product, particularly if it is to be utilized (as are antibiotics) in disease treatment.

Obviously, valid information for testing of this type requires that the compound be in a pure state. However, any indications of toxicity which can be observed early in the screening program will allow the discarding of poor cultures, or possibly the relegation of the compound to use only for topical treatment. In order to test the toxicity of a compound when it is not in a pure state, we must make an educated guess as to the types of contaminating materials that may be associated with the compound, and then provide suitable experimental controls for these contaminants in the toxicity testing.

Secondary screening should reveal whether a product resulting from a microbial fermentation occurs in the culture broth in more than one chemical form, and whether it is an optically or biologically active material. Two or more different compounds also can be products of a single fermentation, although one of the compounds usually accumulates in greater quantities. Thus, one to several intermediate compounds in the metabolic sequence leading to product formation, as well as completely unrelated compounds, may also accumulate in the fermentation broth. These additional major or minor products are of distinct interest, since their recovery and sale as by-products can markedly improve the economic position of the prime fermentation.

Secondary screening should reveal whether microorganisms are able to chemically alter or even destroy their own fermentation products. The microorganisms may, because of a high-level accumulation of product in the culture broth, produce adaptive enzymes that destroy the usefulness of the product. Thus, a microorganism might produce a "racemase" enzyme that will change the L-configuration of an amino acid product to a mixture of the D- and L-isomers, with the D-isomer being of little biological value. A microorganism also might respond to the accumulation of an amino acid by adaptively producing a "decarboxylase" enzyme that removes carbon dioxide from the molecule, leaving an organic amine.

The preceding discussion emphasizes the fact that secondary screening can provide a broad range of information which helps in deciding which of various microbial isolates possess possible usefulness as an industrial organism. Also it is obvious that secondary screening helps in predicting the approaches to be utilized in conducting further research on the microorganism and its fermentation process. There are many possible techniques and procedures that can be applied in secondary screening. To illustrate their application and the sequence of events that may occur in a study of this type, the search for *streptomyces* species capable of producing new and valuable antibiotics will be specifically considered. However, it should be remembered that, while the described methods of screening relate primarily to the study of antibiotic-producing microorganisms, similar screening and analytical methods could be used for the isolation of organisms important in the production of other industrial chemicals.

Primary screening allows the isolation of streptomycetes which, at least on agar media, produce substances toxic to the growth of sensitive test organisms. The next step is to determine the "inhibition spectrum" for the antibiotics produced by each of the streptomycete isolates, that is, the range of types of test organisms sensitive to each antibiotic. The simplest procedure for this determination is the "giant colony" technique (Figure 4.7). The streptomycete cultures are inoculated onto the central areas of Petri plates containing a nutritious agar medium, or they are streaked in a narrow band across the centers of the plates. The plates are then incubated until growth and, possibly, sporulation have occurred. Strains of microorganisms to be tested for possible sensitivity to the antibiotics (the test organisms) are then streaked from the edges of the plates up to but not touching the streptomycete growth. The plates are further incubated to allow growth of the test organisms, and the distance over which the growth of each test organisms has been inhibited by antibiotic in the vicinity of the streptomycete is then measured in millimeters. Obviously, those test organisms, whose growth has been inhibited for a considerable distance from the streptomycete colony, are more sensitive to the antibiotic than are those test organisms that can grow close to the streptomycete colony. Only those streptomycetes that have produced antibiotics with interesting microbial inhibition spectra are retained for further testing.

Some antibiotics are only poorly soluble in water or do not diffuse through the agar to any extent away from the streptomycete colony. An alternate procedure, but one requiring more effort, is used when the presence of these antibiotics is suspected. The streptomycete is first grown in broth culture, and its mycelium is separated by filtration. Various dilutions of the antibiotic filtrate then are prepared and incorporated into melted agar-plating media. The various test organisms are streaked in parallel lines across the surface of the hardened agar, and the plates are incubated. The relative activity of the antibiotic against the various test organisms is evident when the presence or absence of test-organism growth is compared with the amount of dilution that the antibiotic culture filtrate received before its addition to the plating medium.

While further screening can be carried out using growth of the streptomycetes on agar media, it is safer, at about this point in the screening program, to switch to the use of liquid media in flasks. It is at this point, also, that we should start to use a cylinder or paper disk-agar diffusion assay (Chapter 5) with the agar seeded, or inoculated, with a sensitive test organism so that exact determinations can be made of the amounts of antibiotic which are present in samples of culture fluids.

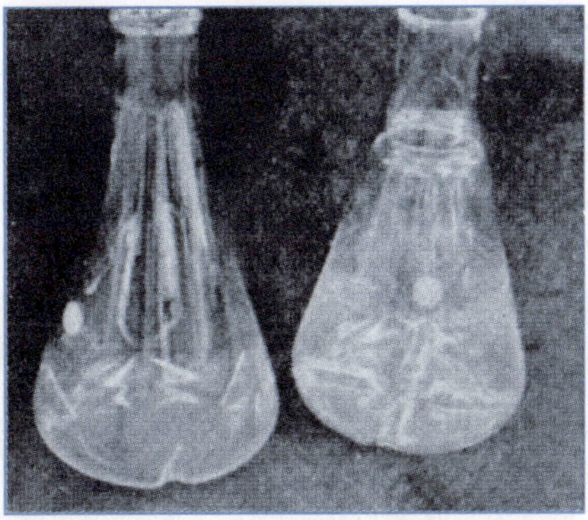

Figure 4.8 Baffle flasks for the shaken liquid culture of microorganisms.

Several different but highly nutritious liquid media are placed in Erlenmeyer flasks. In this regard, flasks with glass baffles projecting into the medium from bottoms or sides (Figure 4.8), provide better aeration characteristics than do conventional Erlenmeyer flasks. The media are sterilized and inoculated with one of the streptomycetes to be tested. These flasks can be incubated stationary or shaken vigorously, but the latter procedure is preferred, because experience has shown that growth and antibiotic yields are usually much greater in highly aerated cultures. The flasks are shaken at a constant temperature, usually near room temperature, and at intervals during growth of the organism, samples of culture fluid are aseptically withdrawn for analysis. In certain instances, as with the polyene group of antibiotics, the antibiotic activity is present not in the culture fluid but within the mycelium of the streptomycete, thus requiring special extraction procedures for recovering the antibiotic from the mycelium. The present discussion, however, will consider only those antibiotics that occur free in the culture fluids.

The samples for analysis are checked for the presence of contamination by microscopic observation and, often, in addition by inoculation into a medium suitable for allowing extensive growth of contaminants. The pH value of the sample also is determined to aid in detecting contamination and to provide information on the growth of the streptomycete during antibiotic production. The latter information can serve as a guide for the redesigning of the medium if unwanted changes in pH values have occurred. The culture samples are further observed for the relative amounts of growth of the streptomycete which have occurred with the various media. The samples then are adjusted to a pH value near neutrality, sterilized by filtration through a bacteriological filter (Figure 4.9), and assayed for antibiotic yields against a sensitive test organism. The assay results point out which medium is best for antibiotic production, and at what point the antibiotic yields are greatest during the growth of the organism on the various media. The results of these assays also demonstrate that the microbial inhibition previously noted for the cultures actually is not artifact, such as may occur with the "giant-colony" screening procedure.

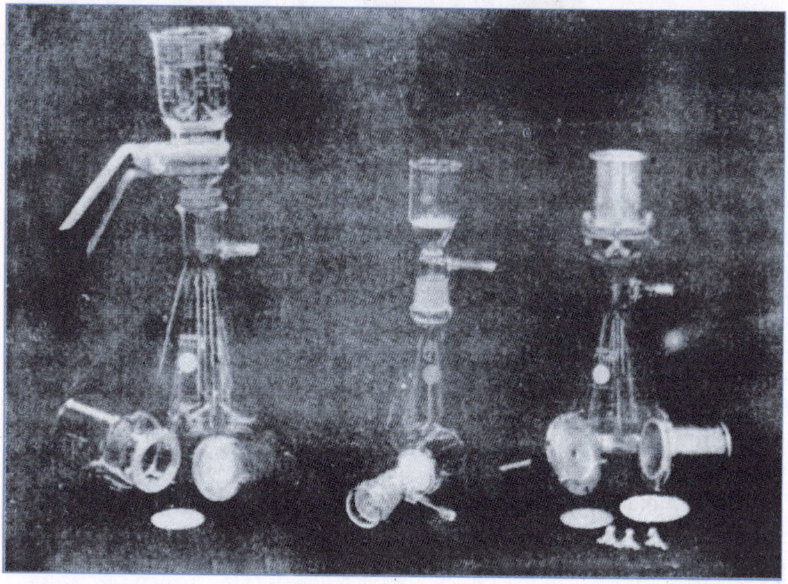

Figure 4.9 Three types of laboratory bacteriological filters. These filters are, from left to right, a membrane filter, a Morton filter with fritted glass disc, and a Seitz filter with asbestos filtration pad. The upper filtration component of each filter also is shown disassembled.

Several additional determinations are made on the antibiotic culture filtrates from the highest yielding media, although, if all media tested should provide low yields, other media should be screened for antibiotic production. Samples are analyzed by paper or thin-layer chromatography to determine whether the antibiotic is similar to previously described antibiotics, whether it is a new antibiotic or, possibly, whether there is more than one antibiotic present in the culture broth. These methods of chromatography utilize bioautograph plates, and the various techniques are described in Chapter 5. An ever-present possibility is that the antibiotic, as produced on agar medium during primary screening, is not the same antibiotic or antibiotics produced in liquid culture. Therefore, it is of interest to compare he microbial inhibition spectra of the liquid- and agar-grown streptomycete cultures. In addition, at this point, we should expand the inhibition spectrum screening to include more test organisms and, possibly, viruses and carcinoma agents.

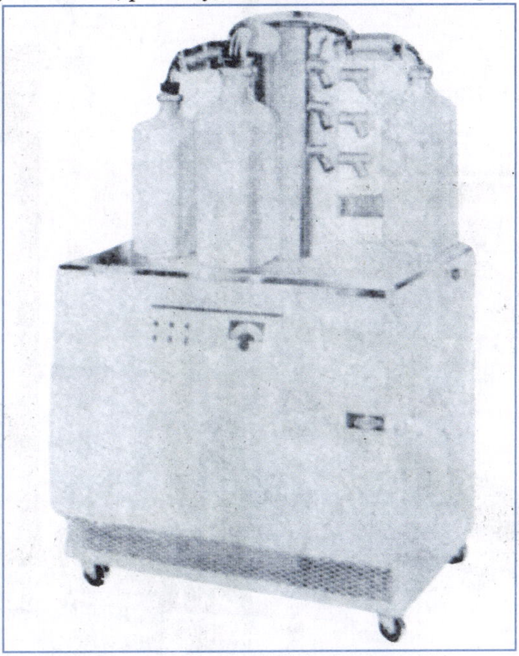

Figure 4.10 VirTis automatic freeze-dryer, Model P-24-MR. The aqueous sample is frozen at low temperature along the walls of the bottles so that the water will sublime on application of a vacuum. At completion of freeze drying, the solids occurring originally in the sample are present as a dry powder. Courtesy of the VirTis Co.

Antibiotic in culture broth also is tested for chemical stability with time, at various pH levels, and various temperatures. Obviously, the relatively stable antibiotics require less precautions in their study than do the less stable antibiotics. Gross instability of an antibiotic should not necessarily cause the antibiotic to be discarded since, in some instances, antibiotics are more stable in the animal or human body than as laboratory preparations.

The solubility of the antibiotic in various organic solvents is determined by solvent extraction of portions of the culture filtrate or by extracting partially purified antibiotic preparations. The filtered culture broth also can be carefully dried, as by freeze-drying or lyophilization (Figure 4.10), so that solvent solubility in the absence of water can be tested. The ability of the antibiotic to adsorb to ion exchange resins or activated carbon is determined

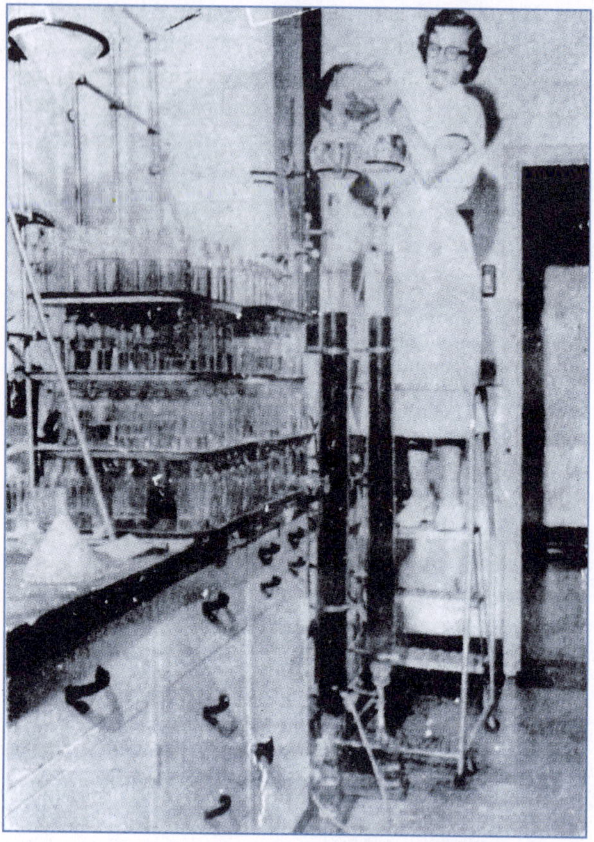

Figure 4.11 Ion exchange column for purification products containing reactive basis or acidic chemical groups. The columns are packed with cation exchange resins to adsorb basic molecules, or anion exchange resins to adsorb acidic molecules. After adsorption, the fermentation products are eluted from the column by passing a dilute acidic or basic solution through the column to displace the corresponding acidic or basic fermentation product. Photo courtesy of Charles Pfizer and Co., Inc.

by mixing the culture broth with these agents or by passing it through columns (Figure 4.11) packed with these materials. If adsorption occurs, then these agents can be employed to remove the antibiotic from aqueous solution followed by recovery from the adsorbant. Antibiotic recovered from any one Inc. of these steps probably will have become partially purified, and a combination of these steps may further aid in purification. Partially purified antibiotic material is tested for toxicity in mice or other small laboratory animals. If the toxicity level proves to be low enough, the antibiotic is further tested against experimental infections of these laboratory animals, as well as for any adverse effects it might have on the well being of the healthy animal (see Figures 4.12 and 4.13).

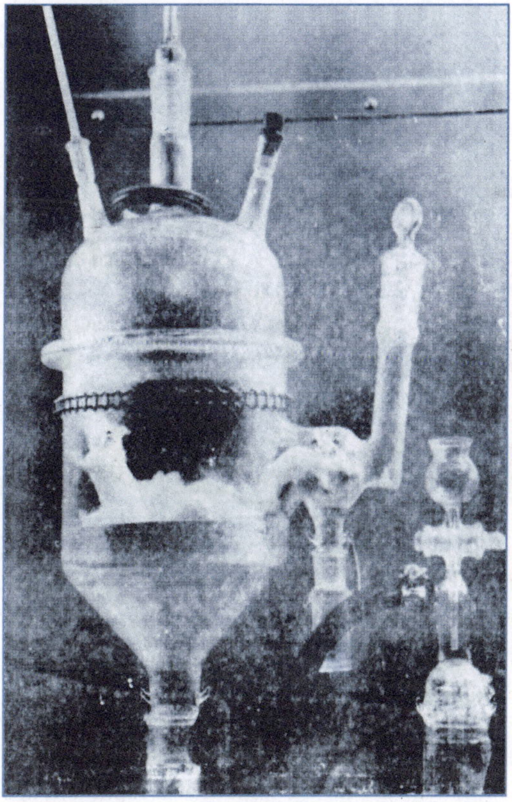

Figure 4.12 Use of mice in the animal testing of new drugs. The apparatus shown records the metabolic rates of the mice. Photo courtesy of Charles Pfizer and Co., Inc.

It would be hoped that most of the streptomycetes not producing valuable antibiotics will have been discarded by this time. Further studies become more specific for the individual organism and its fermentation and, therefore, do not utilize the screening approach as extensively for the discarding of poor cultures. Thus, the further studies that are initiated at this time or possibly later are designed to yield additional information about the fermentation, the organism, and the antibiotic. For example, the effect on the fermentation of incubation temperatures and of inert and crude antifoam agents is determined. The antibiotic is checked to see if it is bacteriostatic or bactericidal against

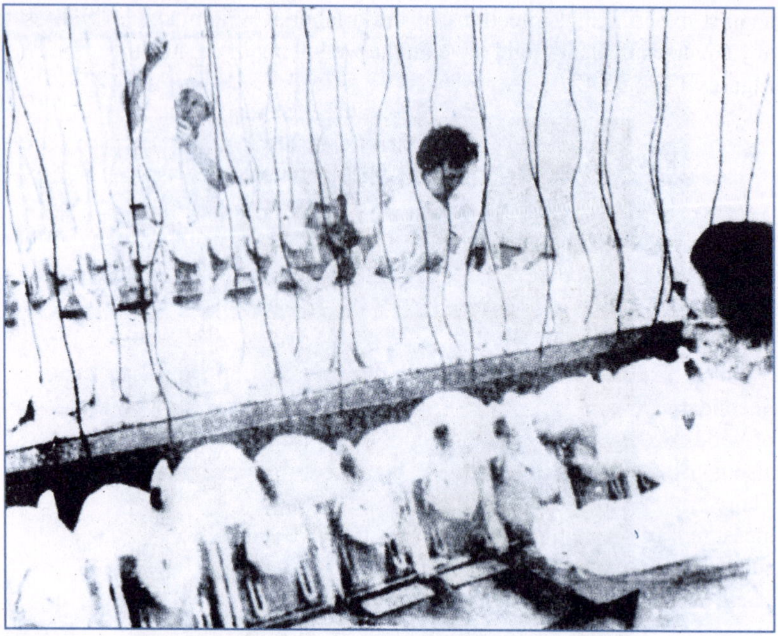

Figure 4.13 Use of rabbits in the animal testing of new drugs. The thermocouple system connects to an instrument that records the temperatures of each of the 30 rabbits. Photo courtesy of Charles Pfizer and Co.,

test organisms, and the rate of resistance build-up among sensitive test organisms is examined. The antibiotic is tested for its ability to precipitate serum proteins, to cause haemolysis of blood, or to harm phagocytes. The organism is further classified as to species, if this is possible. Other assay systems are investigated with the hope that a rapid and specific chemical or physical assay for the antibiotic can be found. Further media are tested (Chapter 7), and the potential for the inclusion in the medium of precursors of the antibiotic molecule is investigated. Also, the possible occurrence of a diauxie phenomenon (to be described later) is investigated for possible improvement in antibiotic yields. Finally, mutation and other genetic studies are initiated.

CHAPTER 5

Detection and Assay of Fermentation Products

Secondary screening and, to a certain extent, primary screening require the use of good detection and assay procedures for the fermentation products. This also is true for most of the fermentation studies at all points of development. These procedures must be quick, simple, reliable, and accurate, and they must measure only the compound of interest in the presence of relatively greater concentrations of various chemical contaminants from the growth medium. These assays usually fall into one of three categories: physical chemical, biological, or chromatographic partition. Sometimes, more than one assay procedure is possible so that the best assay can be chosen, with an alternate assay used periodically to test the validity of the assay of choice.

PHYSICAL-CHEMICAL ASSAYS

There are many types of physical or chemical assays which can be used in conjunction with crude fermentation products, and only a few examples of the more important of these assays will be considered. The actual choice of the particular assay to be used depends on the selectivity of the chemical reaction or chemical analysis involved, since the fermentation broths contain many compounds in addition to those to be determined. In fact, in some instances, at least a partial purification of the fermentation product may be necessary before carrying out the assay.

Titration and Gravimetric Analysis

The amount of an organic acid, such as lactic acid, produced during a fermentation is roughly determined by adding a pH-indicating dye, such as bromthymol blue, to a sample of the fermentation broth followed by titration with alkali of known strength. The pH-indicating dye is not required, however, if electrometric titrations are employed. If the acid, and not other medium components, will form an insoluble salt, it can be precipitated, washed, dried and weighed. Volatile small molecular weight organic acids can be distilled directly from acidified fermentation broth so that the distillate can be analyzed by titration. Organic acids of greater molecular weight can be separated from the fermentation medium for titration, by adsorption onto and elution from a suitable anion exchange resin (Figure 4.10), although the eluting agent, which will probably itself be an acid, will likely need to be removed before titration.

Turbidity Analysis and Cell-Yield Determinations

The determination of packed-cell volumes provides a simple and quick estimate of cell yields if microbial cells are the only insoluble component in the sample. Portions of fermentation broth with their cells are centrifuged in graduated centrifuge tubes, and the volumes of sedimented cells are measured in cubic centimeters (Figure 5.1).

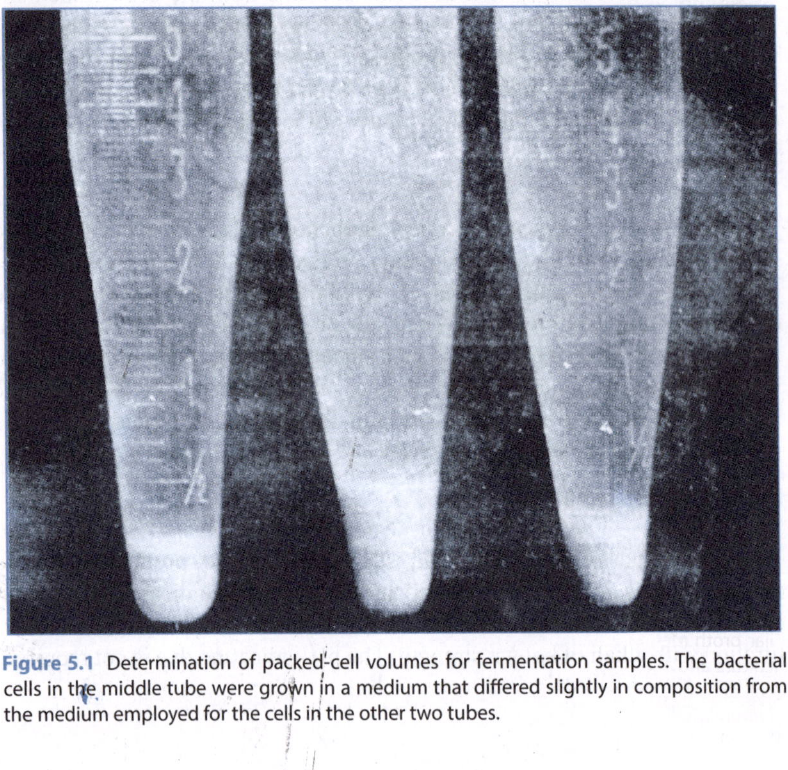

Figure 5.1 Determination of packed-cell volumes for fermentation samples. The bacterial cells in the middle tube were grown in a medium that differed slightly in composition from the medium employed for the cells in the other two tubes.

Turbidity analysis is another method used to measure the cell yield of a fermentation, since the cellular turbidity of a culture broth can be determined if the medium contains little insoluble debris other than the cells. The cells, suspended in their growth medium, are diluted to a turbidity range that can be quantitatively measured as optical density with a simple electric colorimeter or nephelometer (such as the Klett-Summerson, Evelyn, Beckman, or other instruments), by the deflection of light that is caused by the microbial cells when suspended in the light paths of these instruments. These assays utilize the visible range of light, and a filter or monochromator in the instrument is adjusted or chosen, respectively, to selectively eliminate colors associated with the growth medium. As an additional precaution in eliminating apparent turbidity due to light absorption by the growth medium, uninoculated medium diluted to the same extent as for the culture sample can be employed in setting the 100 percent light-transmission value for the instrument. Turbidimetric measurements of cell numbers are usually standardized against some other procedure, such as plate counts, for determining numbers of cells. A standard curve is prepared relating optical density to plate count or other determination of cell numbers by using information from each of a series of dilutions of the cell suspension (Figure 5.2). Once we have prepared this standard curve, we can, in further determinations, easily convert optical density readings to cell numbers.

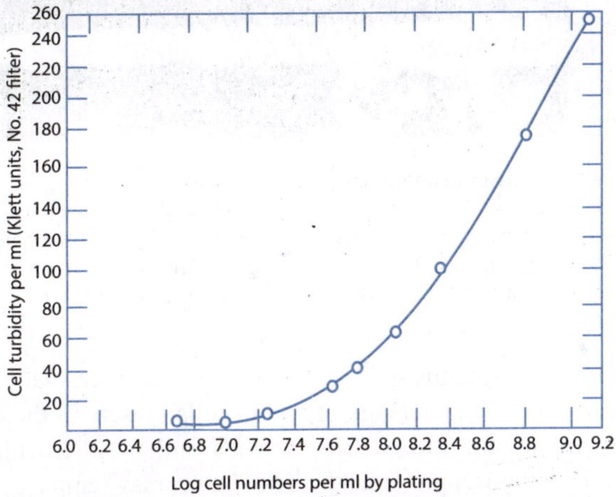

Figure 5.2 Example of a standard curve relating plate-count numbers of microbial cells to optical density. A 20-hour Escherichia coli culture in Bacto AC broth was diluted in fresh similar broth medium, then plated on AC agar for total viable cell counts. Simultaneously, the culture and a sample of uninoculated medium were diluted in water for the determination of cell densities as Klett units in a Klett-Summerson colorimeter. The dilutions of uninoculated culture medium were employed for zeroing the instrument.

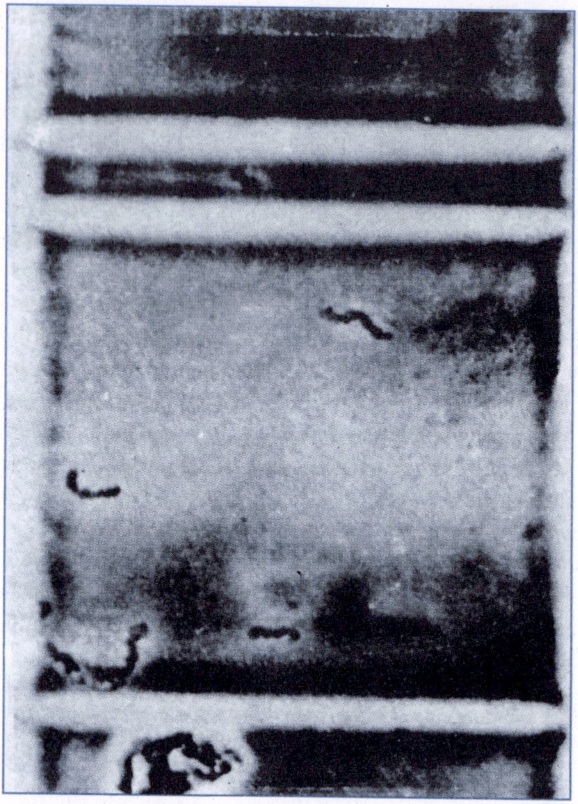

Figure 5.3 Petroff-Hausser counting chamber with spiral-shaped bacteria as viewed with phase-contrast microscopy at a magnification of 1250 fold. The counting chamber is a special microscope slide with many small depressions, each of which contains a defined volume of the sample. The picture shows one of these depressions. The average number of bacteria per depression is multiplied by a factor that relates the volume of sample in each depression to a milliliter of the original culture.

If the medium contains sediment other than the microbial cells, or there is a question as to the percentage of viable cells present in the culture, then we cannot employ the turbimetric methods and must use plate-counting procedures or microscopic counts. The latter may employ the Petroff-Hausser counting chamber (Figure 5.3) or similar microscopic quantitation to determine the total number of microbial cells present. Often, it also is possible to use a fluorescence microscope with the vital, fluorescent stain, Acridine Orange, which will allow microscopic counting of only the viable cells (Figure 5.4).

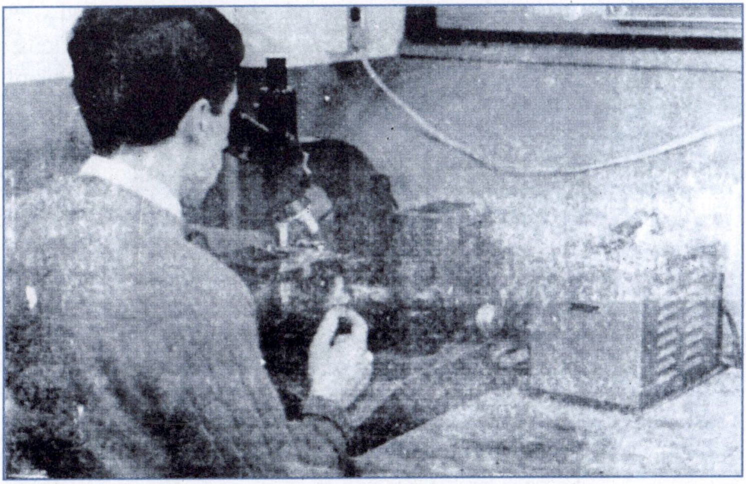

Figure 5.4 Observation by ultraviolet fluorescence microscopy of bacteria vitally stained with Acridine Orange. The power source is at the right of the investigator, and the high-pressure mercury vapor lamp ultraviolet source is attached to the rear of the microscope. The procedure, as outlined by Strugger (1948, *Canadian J. Res.* (C) 26, 188-193), reveals living bacteria as a blue to green color and dead bacteria and insoluble organic media components as a brick red.

Spectrophotometric Assays

Spectrophotometric assays utilize various types of spectrophotometers to measure amounts of absorption of visible light by colored solutions at specific wavelengths in the visible light range, the quantity of ultraviolet light absorbed by a compound in the ultraviolet wavelength range, or the intensity of fluorescence emitted when a compound is exposed to ultraviolet light. Spectrophotometers of the colorimeter type are sensitive to visible light in the range of about 350 to 1000 mμ. They measure the amount of light at a specific wavelength, or narrow band of wavelengths, which is absorbed as a light beam passes through a colored solution; each color absorbs light only over a specific band of wavelengths. Fermentation products, which are in themselves colored, but of a different hue than that of the medium, can be measured directly in the colorimeter or, possibly, after a simple purification step. Thus, the actual wavelength of light to be used is chosen so that the compound being assayed will absorb a maximum amount of light, and so that the extraneous colors from the medium will absorb minimally. Also, the effects of extraneous colors can be minimized by using uninoculated medium, diluted to the same extent as for the sample, to set the 100 percent light transmission value for the instrument. A standard curve is prepared which relates the optical density values observed to the various concentrations of the pure compound, if this compound is available. To be of value, this plot should demonstrate Beer's law; that is, the relationship of color intensity (absorbance) to concentration of the fermentation product as shown by the standard curve (Figure 5.5) should be linear over the range of concentrations that will be analyzed.

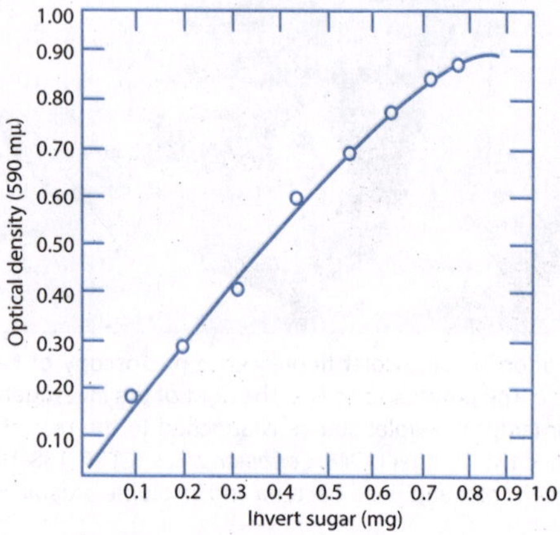

Figure 5.5 Standard curve relating optical density to various concentrations of a colored compound in solution. Beer's law is followed from 0.1 to 0.5 mg. In this particular instance, the color was developed by treatment with alkali, 2- (p-iodophenyl) -3- (pnitrophenyl)-5-phenyltetrazolium chloride and methanol.

The fermentation product may not, in itself, possess a visible color. A colorimetric analysis can still be applied to a product of this type, however, if it can be specifically reacted with a chemical reagent so as to yield a colored product (see Figure 5.5). For example amino acids are not in themselves colored, but they will react with ninhydrin under suitable conditions to yield a purple color that can be measured colorimetrically. Again, it may be advantageous to extract the colored product or to purify it, in some manner, before performing the colorimetric determination.

Somewhat similar spectrophotometric assays can be performed for fermentation products that are not visibly colored, or which do not react with chemical agents to form visible products, if these compounds will absorb or fluoresce when subjected to specific wavelengths of ultraviolet light within the wavelength range of approximately 200 to 380 mμ· Thus, compounds possessing conjugated double bonds, such as are found in the aromatic nucleus, will usually absorb ultraviolet light at one or several wavelengths in the ultraviolet spectrum. In contrast, certain compounds, such as riboflavin, fluoresce at specific wavelengths of ultraviolet light. The principles of analysis are similar to those for visible light determinations, and ultraviolet wavelengths are chosen to allow maximal fluorescence or absorption of the ultraviolet light, as related to the fermentation product, with minimal activity for contaminating compounds. A standard curve is prepared relating ultraviolet absorption or fluorescence to various concentrations of the reference or standard compound, and the usable portion of the resulting plot should follow Beer's law.

The use of spectrophotometric analysis to assay a previously unknown fermentation product is more difficult, because the pure compound may not be available for use as a reference standard in preparing standard curves. The spectrophotometric approach, nevertheless, can still be used on a relative basis in determining visible color, or absorption or fluorescence with ultraviolet light. If the fermentation product is relatively stable, a sample of fermentation broth can be carefully dried (or freeze-dried), refrigerated, and held as a reference standard. An arbitrary number of units is assigned to this standard, and a standard curve is prepared. The results of further analyses are then compared to these arbitrary units of activity as determined from the standard curve. Of course, when pure material becomes available, these arbitrary units can be converted to a weight basis.

During the performance of spectrophotometric analyses, a question may arise as to whether events may be occurring such as the decomposition of the product during analysis, interaction of the product with other components present in the sample, fading of visible color or fluorescence, and so forth. If any of these phenomena are suspected, it is wise to incorporate an internal standard of known concentration in the dilutions of the fermentation sample. Thus, a small but detectable amount of the compound is added to a dilution of fermentation broth containing similar microbially produced product, and this is compared with a similar dilution of fermentation product that did not receive the standard compound. The results of the two determinations should differ only by the amount of standard compound added. If they differ by less or more than this amount, then we must reevaluate the assay. Changes such as a fading in the absorption of ultraviolet or visible light or in the level of ultraviolet fluorescence are detected by performing the determinations at various time intervals after preparation of the sample. A specific time interval is then chosen to allow consistent and reproducible results.

Spectrophotometric analyses that do not yield quantitative results are employed to detect the presence of unsuspected compounds in a fermentation broth and can be used as a descriptive feature for a newly discovered fermentation product. This is particularly true for compounds that absorb ultraviolet light. A dilution of the fermentation broth or of partially purified product is tested for ultraviolet absorption at individual wavelengths over the entire spectrum of ultraviolet light. A recording spectrophotometer is of distinct value for this determination. The spectral analysis will show peaks of ultraviolet absorption at certain wavelengths, and other wavelengths will show little, if any, ultraviolet light absorption. These maxima and minima of ultra violet absorption are associated with specific groupings within the molecule and are characteristic for the particular compound. In addition, further description of the compound is obtained if the addition of alkali or acid to the sample will cause a shift in the positions of these maxima and minima.

Chromatrographic Partition Assays

The advent of partition chromatography on paper and thin-layer plates has allowed marked strides in fermentation research and technology. Before the discovery of this technique, it was difficult to detect, identify or quantitate many types of new fermentation products, particularly if they occurred in only small amounts in the fermentation medium. However, partition chromatography now allows the detection of compounds in either pure or impure states, the identification of compounds if they have been previously described, and the assay of materials that otherwise require some type of preliminary purification. In addition, only small amounts of sample are required.

Paper and thin-layer chromatography are forms of partition chromatography. The solute, or sample, is partitioned continuously between a stationary phase, such as paper or the silica gel of thin-layer plates, and a mobile phase, consisting of a mixture of solvents, as these solvents migrate across the paper or silica gel layer. Paper chromatography has particular application for water-soluble compounds, and thin-layer chromatography for the more hydrophobic compounds. However, water-soluble and insoluble compounds can be separated by both procedures. Thus, paper chromatography will separate water-insoluble compounds if it is used in "reverse phase"; that is, if the sheet is first impregnated with mineral oil, petrolatum, or silicone to make it less hydrophilic.

The procedures for paper and thin-layer chromatography are relatively simple, and there are many variations on these procedures. Paper chromatography utilizes a good grade of chemically clean filter paper, while thin-layer chromatography requires that a thin layer of silica gel, aluminum oxide or other material be applied to the surface of a glass plate (Figure 5.6). A binder compound, such as calcium sulfate or starch, may be incorporated in the chromatographic agent so as to aid in binding the layer to the glass. Small portions of fermentation broth samples are applied as a series of small spots about 3/4 inch apart along a line about one inch from one end of a rectangular sheet of filter paper or thin-layer plate (Figure 5.7). However, the samples also may be applied as bands instead of spots (Figure 5.18). Also, for either procedure, the exact distance of the bands or spots from the edge depends on the particular technique being utilized. In circular paper chromatography, the sample spots are applied around a hole cut from the center of a circular piece of paper (Figure 5.10). The spots or bands are allowed to dry at room temperature or, if the compounds to be assayed are relatively stable, the spots or bands are heated with a stream of warm air or an infrared lamp. Individual spots may be respotted or "over-spotted" with their respective samples if it is desired to increase the concentration of the sample, or a portion of a reference or standard compound may be overspotted on the dry spot of fermentation broth if there is some question as to the identity of the fermentation product.

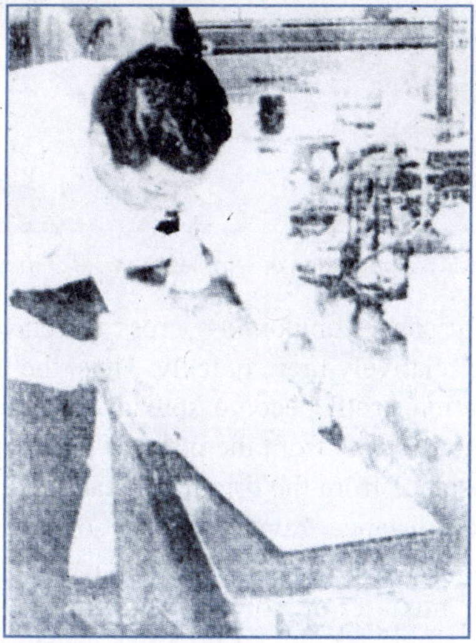

Figure 5.6 Application of thin layers of silica gel to glass plates for use in thin-layer chromatography. The thickness of the silica gel layer is controlled by the applicator device and several plates are placed side by side so that they can be coated in a single operation. Precoated plates also are commercially available for those who do not wish to prepare their own.

After the spots on the chromatograms have dried, a mixture of solvents, or even a single solvent for thin-layer chromatography, is allowed to migrate across the chromatogram starting from the end on which the samples were applied while making sure that the solvents are not allowed to migrate completely across the chromatogram. During solvent migration, the individual compounds that were present in the original spot of fermentation sample partition back and forth between the solvents of the solvent mixture and the stationary phase, in this case, the paper or silica gel. In the process,

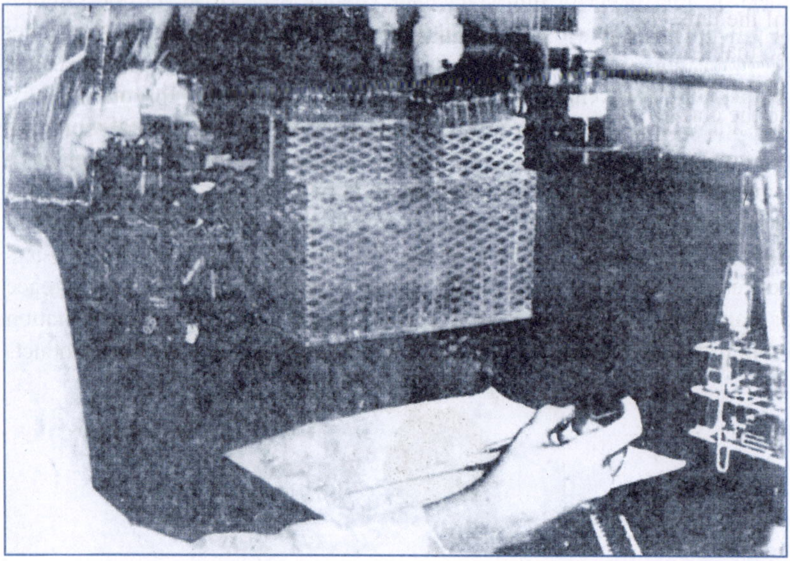

Figure 5.7 Application of samples to paper chromatograms.

the rate of travel of some compounds across the chromatogram is slowed, while others move relatively more quickly. Thus, the individual compounds from the fermentation broth become spread out and separated along the path of travel of the solvents from the point of spot application, or "origin." The ratio of the distance from the origin that each individual compound has traveled to the total distance traveled by the solvent mixture, the "solvent front," provides an "Rf value" which is characteristic for each compound for the particular mixture of solvents and other conditions associated with the chromatography (Figure 5.14.). This value will always be less than one. To identify a fermentation product by this procedure, known or standard compounds are spotted and chromatographed alongside the spots of fermentation products so as to compare their respective Rf values. If the fermentation products and standard compounds actually are the same chemicals, they should present similar Rf values.

In carrying out the solvent migration, the chromatograms are placed in a closed tank so that the atmosphere of the tank becomes saturated with the individual components of the solvent mixture. In "descending" paper chromatography, a trough containing the solvent mixture is placed near the top of the tank, and the spotted end of the sheet is placed in this trough so that the solvents will migrate down the sheet (Figure 5.8). For "ascending" chromatography, the solvent mixture is placed as a shallow layer in the bottom of the tank, and the paper chromatograms or thin-layer plates are suspended so that the spotted end just extends into the solvents (Figure 5.9). In circular paper chromatography, a wick placed in the central hole elevates the solvents to the chromatograph from a reservoir beneath the sheet (Figure 5.10).

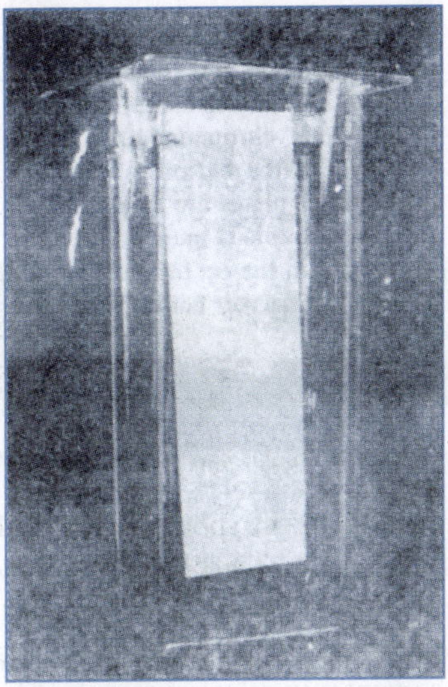

Figure 5.8 Descending-paper chromatography.

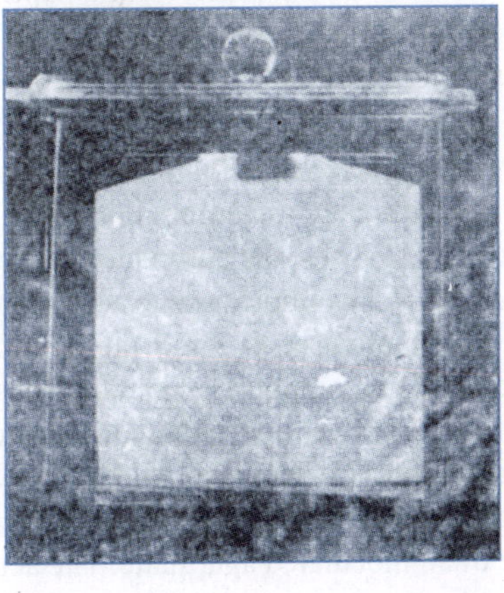

Figure 5.9 Ascending-paper chromatography.

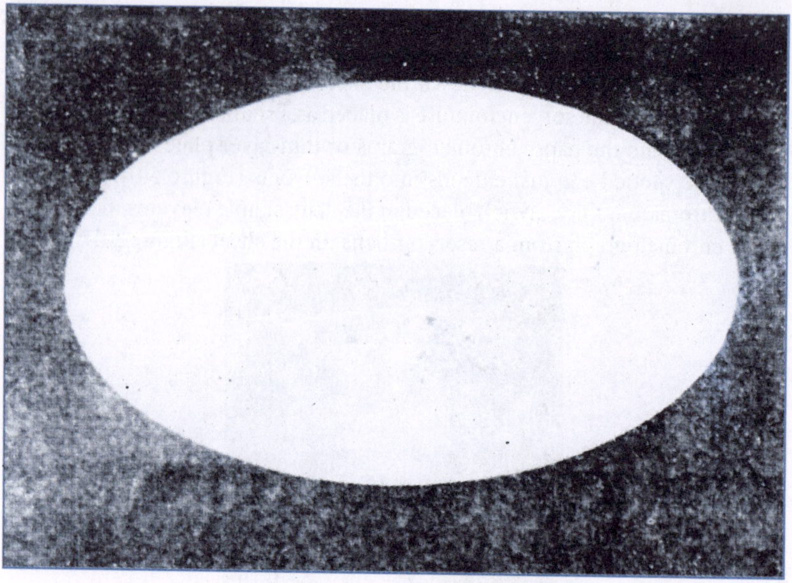

Figure 5.10 Circular-paper chromatography.

In each of these procedures, the spotted area should be far enough from the edge of the paper or plate so that the spots do not become wetted on initial contact of the plate or paper with the solvents; the solvent mixture must travel through the spots. For precise analytical determinations the temperature at which solvent migration occurs must be carefully controlled. When solvent migration has been completed, the paper sheets or thin-layer plates are removed from the tanks and allowed to air dry for removal of residual solvents. In some instances, the dried chromatograms are further heated in an oven.

The compounds being separated on the chromatograms will not be observed at this point, unless they are colored or will fluoresce or absorb in ultraviolet light (Figure 5.11). Thus, the chromatograms usually must be so as to provide a color reaction. For example, amino acids are detected by spraying the chromatograms with ninhydrin to yield purple-colored spots (Figures 5.12 to 5.14). Acidic or basic compounds can be detected by spraying with a solution of a pH-indicating dye, and radioactive materials are located by exposing the chromatograph to X-ray film. Biologically active compounds, such as antibiotics, can be detected by placing the chromatogram for a short period on the surface of an inoculated agar plate. The active material diffuses from its spot on the chromatogram into the agar directly beneath and, on removal of the sheet and incubation of the inoculated agar, the biological activity, such as inhibition of a test organism by an antibiotic, appears on the agar surface (Figure 5.15). The respective Rf values are determined by comparing the chromatogram with its imprint on the inoculated agar surface at termination of the growth or the organisms.

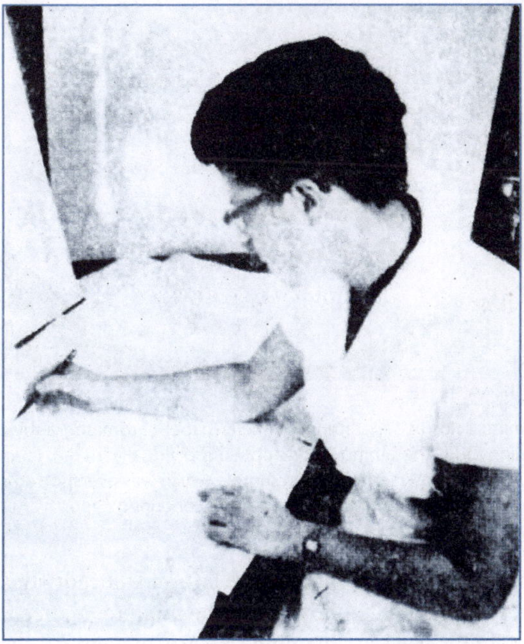

Figure 5.11 Observation of paper chromatographs by ultraviolet light to detect spots that either absorb ultraviolet light or fluoresce in its presence. Photo courtesy of Charles Pfizer and Co., Inc.

At times, we would like to detect all of the organic compounds present in a sample of fermentation broth, regardless of whether these compounds are microbial products or residual medium constituents. This is accomplished by chromatography on silica gel thin-layer plates. The individual compounds are detected either by exposing the plates to iodine vapors in a closed container, which will stain many organic compounds, or by spraying the chromatograms with strong sulfuric acid or other powerful oxidizing agent followed by heating of the plates. This procedure causes charring of the organic compounds to yield brown to black spots (Figure 5.16).

Figure 5.13 Amino acids as separated by ascending-paper chromatography and detected by spraying with ninhydrin. A mixture of L-glutamic acid,

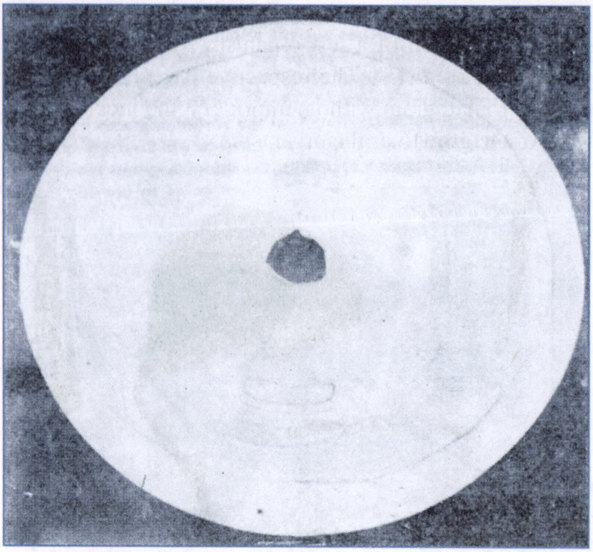

Figure 5.12 Amino acids as separated by circular-paper chromatography and detected by spraying with ninhydrin. The amino acids applied individually were L-leucine, L-lysine and glycine. The fourth spot was a fermentation sample which was overspotted with a mixture of the three amino acids. Notice that the latter sample contained a fourth amino acid different from the standard amino acids.

L-lysine, and L-leucine was applied at the left, and the individual amino acids were applied, respectively, to the right of the mixture. Notice that, under the particular conditions used in obtaining this chromatograph, the L-leucine at the far right moved further from the origin (greater Rf value) than did the L-leucine in the mixture. Also, the L-glutamic acid in the mixture split to yield two chromatograph spots. These results indicate that, with this particular chromatographic system, overspotting would be necessary to be sure of the identity of these amino acids as they occur in fermentation samples.

Chromatography with a single mixture of solvents may not separate the Rf, values of compounds of interest from each other or from other components of the fermentation broth. In this instance, several different solvent mixtures should be tested to find a "solvent system" that will produce a clean separation of the compounds. In fact, it is advantageous to have at our disposal more than one solvent system for separating any specific group of compounds, because at times two or more dissimilar compounds will present similar Rf, values in one solvent system (Figure 5.14) but not in a second system.

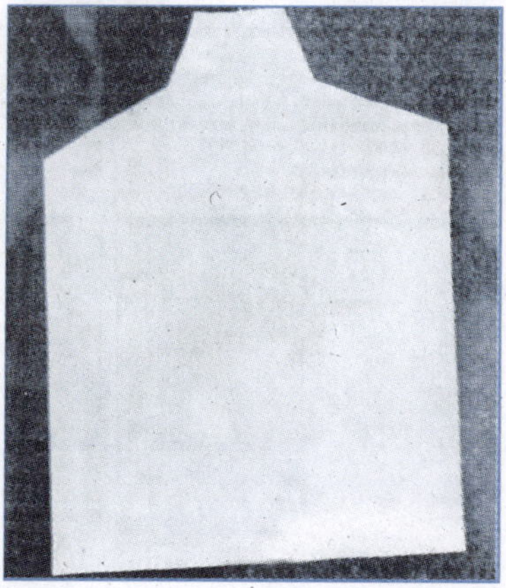

Figure 5.13 Amino acids as separated by ascending-paper chromatography and detected by spraying with ninhydrin. A mixture of L-glutamic acid, L-lysine, and L-leucine was applied at the left, and the individual amino acids were applied, respectively, to the right of the mixture. Notice that, under the particular conditions used in obtaining this chromatograph, the L-leucine at the far right moved further from the origin (greater R_f value) than did the L-leucine in the mixture. Also, the L-glutamic acid in the mixture split to yield two chromatograph spots. These results indicate that, with this particular chromatographic system, overspotting would be necessary to be sure of the identity of these amino acids as they occur in fermentation samples.

Figure 5.14 Separation of ten different amino acids by ascending paper chromatography. The sample at the far left contained two marker dyes. The solvent irrigation system contained N-butanol, H_2O, and propionic acid. The amino acids from left to right are L-lysine, L-aspartic acid, glycine, L-threonine, L-proline, L-valine, L-tryptophan, L-phenylalanine, L-leucine, and L-isoleucine. Notice that this chromatographic system did not separate L-aspartic acid and glycine, nor did it separate L-phenylalanine and L-isoleucine. The Rf value for L-proline (sixth from right) is $\frac{161mm/}{/343mm}$ = 0.47. Chromatograph courtesy of Kunda Sashital.

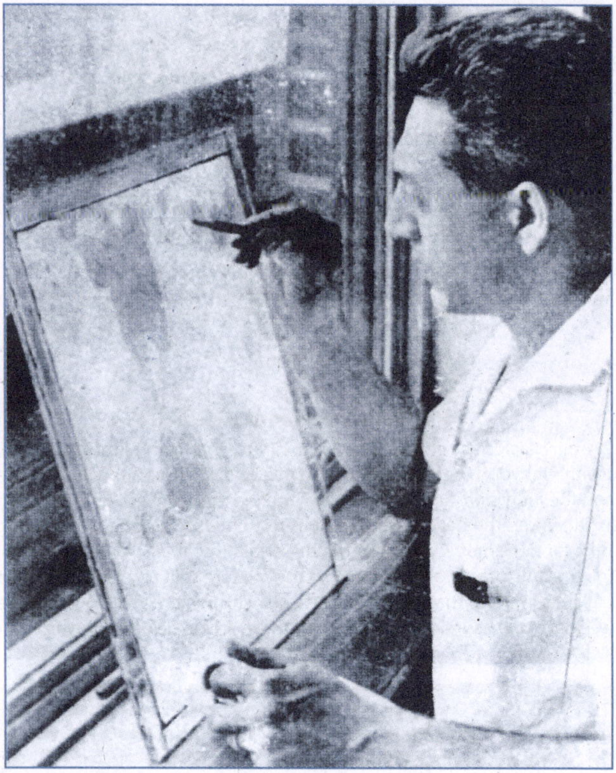

Figure 5.15 A bioautograph plate as used in the paper chromatographic separation of antibiotics. Photo courtesy of Charles Pfizer and Co., Inc.

Sometimes, no solvent system will separate the compounds, or there are so many compounds present that the individual spots on the chromatograph tend to coalesce. In these instances, "two-dimensional" chromatography is of value (Figures 5.16 and 5.17). A single spot, with or without overspotting of reference compounds, is applied at one corner of the chromatogram, and solvent migration is allowed to occur across the chromatogram. This moves out individual compounds along a line from the origin in the direction of solvent migration. The solvents are then evaporated from the chromatogram, and the chromatogram is turned 90 degrees and placed in a different solvent system; thus, the line of travel of the compounds which occurred with the first solvent system becomes adjacent to the surface of the new solvent system. Solvent migration with the second solvent system moves each individual compound across the chromatogram at an angle of 90 degrees from the

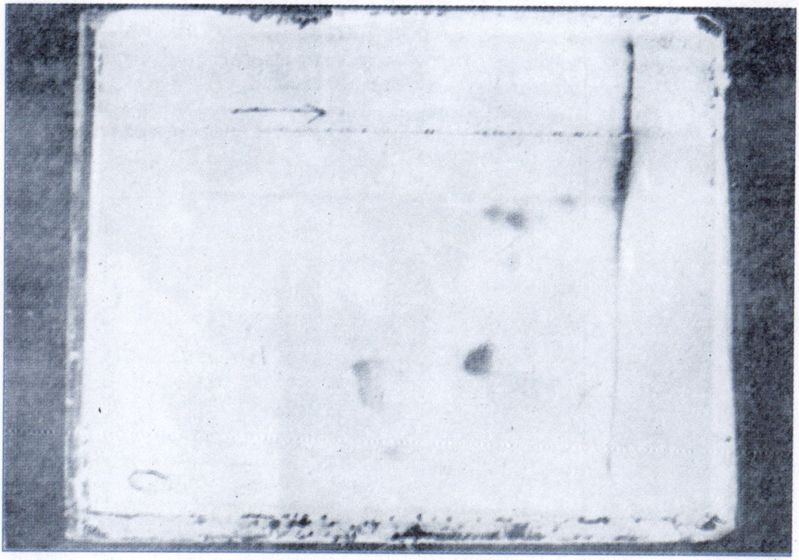

Figure 5.16 Two-dimensional thin-layer chromatographic separation of 19 polar lipids. The spots were detected by applying chromic acid and heat so as to cause charring. The point of original application of the sample is circled. Chromatograph courtesy of S. Patton.

original direction of travel. Two-dimensional chromatography thus allows the use of two different, even contrasting, solvent systems on a single chromatogram, and, it makes use of the whole chromatogram for positioning the separated compounds. However, there are two drawbacks to two-dimensional chromatography. Only a single spot can be applied to the chromatogram, and the Rf values are difficult to interpret since they are associated with two different directions of solvent migration. Nevertheless, this procedure provides considerable information when reference compounds are overspotted on the spot of fermentation broth, so that the final positions of reference compounds and fermentation products on the chromatograms can be compared.

Partition chromatography has uses other than for the separation and identification of fermentation products. It can be quantitated to provide an assay for fermentation products that require a preliminary chemical separation. As such, it will determine the concentrations of products, even when present in only small amounts in the fermentation broth, and only small-size samples are required. Also, if by partition chromatography a newly discovered fermentation product can be separated from contaminating materials of the fermentation broth, it can be assayed even though there is no

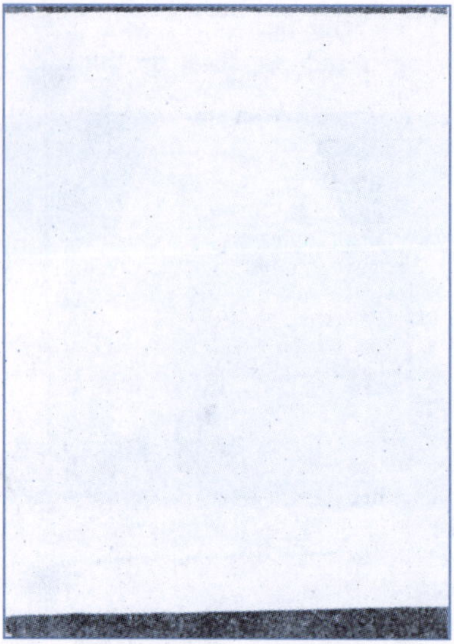

Figure 5.17 Two-dimensional paper chromatography of the ten amino acids shown in Figure 5.14. The origin is at the lower left-hand corner. The first solvent system used (from bottom to top) was a mixture of phenol and water, and the second solvent system (migrating left to right) was similar to that in Figure 5.14. Two marker dyes are shown by squares with crossed lines. Notice that L-aspartic acid and glycine are now separated (the two spots just to the left and below the lower marker dye; also see Figure 5.14), although L-phenylalanine and L-isoleucine again did not separate (to right of upper marker dye). Chromatograph courtesy of Kunda Sashital.

reference compound available. A sample of fermentation broth is carefully dried and then assigned arbitrary units so as to serve as a reference standard until larger amounts of more pure material become available. Depending on the nature of the fermentation product, the actual assay, may be carried out in a number of ways. For these procedures, a definite volume of fermentation broth, such as 100 lambda, is applied as a band, instead of a spot, across one edge of the chromatogram at one band per sheet or thin-layer plate. Various concentrations of reference compound also are applied as bands on other chromatograms. All of these chromatograms are then exposed simultaneously to solvent migration and dried as usual. The compound to be assayed thus moves out as a band on the chromatogram (Figure 5.18). The band is converted to a colored product, then extracted from the chromatogram for colorimetric analysis, or the band is extracted directly without color formation so that other means of quantitation can be applied to the compound. The values obtained for the various concentrations of reference compound are then plotted to yield a standard curve.

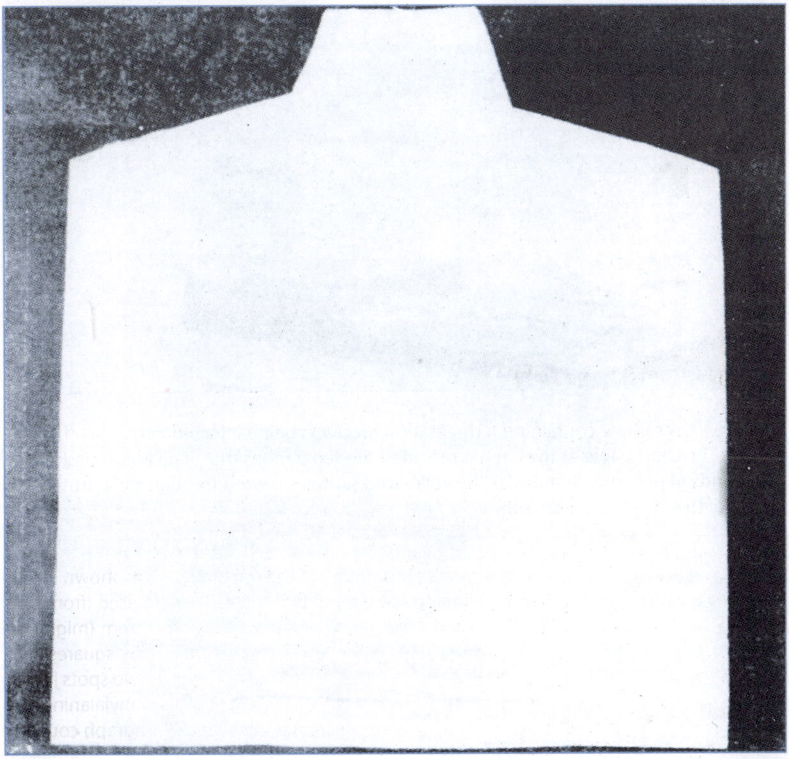

Figure 5.18 Paper chromatography for the assay of fermentation products. A sample (100 lambda) of fermentation broth was streaked along the origin, then the chromatogram was irrigated with solvent. The band that moves out is treated with indicator if required cut from the sheet, extracted and assayed.

Partition chromatography also finds use for small-scale preparative purposes, since the chromatographic separation provides a considerable purification of the fermentation product as it migrates across the chromatogram. Portions of fermentation broth are applied as bands on many paper sheets or thin-layer plates for chromatographic separation. The chromatographed fermentation product is then eluted with appropriate solvent from all the sheets or plates. The eluates containing fermentation product are combined, filtered, and concentrated to yield a solution or residue of purified fermentation product. Obviously, the amount of material that can be purified by this procedure is relatively small. However, this procedure may yield purified or even crystallized fermentation product for further studies before larger scale chemical preparative procedures have been developed.

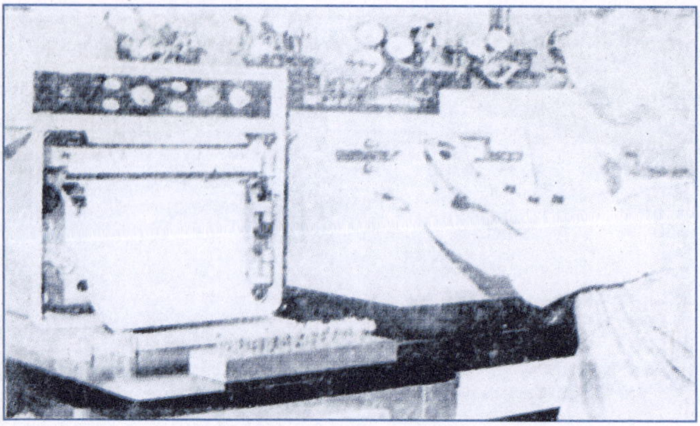

Figure 5.19 A sample containing fermentation products being injected into a gas chromatograph. The chart paper at the left has recorded the separations that were accomplished for compounds in previous samples as the volatilized samples passed through the partitioning column of the gas chromatograph.

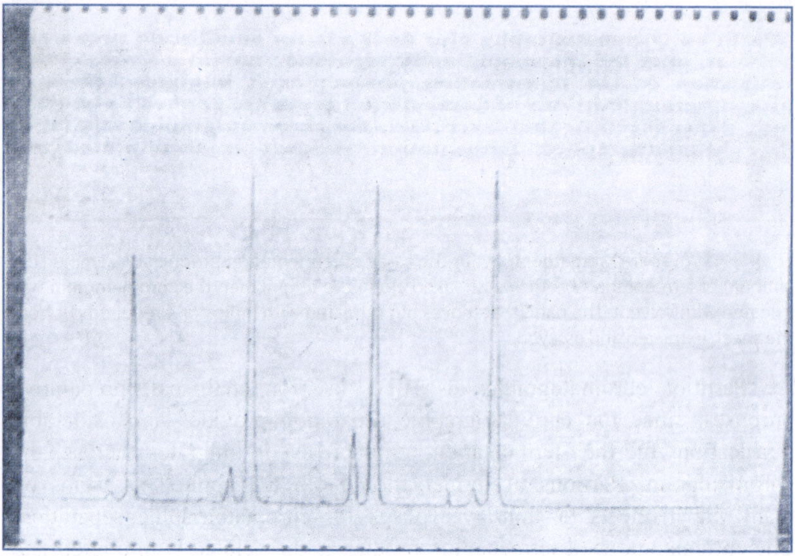

Figure 5.20 Gas chromatographic separations of fermentation products as drawn by the recorder attached to the gas chromatograph. Samples of the hydrocarbon phases from four different flasks in a hydrocarbon fermentation study were injected sequentially into the gas chromatograph. In each instance, from right to left, the hydrocarbon substrate came off the partitioning column first followed by one to two fermentation products in lesser quantities. Notice the greater yield of one of the fermentation products for the sample second from right.

Gas Chromatographic Assays

The gas chromatograph utilizes a form of partition chromatography to volatilize and separate certain types of fermentation products. In most instances, extraction or other preliminary purification is required to remove water and other compounds that cannot be volatilized from the sample. On injection into the gas chromatograph (Figure 5.19) the fermentation product is converted by heat to its gaseous state and in this state is pushed by a stream of inert gas through a partitioning column. Compounds separated during passage through this column are then detected electronically as they emanate from the column and, with the proper detector system, often they can be cooled and collected in a relatively pure state. Fermentation products not volatile with heat also can be analyzed by gas chromatography if volatile esters or other chemical reaction products can be prepared. Quantitative assay is obtained by comparison of the areas occurring under peaks on plots of the data (Figure 5.20) with corresponding areas for various quantities of reference compound.

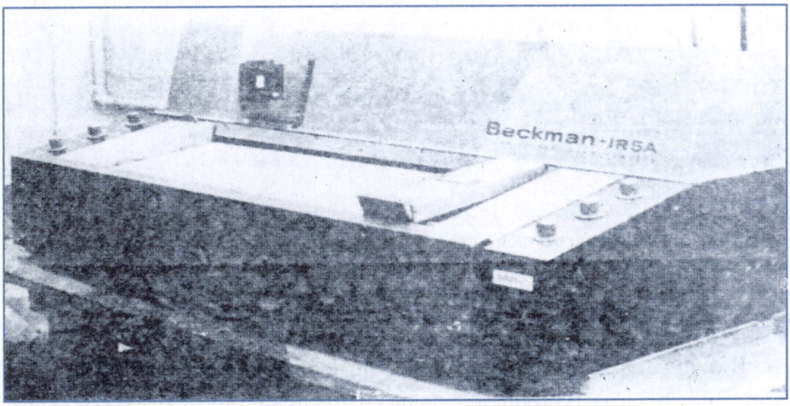

Figure 5.21 Apparatus for the determination of the infrared absorption spectrum of an organic compound. A small amount of the relatively pure fermentation product dissolved in a solvent such as chloroform or carbon tetrachloride is placed between salt plates positioned in a beam of infrared light. In the picture, the sample is visible as the light-colored small rectangle in the darker-colored sample holder at the upper left. The apparatus continuously scans the compound with increasing wavelengths of infrared light and records the infrared absorption at each wavelength.

Other Techniques

Infrared spectroscopy (Figures 5.21 and 5.22), nuclear magnetic resonance, and mass spectrometry are techniques that provide valuable information on the chemical structures of fermentation products, although they find relatively little use as quantitative assays. The fermentation products must be in a relatively pure state for analyses by these techniques. Countercurrent distribution (Figure 5.23) utilizes successive solvent fractionations to purify fermentation products but, again, it is not usually considered to be an assay procedure.

BIOLOGICAL ASSAYS

Biological assays include both those assays in which the compound being quantitated either depresses or stimulates the growth of a sensitive test microorganism, and those assays that employ enzymes.

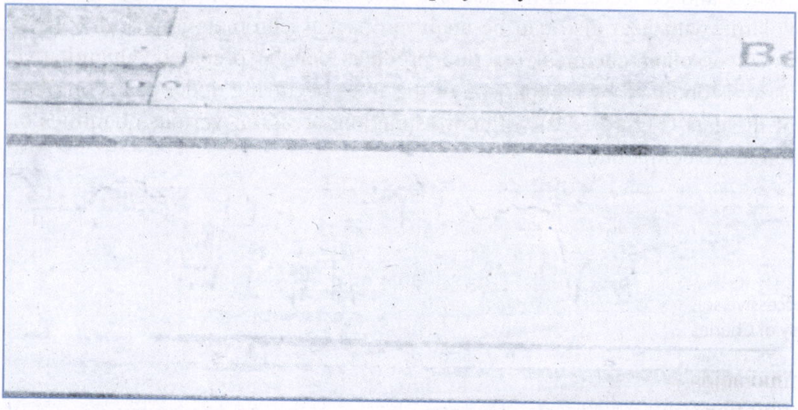

Figure 5.22 Infrared spectrum of 10 percent benzaldehyde in carbon tetrachloride. The infrared absorptions occurring on approximately the left half of the scan are specific for the various chemical groups making up the molecule. Those on the right half are characteristic of the entire molecule.

Biological assays usually are more difficult to perform, provide greater error, and are less reproducible than chemical or physical assays. Thus, careful standardization of every step in the assay procedure is mandatory and, in fact, these assays usually are not used if a good alternative physical or chemical assay is available.

Test organisms for biological assays may be strains normally encountered in nature, or they may be strains that have been artificially mutated for their use in a specific assay. An example of the latter is a microbial strain that has been mutated so that, through lack of an enzyme(s), it requires a certain compound for growth and provides a graded growth response in the presence of varying levels of this compound. The microorganisms employed in biological assays are of various types. Bacteria are used for the assay of

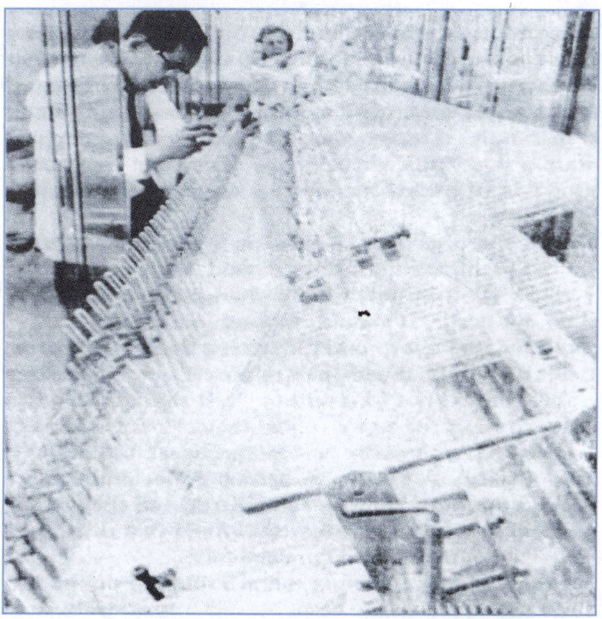

Figure 5.23 Counter-current distribution apparatus. The fermentation sample undergoes successive solvent fractionations as it passes from tube to tube in this apparatus. Photo courtesy of Charles Pfizer and Co., Inc.

amino acids, antibiotics, and vitamins. Yeasts have been used in vitamin and antibiotic assays. Fungi are employed for vitamins, trace metals, antibiotics, and fungicidal and fungistatic materials. A protozoan, *Euglena gracilis*, finds use in the assay of vitamin B_{12}. Thus, virtually any microorganism may be used if it will respond in a graded manner to varying concentrations of the material to be assayed.

Regardless of the organism chosen for a particular assay, it should meet several requirements if it is to be a good test organism. It should be genetically stable so that undesirable changes in response to the test compound do not occur. It should respond in a graded manner only to the test compound and not to other materials that may be present in the solution to be assayed. It should grow relatively quickly on simple media and, preferably, should not be a pathogen. It should grow in a fashion that facilitates reading the assay. Thus, the cells should not clump for turbidimetric assays or swarm across the agar surface for diffusion assays. It should, if possible, be an aerobe or facultative aerobe since anaerobic assays are more difficult to perform, and they require special equipment. Finally, it should grow well at a pH that does not affect the stability or toxicity of the material under assay.

Biological assays fall into four general groups. For the present discussion, these categories have been labelled respectively as diffusion, turbidimetric, metabolic response, and enzymatic assays.

Diffusion Assays

Diffusion assays are carried out on a solid medium, usually an agar medium, which is suitable for growth of the test organism. The compound to be assayed is allowed to diffuse through the medium in a radial fashion from

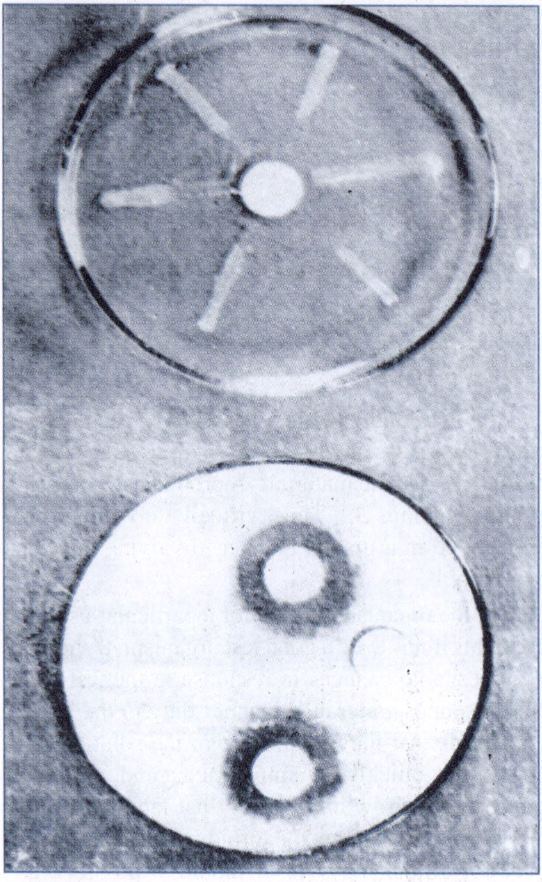

Figure 5.24 Growth inhibition by antibiotic diffusing through an agar medium from a paper disc. The agar in the upper plate was streaked with six different test organisms. The lower plate was seeded with a fungus. A fourth disc on the lower plate is no apparent because of lack of antibiotic activity so that the fungus partially overgrew the disc. Photo courtesy of Charles Pfizer and Co,. Inc.

a pad or cup so that the adjacent growth of the test organism is either depressed, as with an antibiotic (Figure 5.24), or stimulated, as with a growth factor (Figure 5.25). The diameter of this area reflects the concentration of the compound being assayed, and it is compared with similar zones produced by various known concentrations of standard or reference compound. The zone diameters of the standard are plotted against logarithms of the concentrations used, and the linear portion of this standard curve is used for determining the actual concentration of the sample being assayed.

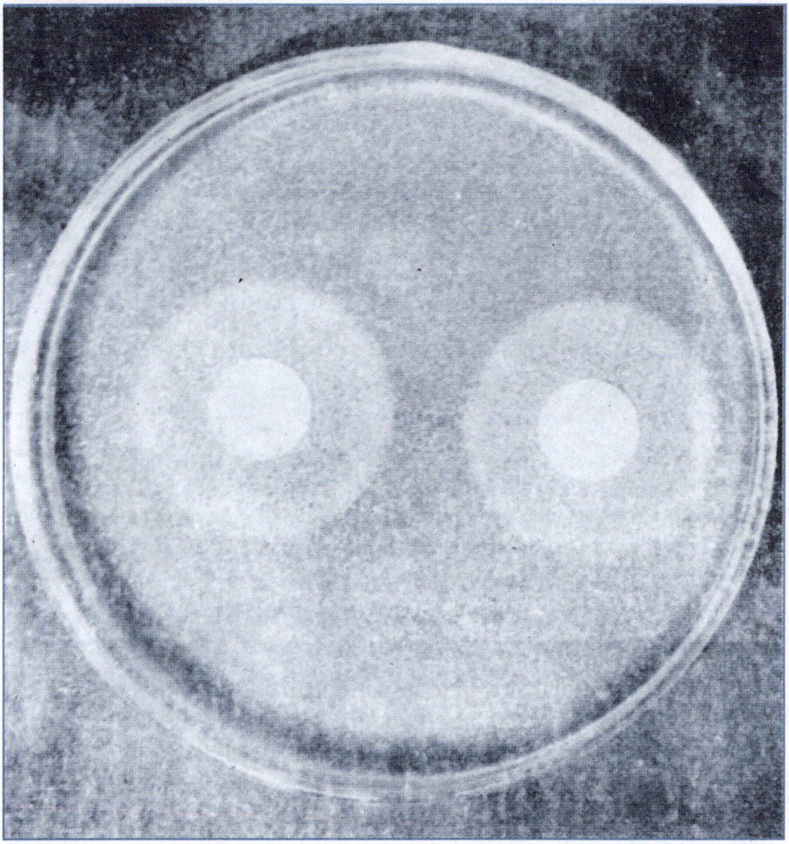

Figure 5.25 Growth stimulation by material diffusing from a paper disc. The entire surface of the agar was seeded with a bacterial test organism. (Casida, 1961. *Soil Sci.*, 92,287,297.)

There are two types of diffusion assay and, although somewhat similar, each has its own particular advantages. In the cylinder method (Figure 5.26), a portion of the antibiotic solution or other fermentation product diffuses

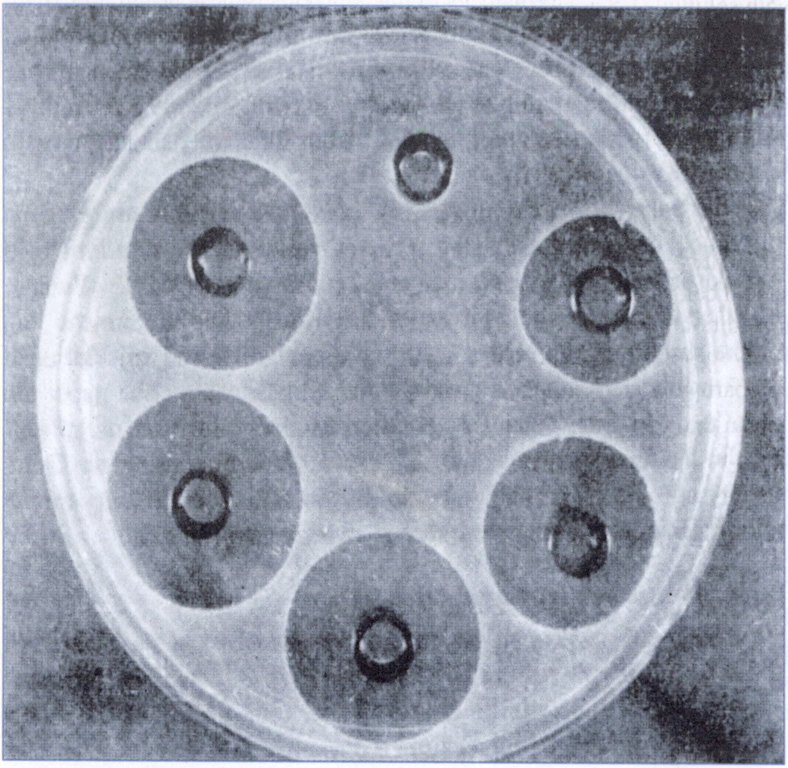

Figure 5.26 Antibiotic diffusion bioassay with cylinders. The cylinders were filled with samples containing various concentrations of antibiotic. Photo courtesy of Merck and Co., Inc.

from a reservoir, or cylinder, into the surrounding agar, while in the paper-disc method (Figures 5.24 and 5.25), only a defined amount of fermentation solution, such as 0.1 ml, is applied to the disc. A standardized amount of agar medium, perhaps 10 ml, is placed in Petri plates and allowed to harden. As soon as this base layer is hard, a standardized amount (usually about 5 ml) of the same or a different agar medium inoculated with a test microorganism is added above the base layer and allowed to harden to form the "seeded agar" layer. Several small metal, glazed porcelain, or glass cylinders are set on the agar surface. A slight preheating of these cylinders helps to seal them to the agar. The numbers of cylinders used per plate depends on the expected sizes of the zones, since the zones should not overlap. In fact, it is often necessary to dilute the samples to hold down the sizes of the zones. The cylinders are filled with appropriate dilutions of the solutions to be assayed or with solutions containing known concentrations of the reference compound, and the plates are incubated for a specified period of time at constant temperature. The diameters of the zones of stimulated or reduced growth are then measured in millimeters, and the concentrations in the solutions under assay are determined by comparison with a standard curve prepared from the inhibition or stimulation zone data for the standards. To obtain valid and reproducible results, each sample of unknown compound and each concentration of reference compound should be replicated several times on different plates so that average values can be calculated. Each assay plate also should contain a cylinder with at least one concentration of standard solution in addition to the fermentation samples, because variability in zone sizes is likely to be greater when comparing values from different plates than when comparing values from the same plate.

In the paper-disc assay, plates of seeded agar medium are prepared and inoculated as for the cylinder assay. However, the solutions to be assayed or solutions of reference compound are added at a volume of 0.1 ml to discs of sterile filter paper, usually 12.8 mm in diameter, laid on the surface of the seeded agar. The incubation and calculation of assay results are similar to those for the cylinder assay. The paper disc assay also finds use when fermentation products dissolved in solvents toxic to the test organism are to be assayed. The solutions are applied to discs lying on a glass plate, and the solvents are allowed to evaporate before placing the discs on the seeded agar medium for assay.

Turbidimetric and Growth Assays

Turbidimetric assays are those in which the effect of the compound under test in liquid culture is measured as an increased or decreased turbidity associated with the growth rate or total growth of the microorganism. A suitable liquid medium is dispensed in a series of tubes, and graded amounts of the material to be assayed are added. Obviously, all media and solutions must be sterile. The tubes are inoculated with a small and constant amount of a vigorous, young culture of the test organism, and then incubated for a predetermined period of time at constant temperature. The length of the incubation period to be used depends on whether the turbidity of the cultures is to be determined at some point during logarithmic growth, for the effect of the compound on growth rate, or during the maximum stationary growth phase, for the effect of the compound on the total growth of the organism which can occur in the particular medium. The relative turbidity produced in the tubes can be determined visually. However, these determinations usually employ a spectrophotometer (Figure 5.27) with a filter or defraction grating to allow the passage of a narrow wavelength band of visible light. The choice of wavelengths is determined by the color of the medium, so that at the proper wavelengths the medium color will have little effect on the assay.

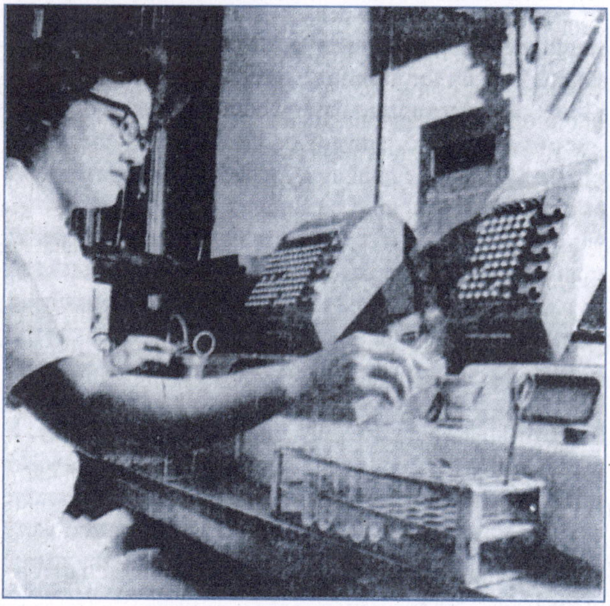

Figure 5.27 Automated turbidimetric bioassay. The technician is in the process of pouring a culture sample into the spectrophotometer. Photo courtesy of Charles Pfizer and Co., Inc.

Readings are made as optical densities, or absorbance. If the particular instrument happens to register only galvanometer deflections (percent light transmission), these are converted to optical density by applying the correction factor of 2-log galvanometer deflection. Some instruments, such as the Klett-Summerson Colorimeter, use a special scale for readings. These readings can be considered as analogous to but not quite the same as optical density determinations. The optical density is plotted against the concentration of standard to obtain a standard curve. Usually a portion of the curve will be linear, although, in some instances, it may be necessary to convert the concentration, optical density reading, or both to logarithms to obtain linearity.

The fermentation product to be assayed is usually added to the assay tubes at several dilutions, although, theoretically, only one dilution is necessary.

This precaution is required when materials are examined which have not previously been routinely assayed. Testing at several levels insures that the optical density obtained for one of the dilutions of the sample will fall on a linear portion of the standard curve. Also, if more than one of the dilutions meet this criterion, then the assay values allow a determination of whether unknown factors in the sample, growth of the organism, or elsewhere in the assay are contributing error. Thus, the final assay values obtained from two or more dilutions of the sample should be similar.

To help in minimizing errors, several tubes are used per dilution of test sample or standard, and these tubes are randomized in their racks. Other precautions also must be taken. All samples must be sterile, and the sample must not alter the pH or other characteristics of the medium. Samples that are themselves highly turbid or colored must receive special attention. The sample must be soluble in water or in a solvent miscible with water which does not interfere with the assay. For assays in which very small amounts of the fermentation product yield a growth response, the glassware must be completely devoid of this material prior to the assay. Test organisms that demand high aeration for maximum response to the test compound often require that the assay tubes be shaken during incubation. Conversely, anaerobic test organisms require special precautions.

End-Point Determination Assays

Microbial growth does not always yield dispersed cells for determination of turbidity. Sometimes, the growth occurs as a pellicle on the surface of the medium, or as a clump of cells at the bottom, which cannot be suitably broken up and dispersed for turbidity determinations. A bioassay is still possible, however, by employing an end-point assay. Thus, for a fermentation product that inhibits growth, such as an antibiotic, a series of tubes of growth medium containing progressively less and less of the compound to be assayed (a dilution series) is inoculated with the test organism. The tubes are incubated for a defined period at constant temperature, and each tube is observed to determine the presence or absence of growth (Figure 5.28). The relative amount of the fermentation product in the original fermentation broth is then determined by the amount of dilution which the fermentation product can withstand in the assay tubes and still be able to inhibit growth of the test organism. In other words, if the last tube that does not show growth in the dilution series is equivalent to a dilution of 1/64 of the fermentation broth, we can say that there are approximately 64 "dilution units" per milliliter of the compound present in the fermentation broth. These dilution units are of value when the fermentation product is newly discovered and standard reference material is not available. If reference material does become available, it can be similarly diluted and assayed to determine just how much is required to yield an inhibition end point similar to that observed with the diluted fermentation product. An endpoint bioassay that employs an agar medium is described in Chapter 4.

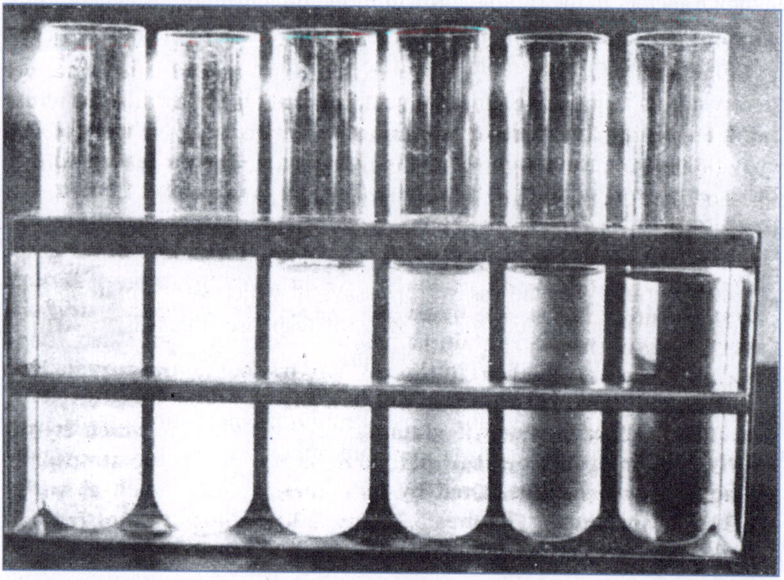

Figure 5.28 Dilution end-point bit assay. In this dilution sequence only the tube at the right, which contained a 1 : 2 dilution of the antibiotic sample, demonstrates a complete suppression of growth. However, notice the progressively decreasing activity of the further dilutions of the antibiotic in the succeeding tubes. Photo courtesy of Charles Pfizer and Co., Inc.

Metabolic Response Assays

Metabolic response assays are similar to turbidimetric assays except that, instead of measuring the effect of the fermentation product on the rate of growth or the total growth of the test organism, we measure its effect on some metabolic reaction that the test organism carries out during growth. A few metabolic reactions used for assays of this type are acid production, carbon dioxide evolution, oxygen absorption, and enzyme dehydrogenase activity.

Enzymatic Assays

Enzymatic assays are highly specific, and they will quantitatively detect minute amounts of a fermentation product, as well as differentiate

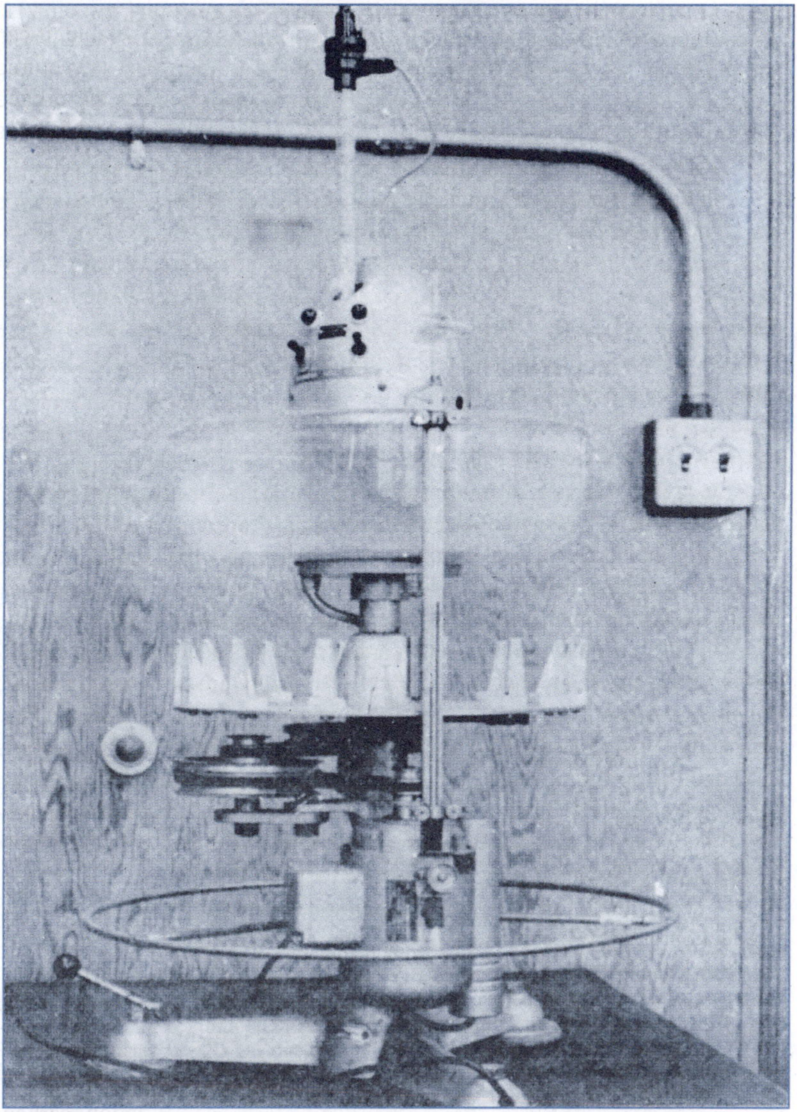

Figure 5.29 Warburg respirometer with a manometer and its attached Warburg vessel. The manometer is itself attached to a reciprocating shaking platform, and the Warburg vessel is suspended in a constant-temperature water bath. The atmosphere In the vessel and in the right side of the manometer is a closed system so that an increase or decrease in the volume of a component of this atmosphere resulting from enzymatic activity registers as a depression or rise, respectively in the manometer fluid.

between biologically active and inactive forms of a compound. An enzyme preparation (from a commercial source, a microbial culture, or other enzyme source) is incubated with a sample of culture broth so as to cause some enzyme-mediated change in the fermentation product, such as a partial decomposition with consequent formation of a measurable product. For example, L-glutamic acid in a small sample of fermentation broth can be assayed by adding washed cells of certain strains of *Escherichia coli* which contain the enzyme "glutamic acid decarboxylase." Toluene also is added to this mixture to liberate the enzyme from the cells, and the assay is carried out at a pH of 5. One mole of CO_2 is liberated from each mole of glutamic acid. The CO_2, which is only poorly soluble in water at this pH value, is evolved to the atmosphere as the gas, and it is measured by manometric means such as with a Warburg respirometer (Figures 5.29 and 5.30). Toluene is not required if the *Escherichia coli* cells are first carefully dried *in vacuo* over $CaCl_2$ or dried by several washings with cold acetone (an acetone powder).

Enzymatic assays must be carefully tested to determine that they actually function properly under the specific conditions being employed. A known amount of the pure chemical product is added as an internal standard to one sample of a typical fermentation broth, but not to another sample. The assay results should quantitatively reflect the amount of added chemical when the assay values for the two samples are compared. If this is not the case, several possibilities should be checked. The pH or temperature at which the assay is being carried out may not be optimal for the enzyme, or the enzyme may be inactive under these conditions. There may be compounds in the sample of fermentation broth, such as metals or alternate substrates, which inhibit the enzyme or compete for its active sites. The enzyme may be inherently unstable or may be unstable under the conditions of the assay. Enzyme from a microbial cell source may have been produced in only small quantities or not at all, since special growth conditions often are required for good production of a given enzyme. Enzyme from a commercial source may have been improperly stored; these preparations should be obtained from a reliable source and stored dry in the cold without being allowed to become too old before use. The specificity of the enzyme may be either too little or too great. Obviously, an enzyme that attacks compounds in the culture broth other than the fermentation product will provide erroneous results. Enzymes are usually specific for stereoisomers. For example, in a mixture of D- and L-isomers of glutamic acid only one of the isomers, usually the L-form, will be degraded. However, a microbial cell enzyme source may contain additional enzymes known as "racemases" which racemize either the D- or L-isomer to a mixture of the isomers, a phenomenon that also can cause erroneous assay results.

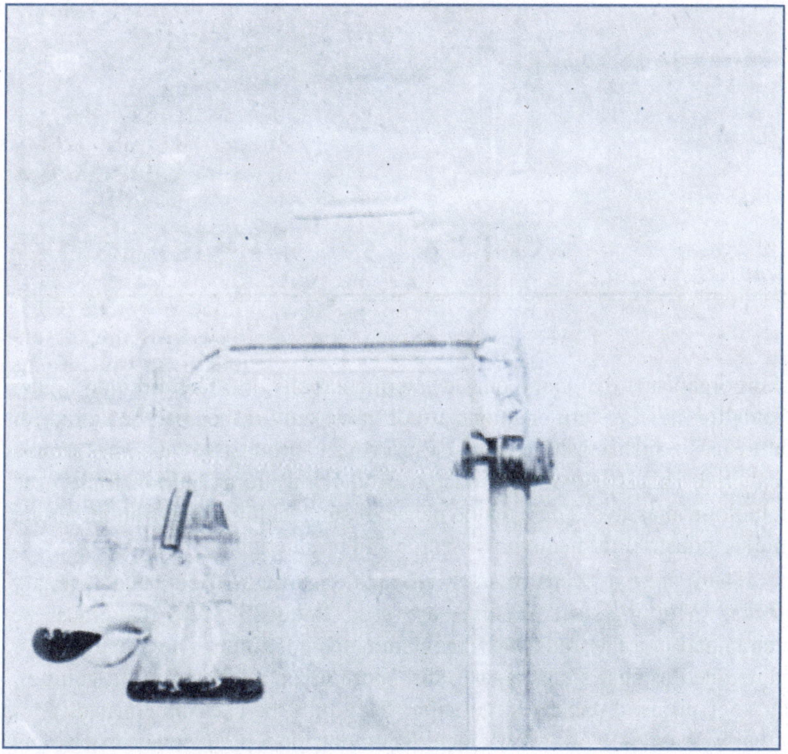

Figure 5.30 Warburg vessel attached to its manometer. The enzyme solution is seen in the main chamber of the vessel and the solution of the compound to be assayed (the substrate) in the side arm. To start the reaction, the substrate from the side arm is tipped into the main chamber. The vessel pictured has KOH and a piece of filter paper in the small center well of the main chamber to absorb evolved CO_2 so that O_2 depletion from the atmosphere can be measured.

The toluene possibly may not release the enzyme from the cells, or it may be inhibitory to the released enzyme. If this proves to be the case, N-butanol or chloroform often can be substituted for the toluene and, in certain instances, the enzyme can be released from the cells by incubation with the respective strain of bacteriophage. Finally, the enzyme source or fermentation broth may contain additional enzymes capable of further degrading the product of the initial enzyme reaction. Sometimes, the activities of these unwanted enzymes can be controlled by allowing the main enzyme reaction to proceed at a pH value unfavorable to the activities of the other enzymes present. You will remember that the assay for L-glutamic acid employed a pH of 5, a pH value too acidic to allow other cellular enzymes to interfere with the assay.

CHAPTER 6
Stock Cultures

Microorganisms that carry out new fermentations or which provide higher yields for existing fermentations are of value only if they can be stored for future use in such a fashion that their growth and productive capacities remain unaltered. This is also true for existing production strains and for strains used in biological assays. Thus, maintenance of stock cultures plays an important role in industrial fermentation research and production.

There are two types of stock cultures, "working stocks" and "primary stocks." Working-stock cultures are used frequently, and they must be maintained in a vigorous and uncontaminated condition. These cultures are maintained as agar slants, agar stabs, spore preparations, or broth cultures, and they are held under refrigeration. They must be checked constantly for possible changes in growth characteristics, nutrition, productive capacity and contamination.

Primary stocks are cultures that are held in reserve for presently practical or new fermentations, for comparative purposes, for biological assays, or for possible later screening programs. These cultures are not maintained in a state of high physiological activity, and they are delved into only rarely. Transfers from these cultures are made only when a new working-stock culture is required, or when the primary-stock culture must be subcultured to avoid death of the cells. Thus, primary-stock cultures are stored in such a manner as to require the least possible numbers of transfers over a period of time. Death of a high percent of cells in a primary-stock culture is not particularly serious, if viable cells can still be recovered for subculture to fresh medium. Primary-stock cultures stored at room temperature are maintained in sterile soil, or in agar or broth that is provided with an overlay of sterile mineral oil. Agar and broth cultures without mineral oil also are refrigerated, and cultures in milk or agar are maintained frozen at low temperatures. Finally, primary-stock cultures are lyophilized, or freeze-dried, and stored at low temperatures. Often, more than one of these procedures is employed to insure against loss of the cultures or changes in the cells.

The maintenance of refrigerated stock cultures on agar or in broth is the least desirable of these procedures. Although the cultures may survive six months or more under refrigeration, usually they are transferred more frequently. These frequent culture transfers and the many cell generations accompanying these transfers allow the possible occurrence of and selection for undesired genetic changes in the organisms. Also, the potential for contamination is markedly increased with frequent transfer of the cultures. Certain microorganisms, such as *Blakeslea trispora* used in β-carotene production, cannot be stored at refrigeration temperatures, because they die out relatively quickly at these temperatures. However, such cultures can be held as agar slants at room temperature with transfers being made to fresh medium when the cultures have become nearly dried out.

Sterile soil has found wide use for the stock-culture maintenance of microorganisms that form spores. In fact, microorganisms that do not form spores also will survive in sterile soil, but they may die out unexpectedly after a period of time. Soil stocks are prepared by mixing enough sand with a rich garden soil to make the soil friable and easy to handle. A small amount of calcium carbonate is added, and the mixture is distributed in screw-capped tubes or in tubes plugged with cotton. The tubes are repeatedly autoclaved until random checks of their contents reveal that sterility has been accomplished. A small volume of a thick suspension of spores or of an actively growing nonsporulated culture is then added to the sterile soil, and the moisture is quickly removed by placing the tubes under reduced atmospheric pressure over a drying agent. Soil stocks, thus prepared, are stored at room temperature with the cotton plugs or screw caps protected from dust.

Agar slant and stab cultures of many microorganisms will survive several years at room temperature if the growth is submerged under sterile mineral oil. The oil overlay provides dissolved oxygen, prevents drying of the agar, and apparently decreases the metabolic activity of the cells to an almost negligible rate. However, genetic changes do occur in cultures stored in this manner.

The most widely used method for culture preservation is by lyophilization, also known as freeze-drying (Figure 6.1). In this procedure, cells in glass ampules are suspended in a carrier or protective agent such as sterile bovine serum, rapidly frozen at low temperature, and dried in a high vacuum. The ampules are then sealed and stored at low temperatures. If properly prepared and stored, most lyophilized cultures will remain viable for long periods without the occurrence of genetic changes. When needed, the cultures are recovered from the ampules by suspending the lyophilized cells in a minimal amount of growth medium and then incubating.

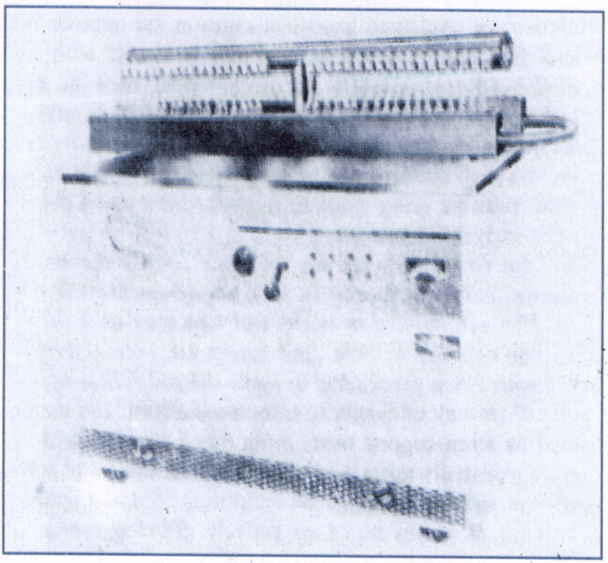

Figure 6.1 VirTis Freeze-Mobile with 72 port manifold, Model 10–45 MH–72. Freeze-drying apparatus for stock cultures. This particular machine dries 72 cultures simultaneously. Courtesy of the VirTis Co.

Regardless of the method or methods chosen for preservation of primary-stock cultures, it is of utmost importance that good, descriptive records be kept on these cultures and that the cultures be well labelled. If little is known or recorded about a newly isolated microbial strain, we cannot hope to be able to recognize changes that may have occurred in that culture after a prolonged storage period.

CHAPTER 7

Fermentation Media

MEDIA COMPOSITION

The choice of a good medium is virtually as important to the success of an industrial fermentation as is the selection of an organism to carry out the fermentation. The medium supplies nutrients for growth, energy, building of cell substance, and biosynthesis of fermentation products. Of particular importance are the sources of carbon and nitrogen in the medium, since microbial cells and fermentation products are composed largely of these elements. In addition to the carbon and nitrogen compounds, a medium contains inorganic salts, water, vitamins, and other growth factors, precursors of fermentation products, dissolved oxygen and other gases, buffers, antifoam, lysate of dead cells, and fermentation products. All of these can be considered as nutrients. In addition to the nutrients, a medium also may contain various inhibitors of microbial growth and biosynthesis and, if it has not been sterilized, it may even contain active enzymes added as components of certain of the medium constituents. A poor choice of medium components can cause limited cellular growth and little if any yield of fermentation products. Also, a poor medium can alter the types and ratios of products from among those for which a particular microorganism has biosynthetic capability. Thus, the types and amounts of the nutritive components of a medium are critical.

Microbial growth under industrial fermentation conditions usually utilizes a "luxury metabolism" of the organisms. Thus, good yields of fermentation products occur only if relatively large amounts of carbon, and possibly nitrogen, are channeled through the metabolic pathways of the microorganism. The microorganism provided with an excoss, of nutrients under ideal growth conditions becomes greedy, and it utilizes far more substrate than it would normally use in its natural environment or under the usual minimal conditions of laboratory growth. A part of the carbon substrate is utilized for the synthesis of cell components: other carbon is degraded during cellular respiration and, as such, is evolved as carbon dioxide and water. The remaining carbon is channeled to those enzymatic sequences that, for one reason or another, yield products not required or used completely by the cells. Thus, through the latter reactions, excess carbon is drained from the metabolism so that it does not interfere with those enzymatic reactions associated with vital metabolic pathways.

The particular composition of a fermentation medium can be simple to complex depending on the particular microorganism and its fermentation. Autotrophic microorganisms require only the simplest of inorganic media. They require a few inorganic salts, water, and a nitrogen source; their carbon requirement is fulfilled by the carbon dioxide of the air or by carbonates. Thus, from simple inorganic nutrients, autotrophs are able to synthesize all of the complex organic compounds required to sustain life and to allow growth and multiplication of their cells, and they meet their total energy requirements by oxidation of some particular inorganic component of their medium. At the opposite end of the scale are the highly fastidious microorganisms, such as some of the lactic acid bacteria, which lack the ability to synthesize many of their sustenance and growth requirements. These organisms require the presence of many types of simple to complex preformed nutrients in the medium, and they must have an organic carbon supply to provide for synthesis of cell substance and release of metabolic energy. These are the two extremes and, obviously, microorganisms exist with requirements intermediate between these extremes. However, in addition to these considerations, fermentation growth conditions impose a metabolic stress on microorganisms, as for instance, the high aeration rates and high substrate levels commonly employed, so that additional nutrients and growth factors may be required as compared to the usual laboratory culture of the organisms. Thus, enzyme systems that normally are not limiting factors in metabolic sequences, because of a lack of sufficient levels of coenzymes or for other reasons, may become limiting under the stresses of fermentation growth: under these conditions more complex media are required than would normally be employed.

Simple and complex media are further subdivided into two categories: "synthetic" and "crude." A synthetic medium, at first glance, would appear to be the medium of choice. It is a medium in which all of the constituents are specifically defined and known compounds. Every constituent is a relatively pure compound, and the exact amounts incorporated into the medium are known. Thus, an example of a synthetic medium would be one containing inorganic salts, water, purified sugar, and an ammonium or nitrate compound or an amino acid to supply combined nitrogen. Obviously, if the nitrogen requirement were to be met with something like dried blood, we would not know the exact components and their amounts in the medium.

Synthetic media present distinct advantages for certain types of studies. Since the amount and chemical structure of each component are known, the concentration of anyone component or of several components can easily be varied to determine its specific effect on cell growth and product yield. Also, individual components are easily deleted or added. These considerations allow the redesigning of a medium to obtain the greatest possible yield of product, and they also allow a study of the metabolic processes leading to or governing product formation. Studies of this type can yield additional information if one of the substrates or a part of the molecule of one of the substrates contains a radioactive or heavy isotope. Isotopes allow us to determine which nutrients or parts of nutrients end up as an integral part of the product. Thus, information of the latter type may allow us to predict alternate substrates or other means for further manipulation of the medium to increase yields. Synthetic media also provide other advantages. Because they are completely defined media, they aid in obtaining reproducibility of growth and product yield from one fermentation run to another so that error due to medium composition is held at a minimum. Foaming usually is not a problem with synthetic media, because they do not contain any protein or relatively high molecular weight peptides. The recovery and purification of fermentation products are relatively simple with these media, because extraneous organic compounds are not included in the medium, and because most of the compounds that might interfere with recovery are known. With advantages such as these, we might assume that synthetic media would find great use in industrial fermentations. However, this is not the case. These media can be expensive, because of the cost of the relatively pure ingredients used, and the yields derived from these media are relatively low. In regard to the latter point, the metabolic stress on the microorganism brought on by fermentation conditions may induce requirements for growth or biosynthesis factors which are not normally associated with the particular organism being employed, or for growth factors that are, as yet, unknown in relation to microbial metabolism.

The alternative is the nonsynthetic or "crude" medium, which usually allows much higher yields of fermentation products than does a synthetic medium. An example of a crude medium is one containing soybean meal, blackstrap molasses, cornsteep liquor, $(NH_4)_2SO_4$, $CaCO_3$ and K_2HPO_4. It also may supply precursors for the biosynthesis of the fermentation product, and it can allow the use of crude antifoam agents without radically changing the nutritive balance of the medium. Thus, crude media contain crude or ill-defined sources of nutrients and, as such, they provide an excess of both nutrients and growth factors. However, it is assumed that a medium such as this does not contain metals, inorganic salts, or organic compounds toxic to the organism or to its product formation. Also, it is assumed that the crude carbon and nitrogen sources in such a medium are in a form that the organism can use. For example, the medium should not provide a pentose sugar for an organism that can only use a hexose, protein for an organism that does not have proteolytic activity, or starch for an organism that lacks amylase.

Crude media, and to some extent synthetic media, must at times meet requirements in addition to providing nutrients for growth and product formation. These requirements include buffering capacity, lack of foam production, control of oxidation-reduction potential, inhibition or slowing of the growth of contaminating microorganisms, neutralization of acidic or alkaline growth products, contribution to maintenance of the genetic stability of the microorganism, promotion of vigorous aeration and agitation, allowing of recovery of the fermentation product without resort to complex recovery procedures, withstanding of sterilization without adverse interaction of nutritive constituents, allowing the growth of the organism in its proper morphological state, provision of precursors if required, allowing or preventing sporulation, provision of specific metabolic inhibitors if such are required, and provision of alternate substrates for a possible diauxie phenomenon. In addition, the medium must be economically feasible for the particular fermentation.

Constituents for fermentation media, particularly crude media, are obtained from a range of sources. Regardless of the source, however, the primary requirement is that these nutrients be inexpensive. In this regard, the by-products of agriculture have always provided the cheapest source of medium components and particularly of carbon substrates. However, the component found in greatest amount in fermentation media is not an agricultural by-product and, in fact, is one that is often overlooked. This component is water, since microorganisms live in an aqueous environment in which most of their nutritive requirements are dissolved. Media usually contain more than 70 percent and often greater than 90 percent water. This water supplies trace minerals, metals such as copper, molybdenum, zinc, and boron, and other substances that may be required in minute quantities by microorganisms or, in contrast, may be inhibitory to their activities. The water used in media make-up also can affect the quality of the product, for instance, the flavor of a beverage product. Thus, as a medium component, the quality of the water can be critical. Water also is used in cooling and in steam production, in the cleaning of equipment, and in product recovery. Therefore, a supply of good cool water of constant composition is essential to the fermentation industry. In fact, the location of production facilities may be dictated by the availability of good water.

Inorganic nutrients usually present little problem when crude media are employed, because the common anions and cations occur in sufficient quantities in the crude medium components. However, major requirements, such as for phosphate, sulfate, magnesium, and possibly ammonium ions, can be met by adding potassium phosphate, magnesium sulfate, and ammonium sulfate or phosphate. Calcium carbonate is sometimes added to neutralize acidic fermentation products or to halt drastic decreases in pH which can occur during microbial growth. Crude media are more likely to provide excesses of toxic ions than to be deficient in required ions. Thus, it is possible that various components of the medium or the complete medium may require a pretreatment with ion exchange resins or some other procedure to remove toxic quantities of certain metals, such as copper, which can poison sensitive microbial enzyme systems.

Carbon sources for fermentation media can be simple or complex carbohydrates, sugar alcohols or other alcohols, organic acids, proteins, peptides, amino acids, and even hydrocarbons. These carbon sources are usually used in a crude form, although semipurified sugars, sugar alcohols, polysaccharides, or hydrocarbons may be required for specific fermentations. Crude sources of simple sugars include beet and cane molasses, corn molasses or "hydrol," whey, sulfite waste liquor, cull fruits, cannery wastes, and so forth. Polysaccharides such as starches are supplied by corn, wheat, rye, milo, rice, potatoes, sweet potatoes, and other agricultural products. Cellulosic by-products also are usable as carbon sources, but they usually require costly saccharification by a procedure such as acid hydrolysis. For example, the following contain approximately 50 percent cellulose: wood wastes, oat hulls, corn cobs, and straw. Hydrocarbon substrates are usually mixtures of various hydrocarbon components and are relatively inexpensive. The pure hydrocarbon compounds or hydrocarbon fractions, however, are more costly.

Even in crude media, inorganic nitrogen-containing salts of nitrate, ammonia, or urea may be added to meet the nitrogen growth requirements of the microorganisms. This is particularly true when the organisms do not demonstrate proteolytic activity. However, crude proteinaceous animal and plant materials more often compose the main nitrogen sources of these fermentation media. Examples of these sources include corn steep liquor, distillers solubles, casein, cereal grains, peptones, tankage, fish meal, stick liquor, meat scraps, soybean meal, yeast and yeast extracts or autolysates, cotton seed meal, linseed oil meal,.and peanut oil meal.

Several of the better crude nutritive sources for fermentation media are in themselves complex mixtures of nutrients, supplying carbon and nitrogen compounds as well as microbial growth factors. Specific examples are molasses, cornsteep liquor, and sulfite waste liquor.

Molasses

Beet and cane molasses are by-products of the sugar industry. These molasses are the concentrated syrups or mother liquors recovered at any one of several steps in the sugar-refining process, and different names are applied to the molasses depending on the particular step from which .it was recovered. Of these, blackstrap molasses prepared from sugar cane normally is the cheapest and the most used sugar source for industrial fermentations. In the commercial production of sugar, the juice from crushed sugar cane is concentrated to allow crystallization of its sucrose. The crystallized sugar is then separated from its mother liquor, and the mother liquor is further concentrated to allow recovery of additional crops of crystalline sugar. This procedure is repeated several times until crystallization inhibitors accumulate to such a concentration that further recovery of sucrose is not economical. At this point, the mother liquor still contains approximately 52 percent total sugars calculated as sucrose (30 percent sucrose, and 22 percent invert sugars) and is known as black-strap molasses. When this molasses is used as a fermentation medium component, it is considered to contain 50 percent fermentable sugars. Refinery blackstrap molasses is a similar product that differs from black-strap molasses only in that it is the residual mother liquor that has accumulated in the recrystallization refining of the crude sucrose.

High-test or invert molasses contains approximately 70 to 75 percent sugar, and it is produced in a manner different from that previously described the whole cane juice is partially inverted to prevent sugar crystallization; that is, the sugar is partially hydrolyzed to monosaccharides with heat and acid then neutralized and concentrated without removal of any of the sugar. Thus, high-test or invert molasses contains much of the original sugar of the cane juice, although it has been partially hydrolyzed to D-glucose and D-fructose. It is preferred to blackstrap molasses because of the lower shipping charges on a sugar concentration basis and because of its lower levels of nonfermentable solids including salts and unfermentable sugars. In blackstrap molasses, the unfermentable sugars result from the action of heat on the sugars, particularly fructose, during the refining process. High-test molasses is produced only during years of sugarcane over-production and, hence, its availability at anyone time may be somewhat questionable.

Beet molasses are produced by procedures resembling those for sugar cane. However, beet molasses may be limiting in biotin for yeast growth so that a small amount of cane blackstrap or other source of biotin should be added for growth of these microorganisms. "Hydrol" is a molasses resulting from the manufacture of crystalline dextrose from corn starch. It contains approximately 60 percent sugar, but it also contains a relatively high salt concentration that must be considered if this molasses is to be used as a medium component.

In addition to sucrose, blackstrap molasses contains small amounts of complex polysaccharides and invert sugars. The presence of the invert sugars is attributed to the action of the "invertase" enzyme present in the original cane juice. Blackstrap molasses also contains various noncarbohydrate materials. Thus, dark colored, nitrogen-containing polymeric substances result from "browning," a reaction of the sugars with amino acids because of the heat and alkali used in processing. Inorganic ions are present in high concentrations and include most of the ions of the original cane juice which were concentrated in the mother liquor during sugar crystallization. Calcium, also is present, being added during processing. Organic-acid constituents include aconitic, malic, citric, lactic, formic, acetic and propionic acids. The nitrogen-containing compounds (other than the polymeric forms) are mainly amino acids and, particularly, aspartic and glutamic acids resulting from the damidation of the asparagine and glutamine of the cane juice. A few heat and alkali stable vitamins are present, such as myo-inositol, niacin, pantothenic acid, riboflavin, and small amounts of biotin. Also present are organic phosphorus compounds such as inositol hexaphosphate and its calcium-magnesium salt known as "phytin."

The overall compositions of the various molasses differ according to the specific geographic areas of production. This is particularly true for their contents of certain metal ions and, in fact, for certain fermentations, such as that for citric acid, the molasses is pretreated with cation exchange resins or potassium ferrocyanide before use so as to remove interfering cations.

Cornsteep Liquor

Cornsteep liquor is the water extract by-product resulting from the steeping of corn during the commercial production of corn starch, gluten, and other corn products. The used or spent steep waters are concentrated to approximately 50 percent solids, and this concentrate, known as cornsteep liquor, is used in the commercial manufacture of feedstuffs and as a medium adjunct in the fermentation industry. It was first extensively employed in fermentation media for the manufacture of penicillin. Of the 50 percent solids of cornsteep liquor, approximately half is lactic acid. The rest includes amino acids, glucose and other reducing sugars, salts, vitamins, and precursors such as those for the penicillin molecule. Although cornsteep liquor does contain this high lactic acid content, the acid is not necessarily utilized by microorganisms during growth in industrial fermentation processes. The high lactic acid content of cornsteep liquor results during its manufacture from the growth of lactic acid bacteria and of mycoderms, which are film-forming, asporogenous, yeast like fungi. Thus, the lactic acid is not a component of corn but results from a natural fermentation of the cornsteep liquor. In other words, cornsteep liquor in itself actually is a natural fermentation product and, as such, it can vary greatly in composition for lots from a single supplier, or between lots received from various suppliers. This variation in composition, at times, can lead to poor reproducibility of an industrial fermentation. Thus, if the cornsteep liquor is supplying certain medium components (such as a particular amino acid, vitamin, or precursor) at low but critical levels, it may be necessary to determine the specific level of this compound as it is present in each lot of cornsteep liquor that is to be used.

Sulfite Waste Liquor

Sulfite waste liquor is the spent sulfite liquor from the paper-pulping industry. It is the Fluid remaining after wood for paper manufacture is digested to cellulose pulp with calcium bisulfite under heat and pressure and, as such, it presents a serious disposal problem for the paper-pulp manufacturers. Disposal in streams, as is the usual practice, causes stream pollution, and in several states legislation has been enacted against this method of disposal. Sulfite waste liquor can be employed as a dilute fermentation medium, being used in the production of ethanol by *Saccharomyces cerevisiae* and in the growth of *Torula utilis* cells for feed. The economics of these fermentations dictate that the fermentation plant be located in close proximity to the pulping operation so that the cost of transporting the waste liquor is not a factor. The waste liquor contains 10 to 12 percent solids of which sugars make up about 20 percent. Thus, sulfite waste liquor is a dilute sugar solution containing approximately 2 percent sugar. These sugars include the hexoses D-glucose, D-galactose and D-mannose, and the pentoses D-xylose and L-arabinose. However, the relative amounts of these sugars present in sulfite waste liquor depend, to some extent, on the woods being digested, with soft woods being higher in hexoses and hardwoods higher in pentoses. This is important if a yeast such as *Saccharomyces cerevisiae* is to be employed as the fermentation organism, since it uses only hexoses. *Torula utilis*, however, can ferment both hexoses and pentoses. In any event, regardless of which type of organism is being considered, the sugars of sulfite waste liquor cannot be fermented directly; the free sulfur dioxide or sulfurous acid of the waste liquor must first be removed by steam stripping or precipitation with lime.

Wood-waste residues hydrolyzed by acid provide sugars similar to those of sulfite waste liquor. The hydrolyzed material is partially neutralized and filtered before use in a fermentation medium. Thus, wood wastes are a virtually untapped source for fermentation carbohydrate nutrients.

Growth Factors

The growthfactor requirements of industrial fermentation microorganisms are usually provided by the crude constituents of the fermentation medium. As stated previously, preliminary determinations of the levels of these factors may be necessary if the particular requirement for them are critical. Yeast products such as cell hydrolysates or autolysates are particularly good sources of microbial growth factors if additional media sources are required.

Precursors

Precursors required in certain industrial fermentations are provided either through crude nutritive constituents, such as cornsteep liquor, or by direct addition of the more pure compounds. Precursors are defined (Lee, 1951) as "Substances added prior to or simultaneously with the fermentation, which are incorporated without any major change into the molecule of the fermentation product, and which generally serve to increase the yield or improve the quality of the product." Thus, the principal criterion is that the precursor becomes incorporated into the fermentation product. Specific examples of the use of precursors are the addition to the medium of phenylacetic acid as a precursor for penicillin G, and the addition of inorganic cobalt for production of vitamin B12. It should be pointed out that the precursor can also dictate as to which product from among several possibilities will be produced in greatest amount during a fermentation. Thus, with cornsteep liquor in the penicillin fermentation up to six different penicillins are possible products but, on addition of phenylacetic acid, the major product becomes penicillin G.

Buffers

Fermentation media contain buffers to retard gross changes in pH values during microbial growth. These buffers can be specifically added for their buffering capacity, or they may be normal constituents of a medium, serving a dual function as both buffer and nutritive source. During microbial growth, pH changes can occur for one of several reasons. Obviously, an acidic or alkaline fermentation product can alter the pH picture. Also, an inorganic salt component of the medium can cause pH changes; for example, ammonium sulfate supplying nitrogen as the ammonium ion for growth will leave behind the sulfate ion as sulfuric acid, thereby making the medium more acidic. Decarboxylation of organic acids or deamination of strongly basic organic amines from among the medium constituents will raise or lower the pH, respectively. Also, deamination and utilization of proteins, peptides, or amino acids can raise the pH value. Calcium carbonate often is incorporated in fermentation media to provide neutralization of acidic fermentation products, although it is a relatively poor buffer : its poor solubility in water allows only slow reaction with acidic products. In fact, the pH value of the medium may decrease to 4 or 5 before the calcium carbonate has much effect. Media containing considerable quantities of proteins, peptides, and amino acids possess good buffer capacity in the pH range near neutrality. Additional buffering capacity in this pH range also is provided by phosphates such as the system of mono- and dihydrogen potassium or sodium phosphates. At lower pH values, acetic acid and other organic acids provide buffering capacity. In contrast to the foregoing discussion, at times it may not be desirable to employ a medium strongly buffered at the pH values initially provided at medium make-up. Thus, an increase or decrease in pH during the fermentation can allow increased yields of certain fermentation products because of specific effects of acidity or alkalinity on the metabolism of the microorganism.

Antifoam

Antifoam agents of the crude types must be considered as potential nutritive sources of alcohols and fatty acids for fermentation media. A discussion of these agents is presented in Chapter 3.

Oxidation-Reduction Potentials

Certain components of fermentation media tend to "poise" or hold the medium within specific ranges of oxidation-reduction potential. These agents usually present little problem in highly aerated fermentations, but they must be considered in anaerobic fermentations. Amino acids such as L-cysteine, peptides such as glutathione, and organic acids such as thioglycolic acid will poise the medium at relatively low oxidation-reduction potentials for growth of anaerobic or microaerophilic microorganisms. In addition, the medium is heated and cooled just before inoculation to drive out dissolved oxygen.

Certain media, such as cooked corn mash for the anaerobic clostridia, further reduce oxygen penetration by their gel-like properties.

Restricted Nutritive Levels

Media conducive to rapid microbial growth and high cell yields are not always the best media for production of fermentation products. Sometimes, media allowing only restricted growth of microorganisms provide high product yields, because relatively greater amounts of carbon and other nutritive components of the medium are shunted into fermentation products instead of to growth. In the production of organic acids by fungi, the yields for some acids are greater if the growth, because of low pH or for other reasons, is relatively poor. Also, the control of the combined nitrogen level of a medium to retard microbial growth is beneficial in fermentations such as that for fat production by the yeast *Rhodotorula gracilis* (Chapter 19). Replacement culture with fungal mycelium is another good example of the use of a restricted growth medium. A fungus, such as *Aspergillus niger* for gluconic acid production (Chapter 21), is first grown on a medium that provides good growth as well as product formation, then the mycelium is separated from its medium and placed in fresh medium high in carbon substrate (sugar), but lacking combined nitrogen so that additional growth cannot occur. Further fermentation occurs enzymatically, in this case, by the glucose oxidase of the mycelium.

MEDIA STERILIZATION AND CONTAMINATION

Media for industrial fermentations usually are sterilized. In certain instances, however, the economics of the fermentation do not allow a sterilization expense, but the fermentation can still be conducted on an industrial scale. Such fermentations employ low pH values and, possibly, other contamination inhibitors (such as lactic acid) to hold in check the levels of contaminating organisms. Alternatively, as with *Candida lipolytica* growing with hydrocarbon as its carbon substrate, sterilization of the medium is not required if the medium components are poorly usable by potentially contaminating microorganisms. We might assume that antibiotic fermentations would not require sterilization of the medium, but this has not proven to be the case. Antibiotic production usually requires a rich growth medium, and the antibiotic accumulates only relatively late in the fermentation. Even with the use of a relatively high inoculum level, antibiotic-producing organisms usually do not outgrow contaminants, and strongly contaminated antibiotic fermentations produce little antibiotic, or the antibiotic is destroyed by the contaminants. Fermentations by most other types of microorganisms also usually cannot withstand more than trace amounts of contamination. Contaminating microorganisms use up or change the chemical nature of nutrients. They cause changes in the pH of the medium and bring on foaming problems with attendant poor aeration. Contaminants produce metabolic products that inhibit or slow the growth rate of the fermentative microorganism. They alter the oxidation-reduction potential of the medium, and they may racemize or even destroy the fermentation product.

Fermentation media are sterilized by boiling or passing live steam through the medium, or by subjecting the medium to steam under pressure (autoclaving). Sterilization of large batches of medium by passage through heated retention tubes containing steam jet heaters is described in Chapter 3. Synthetic media require relatively shorter sterilization times. The more crude media, however, often require considerably longer sterilization times, because the greater viscosity of these media impedes heat penetration, and because relatively heat-resistant bacterial spores may be present in some of the crude medium components. In any event, the minimal sterilization time required to obtain sterility, without overcooking the medium, should be determined. Thus, both the amount and duration of heat application are critical factors for some media. Prolonged heating of a medium will carmalize sugars. Also, with excessive heat, sugars in the medium react with phosphates, and this may require that either the sugar or the phosphate be sterilized separately before addition to the sterile medium. Various medium components undergo degradation or chemical change with heat much more rapidly at low or high pH values. For media containing these materials, a shorter sterilization period or sterilization by filtration or other means may be required, although, if the medium components can stand it, conditions of low or high pH can aid in achieving sterility and, in themselves, will help to inhibit the growth of contaminating microorganisms. Low or high pH media containing materials heat sensitive at these pH values can be autoclaved for normal periods of time, however, if the medium is first adjusted to neutral pH and then, after sterilization, is readjusted to the required acidic or alkaline condition by addition of sterile acid or alkali. Certain medium components, such as some of the vitamins and enzymes, cannot be sterilized by heat and are destroyed during normal heat sterilization of media. These materials should be sterilized separately by passage through a bacteriological filter, such as a Seitz filter, before addition to the previously sterilized medium. Volatile medium components also are lost from the medium by heat sterilization, but these compounds may be sterilized by bacteriological filtration if their volatility level is low enough. Thus, we can see that each individual medium must be evaluated to determine its particular requirements for sterilization.

INOCULUM MEDIA

Inoculum media usually differ in composition from production media. Inoculum media are compounded to quickly yield large numbers of microbial cells in their proper physiological and morphological states, but without sacrificing genetic stability of the cells. If the utilization of some component of the production medium requires that the cells be enzymatically adapted to this substrate, then this particular component should also be included in the inoculum medium. This precaution prevents deadaptation, if the cells already are adapted, or eliminates the lag period during the initial stage of production which may occur while adaptation is being accomplished.

We are not interested in the accumulation of a fermentation product other than cells in the inoculum medium and, hence, the inoculum medium is not balanced for product formation. Thus, inoculum media are usually less nutritious overall than are production media, and they usually contain a considerably lower level of the main nutritive carbon source. For some fermentations, the cells are separated from the inoculum medium before being added to the production medium, and this fact should be considered in the design of the inoculum medium for these fermentations. For example, a carbon source in the inoculum medium which becomes exhausted just before harvest of the inoculum can cause certain bacteria to flocculate and settle from the medium; thus, the cells can be drained from the bottom of the tank or the supernatant fluid can be siphoned off. However, when inoculum cells are separated from the medium by sedimentation or centrifugation, any particulate components of the medium also separate with the cells. Thus, if inoculum cells devoid of adhering inoculum medium components are desired, then completely soluble components are of value.

MEDIA ECONOMICS

Costs associated with production media can comprise a considerable portion of the total cost of an industrial fermentation. Industrial fermentation media are characterized by their high contents of carbon-containing and nitrogen-containing substrates, a fact that requires utilization of the cheapest possible usable sources of these materials. Thus, potato and grain starch sources, molasses, corn steep liquor, and defatted meals of soybean, cottonseed, and so forth, have found extensive use as fermentation nutrients. These materials, in a broad sense, are agricultural products or by-products and are subject to the well-known price fluctuations associated with the supply and demand features of the agricultural economy. In addition, the availability and prices of these materials are strongly affected by governmental, policies of price support for agricultural products. Also, international bickering between governments as well as tariff laws can make far too expensive or can even cut off the supply of those substrates, such as cane blackstrap molasses, which normally are largely imported into the United States. Industrial fermentations are usually designed to use a specific microorganism and medium, with only a narrow range of alternatives for carbon and nitrogen supplying substrates. Therefore, an increase in cost or decrease in availability of these specific substrates can render a fermentation no longer economically competitive. Substitution of cheaper or more readily available substrates may make the fermentation again economically competitive, but this may call for the use of a microorganism with slightly different nutritive requirements and synthetic capabilities. The most serious situation exists in those instances in which a microorganism and its fermentation utilize a monosaccharide or disaccharide nutrient (such as blackstrap molasses) and, for lack of amylase activity or for other reasons cannot be switched to utilization of starchy substrates. There are relatively few alternatives should this situation arise. We can employ malt or some other source of amylase activity as a pretreatment step to hydrolyze the starchy component of the medium, but such a treatment adds expense and can markedly change the nutritive balance of the medium. We can test organisms similar to the organism normally employed in the fermentation so as to find an alternate organism which possesses amylase or other enzymic activity, or we can start anew and screen for a different organism to carry out the fermentation. Finally, we can attempt to mutate the organism normally used in the fermentation with the hope that the derived mutant will retain all of its growth and synthetic abilities but, in addition, acquire amylase or other enzymic activity. Obviously, these alternatives are expensive, and the chances for success are not great.

Certain fermentations require a specific carbon source in the presence of other nonspecific carbon sources in order to allow microbial accumulation of economically feasible levels of product. An example of a fermentation of this type is that producing $\alpha,\in$-diaminopimelic acid and utilizing a mutant of *Escherichia coli* with glycerol as the prime carbon source. The economics of this fermentation depend strongly on the price and availability of glycerol. However, the use of the relatively high-cost glycerol has been circumvented by further mutation of the primary *Escherichia coli* mutant so that it still produces high yields of α,ε-diaminopimelic acid, but now utilizes beet molasses plus lactose instead of glycerol.

Sulfite waste liquor as a carbon nutritive constituent of media is unusual in that it is a waste product which, in many instances, by legislation cannot be disposed of in streams. Its disposal, therefore, provides additional costs for the paper-pulp manufactures, and they are glad to find some commercial use for it. Thus, the prime carbon source for an industrial fermentation such as growth of Torula yeast (Chapter 23) provides little additional expense to the fermentation so long as the sulfite waste liquor is not shipped any distance from the site of the paper-pulping plant. However, expense is incurred to remove the sulfite or sulfurous acid from this substrate.

Hydrocarbon carbon substrates (such as kerosene or furnace oil) are inexpensive, and the supply of these materials does not fluctuate to any extent. Such substrates should find much greater use in industrial fermentations when their potential has received more study, and when the physical problems of handling these substrates have been solved. Many of the more pure hydrocarbons or hydrocarbon fractions are too costly for general fermentation use, but there are indications that new refining and fractionation techniques of the petroleum industry will allow drastically reduced prices for these materials.

An inexpensive potential source of nutrients in the form of spent fermentation broth and spent microbial cells (particularly streptomycete and fungal hyphae) presents the possibility for better economic situations for the fermentation industry. At present, these materials are usually drained into the sewer, but with proper study and with little additional expense could yield growth factors and, in some cases, carbon and nitrogen medium components. It is probable, however, that the mycelium of these organisms will require some form of hydrolysis or lysis before use as a medium component.

Nitrogen-containing components of fermentation media provide an expense element for the fermentation, but they usually do not produce the economic problems associated with carbon nutrients. Principally, this is because there is greater flexibility in most fermentations for substituting one nitrogen source for another if demanded by the prevailing economic conditions or supply factors. However, a protein nitrogen source cannot be substituted for other nonprotein forms of nitrogen if the microorganism lacks proteolytic activity.

As previously mentioned, sterilization of media for some fermentations is not economically feasible. Media for these fermentations employ low pH, poorly available substrate, lactic acid, and other inhibitors, or some other means for inhibiting or delaying growth of contaminating microorganisms. In contrast, certain fermentations utilize sterilized media which, because of their inherent capacity for foam production, are excessively prone to contamination. The cost picture for a fermentation is indeed poor if even a small percentage of the fermentation tanks must be sewered routinely because of contamination attributed to excessive foam, or if large amounts of antifoam added to the fermentation later interfere with product recovery.

The expense associated with the recovery of fermentation products or microbial cells from spent fermentation medium is directly related to the physical and chemical characteristics of the medium. For example, a medium from which a fermentation product is to be recovered by distillation should not contain medium components distilling at a temperature range similar to that of the fermentation product. Thus, also, excessively high salt levels in a medium interfere with product recovery by ion exchange resins, and the presence of high levels of ions that form relatively insoluble salts makes difficult the recovery of a product by precipitation or crystallization. From an overall standpoint, each step in recovery and purification usually involves a small to large loss of the fermentation product. A complicated recovery and purification procedure dictated by the chemical and physical nature of the fermentation medium thus can add up to considerable losses of fermentation product. The obvious answer is to simplify or change the fermentation medium so that recovery becomes simpler and with less loss of product. However, this is not as simple as it sounds since fermentation yields are closely tied to the medium being used, and since a change in the medium may well cause decreased fermentation yields. Thus, we must balance the total yields that can be obtained from various media against the losses that will occur during product recovery because of the characteristics of these media. In other words, a relatively lower yielding medium may well be economically more acceptable, if the final recovered yields of product are greater than for a higher yielding medium with poor product recovery characteristics.

SCREENING FOR FERMENTATION MEDIA

All of the previous points in relation to fermentation media must be considered when we attempt to compound a high-yielding medium for an existing or a new fermentation. Various media of differing types are tested, along with variations on these media known to provide growth of the particular microorganism under study and elaboration of its fermentation product. The cell and product yields are determined for each medium, as are the rate of product formation and the fluctuations in pH values during the fermentation. High-yielding media are then studied individually to determine what effects varying the levels of individual components will have on these fermentation parameters. These studies should yield one or two good media. However, alternate carbon and nitrogen sources also should be tested ıor these media as a hedge against changes in the availability and economic pictures for these substrates. The media selected are then studied from several further points of view. The initial pH value and the buffer capacity of the medium are varied so as to determine the effects of pH on cell and product yields and on the rate of product formation. Residual medium components are quantitatively assayed during the fermentation to determine whether critical carbon or nitrogen nutrients become exhausted too quickly or are present in great excess. This information can indicate either that higher levels of these components should be added at medium make-up or during the fermentation, or that certain components should be decreased in concentration. This information also can reveal whether, during the fermentation, a diauxie phenomenon is occurring in which one carbon source of the medium becomes exhausted before a second carbon source requiring enzymatic adaptation is utilized.

If a fermentation product has a chemical structure that is known to the investigator, it may be possible by study of this structure to predict the possibility for adding a portion of the molecule to the fermentation medium to serve as a precursor. Often, however, determination of the chemical structure of a fermentation product postdates the development of the fermentation. Also, the vast majority of fermentation products are not amenable to employment of precursors.

Most of the above studies are carried out without the addition of antifoam, or, if antifoam is required, it is supplied as the inert silicone type. Further studies utilize crude antifoams to determine a possible interference with or stimulation of product formation by the antifoam agent. The fermentation is next carried out in small fermentors to detect interaction of the medium and microorganism with aeration and agitation conditions. Also, other parameters of the fermentation as described previously, are rechecked for changes that may occur under conditions of tank fermentation. Completed fermentation broths containing high yields of fermentation product are examined for quantitative recovery and purification of the product. If recovery yields are low and with little promise for increase, alternative media for the fermentation must be tested. Finally, cost determinations are made for the economic status of the fermentation based on the expense of medium components, duration of the fermentation, recovery yields, and overhead. If these determinations present an adverse economic picture, the fermentation will need reevaluation, particularly from the standpoints of the choice of medium and microorganism.

References

Anonymous, 1958. Need some sugar? *Chem. Eng. News,* July 14, 40–41.

Binkley, W. W. and M. L. Wolfrom, 1953. Composition of cane juice and cane final molasses. *Scientific Report Series,* **15**, Sugar Res. Foundation Inc., New York.

Bowden,. J. P. and W. H. Peterson, 1946. The role of cornsteep liquor in the production of penicillin. *Arch. Biochem.,* **9,** 387–399.

Hajny, G. J., 1959. Review of developments in microbiological utilization of wood sugars. *Forest Prod. J.,* **9,** 153–157.

Lee, S. B., 1950. Fermentation. *Ind. Eng. Chem.,* **42,** 1672–1690.

Lee, S. B., 1951. Fermentation. *Ind. Eng. Chem.,* **43,** 1948–1969.

Underkofler, L. A. and R. J. Hickey 1954. *Industrial Fermentations,* Vol. 1, pp. 1–13. Chemical Publishing Co., Inc., New York.

CHAPTER 8

Inoculum Preparation

Inoculum production is a critical stage in an industrial fermentation process. Obviously, if a fermentation in a 30,000 gallon tank should receive only one loopful of inoculum, a prolonged period would be required before visible growth would be evident and a much longer period before product formation could be detected. Thus, inoculum is prepared as a stepwise sequence employing increasing volumes of media. All steps, except that of the initial inoculation from a stock culture, require the transfer of approximately 0.5 to 5 percent inoculum by volume from the preceding step in the sequence. At each step, the organisms should grow quickly and in high numbers so that the period of incubation required is relatively short. Little if any fermentation product should accumulate during the inoculum stages, because the cells should be transferred to larger batches of media while still in their logarithmic growth phases and before accumulation of product would normally occur. In fact, inoculum media usually are balanced for rapid cell growth and not for product formation.

The inoculum level introduced into a production tank also usually is in the 0.5 to 5 percent range, but at times it may be as high as 20 percent or greater. These high inoculum levels are employed under conditions in which the presence of growth inhibitors or of poor energy recovery to the cells as in the bisulfite-yeast-glycerol fermentation (Chapter 19), do not allow extensive growth of the microorganism in the fermentation production medium. A similar condition exists when pregrown inoculum is utilized for enzymatic conversions. The latter is exemplified by the use of *Aerobacter* aerogenes cells to provide α,ε-diaminopimelic acid decarboxylase enzyme for decarboxylating α,ε-diaminopimelic acid to L-lysine (Chapter 20). These various high-level inoculum additions to fermentations may require that the inoculum cells be sedimented, centrifuged, or in some other manner separated from the inoculum growth medium so that the addition of a high level of cells does not concurrently cause excessive dilution of the production medium, unwanted pH changes, or carry-over of unwanted nutrients or metabolic waste products.

The quality and reproducibility of the inoculum are critical factors in reproducing high yields from one production run to another and in obtaining valid experimental results in smaller tanks used in research studies. For these studies, enough inoculum should be available in a single batch that it can be split uniformly so as to allow each tank to receive similar inoculum. Thus, experimental results from variables being studied in fermentation tanks are somewhat meaningless if the tanks receive differing amounts of inoculum or inoculum of a differing quality.

It is evident that many generations of microbial cells must occur during inoculum production between the starting point of a stock culture and the termination point of a suitable inoculum for a large production tank. We assume that, during this cellular multiplication, the microorganism does not change physiologically or genetically. However, mutations do occur among these cells, although the occurrence of a particular mutation usually is infrequent and, when it does occur, it usually is lethal to the cell or provides no selective advantage to the cell in its growth competition with nonmutated cells. Thus, the occurrence of a mutation is not serious in inoculum build-up unless it provides the microorganism with a distinct growth advantage and, at the same time, with an altered ability to produce the fermentation product. A serious problem can exist, however, if the organism used for the fermentation is in itself a mutant strain. Mutations are not always stable, and the frequency of occurrence of "back mutation," or loss of a particular mutation, can be rather high; thus, inoculum for production tanks can contain a considerable portion of back mutants. Obviously, fermentation and media conditions tending to select for growth of the mutant fermentation strain or against growth of the back mutant are of definite benefit in inoculum production for this type of organism. For example, an *Escherichia coli* mutant strain requiring L-lysine for growth should not be allowed to exhaust the supply of this amino acid in the medium during inoculum production (Chapter 20). Should this occur, the mutant could not complete in growth with the nonlysine-requiring back mutant, and this back mutant would become dominant in the inoculum. Obviously, stock-culture maintenance of mutated fermentation strains should be rigorously controlled so that the least possible numbers of back mutants will find their way into inoculum production.

Enzymatic adaptation in microorganisms resembles a mutational change, but it is not an inherited characteristic. A microorganism does not continuously produce high levels of enzymes to attack all of the possible substrates for which it has the inherent capability. It produces in quantity only those enzymes that it really needs. Some of these enzymes may be "adaptive enzymes" produced only in response to the presence of a substrate that the organism wishes to utilize for energy and growth. If such a substrate is deleted from the medium or becomes exhausted, the microorganism in succeeding generations decreases its output of the respective adaptive enzyme. Industrial fermentations often utilize the activities of the adaptive enzymes of microorganisms and, hence, these enzymes should be present in the highest possible quantities during production. Therefore, provision should be made that the "inducing" substrate be present either in all the steps of inoculum build-up or, at least, in the final stages. If this consideration is not met, a distinct lag in growth may be observed in the production tank immediately after inoculation while the microorganisms are adaptively forming enzymes to allow utilization of the inducing substrate.

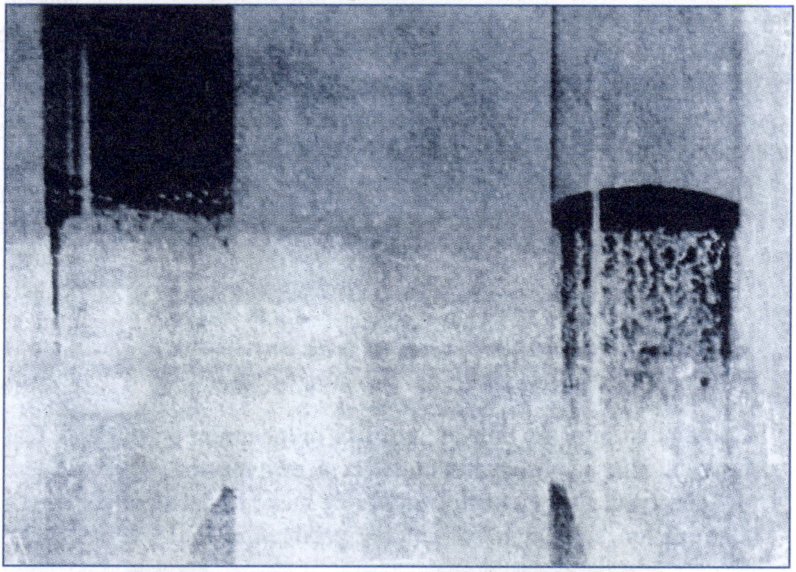

Figure 8.1 Effect of adding a wetting agent to suspensions of hydrophobic fungal spores. The tube on the left did not receive wetting agent, and the spores all are either floating or have crept up the inner wall of the tube. The tube on the right received a small amount of sodium lauryl sulfonate, and the spores are either suspended in the liquid or will easily become suspended with slight shaking of the tube.

The transfer of microbial growth from stock cultures to liquid media, and the initiation of growth in the liquid media at times present special problems as regards the initiation of inoculum build-up. Vegetative cells and spores of bacteria are suspended in a sterile diluent, such as tap water, for addition to the broth medium but, in addition, the bacterial spores and, particularly, those from the genus *Clostridium*, often require a heat treatment, or "heat shocking," to allow germination of a high percentage of the spores. For example, the highly heat-resistant spores of *Clostridium acetobutylicum* for the acetone-butanol fermentation (Chapter 18) are placed in boiling water for approximately 90 seconds before delivery to the bottom of freshly steamed liquid medium. On the other hand, spores of actinomycetes and fungi are not particularly heat resistant and will not withstand heat shocking. Thus, it may be necessary to "pregerminate" spores of these organisms in a special medium if there is some question as to whether the spores will germinate in the normal inoculum medium. Usually, however, pregermination is not required. Spore suspensions of actinomycetes or fungi are prepared by adding a suitable diluent, such as sterile tap water, to sporulated agar growth, followed by scraping loose of the spores with a sterile loop so that the spores become suspended in the diluent. With certain organisms, however, the spores do not become wetted by water and tend to remain as a film on the surface of the hyphae, or they float on the liquid surface and creep up the inner wall of the growth vessel without suspending in the diluents (Figure 8.1). This condition is corrected by adding a small amount of a nontoxic wetting agent, such as sodium lauryl sulfonate to the dilution fluid. In contrast, certain stationary

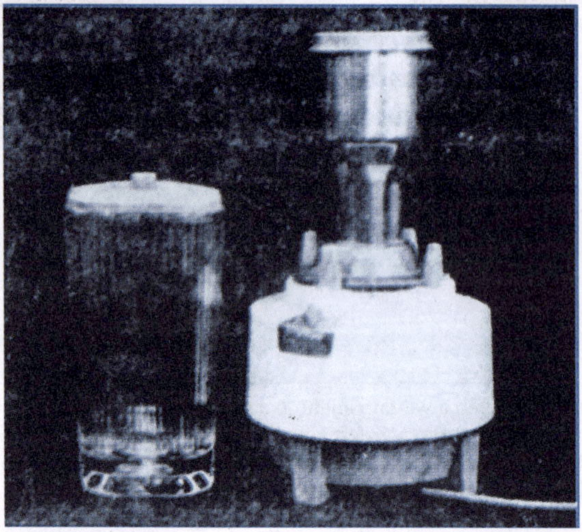

Figure 8.2 Waring blender with heads for macerating small or large quantities of mycelium.

fungal fermentations, such as the *Aspergillus niger* citric acid fermentation (Chapter 26), require that the fungal spores be floated on the surface of the liquid medium so that germination and growth of the spores will yield a floating mycelial mat. This is accomplished by carefully draining the spore suspension down the wall of the culture vessel so that the spores float out across the surface of the liquid medium, or by spraying the spore suspension across the surface of the medium with a atomizer. Non-sporulating or poorly sporulating actinomycetes or fungi are handled in a different manner so that fragmented hyphae are transferred to the broth inoculum medium. The hyphae are broken up by vigorously scraping the agar surface with a loop to provide an aqueous hyphae suspension, or the hypha can be torn apart in a Waring blender (Figure 8.2) or similar macerating device.

Contamination is an ever-present risk in inoculum production. Contamination may be present but undetected, or it may be so gross as to be easily observed. Every attempt should be made to detect either level of contamination so that inoculum for production tanks is completely devoid of contamination. With fermentations employing the hyphae of actinomycetes and fungi, high-level bacterial contamination is sometimes easily observed as general turbidity and even foaming. Usually, however, contamination is detected by resorting to microscopic observation of wet mounts or stained preparations and by culturing samples of the inoculum on a medium that allows growth of suspected contaminating microorganisms. Inoculum for anaerobic fermentations should be tested for contamination by culturing under both anaerobic and aerobic incubation conditions so as to detect the presence of facultative anaerobes. For some fermentations, such as the *Clostridium acetobutylicum* acetone-butanol fermentation (Chapter 18), there are characteristic fermentation patterns which provide a clue to the presence of contamination. During growth of this organism, there is an initial production of acetic and butyric acids accompanied by adaptive enzyme formation for the conversion of these acids to acetone and butanol. Concurrent with the production of the latter solvents, the levels of acetic and butyric acids decrease markedly—the "acid-break"; this phenomenon can be observed by titrating successive samples of inoculum or production culture with dilute alkali. Inoculum of this organism should be used only after a decisive acid-break has occurred, since contaminating microorganisms prevent the detection of a sharp acid-break.

CHAPTER 9

Scale-Up of Fermentations

The experimental fermentation conditions, as determined in flasks or small fermentors in the laboratory, are employed on a more grand scale for the operation of the large production fermentors. However, small to great differences occur between the designs and efficiencies of small-and large-scale fermentation equipment, and these differences often are enough to require at least small changes in a fermentation process before it can be employed successfully on a large-scale production basis. Thus, the determination of the proper incubation conditions to be employed with large-scale production tanks as based on information obtained with various-sized smaller tanks is known as "scale-up." It would seem that the best way to obtain fermentation information for production tanks would be to carry out fermentation studies directly in the large tanks. However, this usually is not possible for a new fermentation, and it is not particularly feasible for variation studies on a fermentation already in production. Production tanks are in continuous use for commercial production of fermentation products, and the utilization of a production tank for an experimental determination removes this tank from the normal production capacity of a company. Moreover, valid experiments cannot be carried out with only a single tank; one or more tanks are required as experimental controls. Aside from these considerations, the various costs, including media, associated with the use of these large production tanks are far too great for their extensive utilization for experimental studies. The commonly accepted alternative is to obtain the most possible information during scale-up studies with the hope that this information will be valid at the production level.

Erlenmeyer flasks are the conventional vessels for fermentation studies during secondary screening or laboratory process development. However, these flasks, even when shaken on a reciprocating or rotary mechanical shaker, provide a poor estimate of the fermentation potential for a microorganism and its medium because of the relatively poor aeration characteristics associated with these vessels. Similar flasks with small glass baffles mounted in the bottom (Figure 4.8) provide better aeration but do not provide the favorable aeration conditions obtainable in a fermentation tank. Small laboratory fermentation tanks of 1 to 10 or 12 liter sizes are more ideal for these studies, since their aeration and agitation conditions can be varied, and since the overall fermentation conditions of these tanks more closely resemble those of the larger production tanks. Although these laboratory-scale tanks do provide considerable information, it still is necessary to study a fermentation in larger experimental tanks (25 to 100 gallons or slightly larger) such as are found in a "pilot plant." These tanks allow fermentation studies on a scale that has meaning in relation to production-tank conditions, but without too great an expense for media, labor, power input, and so forth. Also, at times yet larger tanks intermediate in size between the latter tanks and production tanks are employed to gain additional information on a particular fermentation before it is carried out in production fermentors. Various attempts have been made to mathematically predict the fermentation conditions for a large-scale production tank based on information obtained from laboratory or small pilot-plant tanks. In general, this approach has failed, and it must be said that experience with particular fermentation equipment and previous fermentations is the only real guide in translating scale-up information to production tanks.

Experimentation in production tanks is not completely ruled out. All fermentations, new or old, require some production-scale experimentation at the time of fermentation process development and during later production. Various schemes have been proposed for applying experimental variations to one or two production tanks with the remaining production tanks serving equally as experimental controls and for commercial production of the fermentation product. These procedures usually allow the recovery of at least minimal amounts of valuable information, but the success of this approach again depends, to a large extent, on previous experience with the particular fermentation being studied, with other fermentations, and with the fermentation equipment itself.

Chapter 10

Increasing Product Yields

In order to obtain or maintain a competitive economic position for new or existing fermentations, respectively, it often is necessary to find a means for increasing the yields of the fermentation product, regardless of whether the fermentation product is a chemical compound or microbial cells. It is assumed that the various stages of screening, fermentation process development, and scale-up will have provided the proper organism, medium, aeration, agitation, antifoam, precursor if required, pH control, and so forth, associated with the accumulation of high yields of the fermentation product. Nevertheless, further increases in yields during production sometimes will accrue by additional adjustments in aeration and agitation rates, by small to large changes in the relative concentrations of certain media components, by slight to moderate changes in the control of the pH picture of the fermentation, by adjustment of the inoculum level and the type or quality of inoculum used, by examination of the precise harvest time to be sure that it is occurring at the point of highest possible yields, and by adjustment of the fermentation conditions during inoculum build-up and production for the greatest possible genetic stability of the microorganisms. The latter consideration often is difficult because of a lack of knowledge of the factors actually controlling the genetic stability of the organism, and we may have to rely on trial and error combined with close observation of the fermentation. As mentioned previously, an improvement in fermentation-product recovery can be as important to the overall economics of the fermentation as is increasing the fermentation yields. Thus, revision of the technique of product recovery so that fewer steps are involved and so that less product is lost at each step is of distinct benefit to total recovered-product yields.

The above considerations may well not provide the needed increase in overall recovered product yield for a fermentation. This situation calls for an attempt to alter the genetic make-up of the microbial cells so that more carbon and, possibly, other metabolites are shunted through the metabolic sequences leading to fermentation-product formation. The genetic make-up of the cell can be altered by mutation, sexual recombination, transduction, transformation, phage conversion, and so forth. Of these, the mutation approach, to date, has found most extensive use for industrial organisms. In fact, a continuous program of mutation and selection often is required during process development and even during the commercial life span of the fermentation so as to maintain its economic position.

Before initiating a mutation and selection program, we first should settle on a high-yielding microbial strain and on the best possible production medium on which to superimpose the hoped—for increased yield capacity of a mutant. We also should be sure that we are working with the best possible representatives of the normal population of the microorganism. Thus, by analogy, among a population of humans, there are only a very few individuals capable of running a 4-minute mile. If we were to attempt to mutate humans to obtain an individual that could run a 3-minute mile, we ought first to start with the genetic material of those running the 4-minute mile. In a microbial mutation and selection program we should, therefore, be sure that the selection part of the mutation program is actually selecting newly derived mutants and not merely selecting those members of the normal population which naturally possess a higher yield capacity or are naturally occurring mutants. This means that the normal microbial population should be initially broken down into individual cells (or colonies derived from these cells) with testing of each for fermentative ability so as to select the naturally higher-yielding variants.

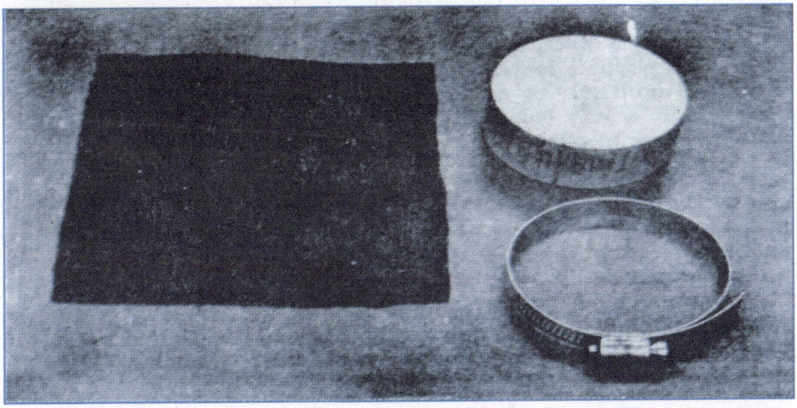

Figure 10.1 Velveteen pad and an example of a mounting frame for use in replica plating (see Figure 10.2).

Mutation and selection programs employ ionizing radiation ultraviolet light, alkylating agents, nitrous acid, purine and pyrimidine analogues, or other mutagenic agents to adjust or change the hereditary material of the cell. The ultraviolet light (2537 Å) and ionizing radiation (but not necessarily other mutagenic agents) are employed at lethal levels and are adjusted so that approximately 90 to 99 percent of the population is killed. This kill is caused in part, by the lethal action of these mutagenic agents and, in part, by the occurrence of lethal mutations to the cells; that is, mutations that prevent formation of critical components of the cell's metabolic machinery. The survivors are not necessarily all mutants, and only a very small percentage, if any, of the mutants will have taken on any real value for the fermentation. Thus, it is necessary to select from among the survivors only those few cells that may have acquired the particular high-yielding mutation of interest. This selection is the most difficult part of a mutation program because of the problem encountered in detecting that cell which has acquired an interesting mutation from among the many other cells exposed to the mutagenic agent. The problem is less acute if the mutation program has been designed merely to select an auxotroph from among a "wild-type" or normal parent population without particular regard to the yield capacities of the auxotrophs. An auxotroph is a microbial cell that, through mutation, has lost the ability to synthesize enough of some metabolite to meet its own requirements for growth. Thus, an auxotroph has gained a growth requirement for some

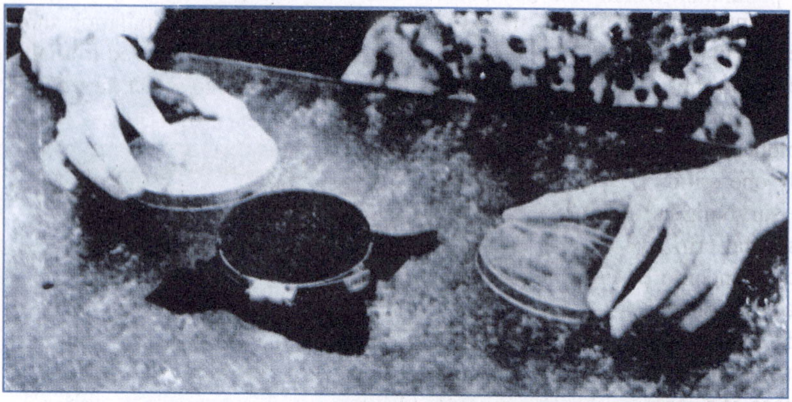

Figure 10.2 The imprinting of colonies during replica plating. The colonies on the agar surface have just been printed onto the velveteen pad. Fresh test plates of agar medium next are pressed lightly against the velveteen to allow an exact replication of the positions of the colonies on the latter plates.

metabolite, and this metabolite, therefore, must be supplied as a medium component. These auxotrophs are of interest, because various intermediate compounds associated with the pertinent biosynthetic route tend to accumulate behind the metabolic block in these organisms. An example of this condition is provided by a mutant of *Escherichia coli* which, through mutation, has lost the ability to enzymatically decarboxylate its own α,ε-diaminopimelic acid to L-lysine so that L-lysine, at least in minimal amounts, must he supplied in the medium (see Chapter 20). Because of this inability, the *Escherichia coli* mutant accumulates α,ε-diaminopimelic acid behind the metabolic block and elaborates considerable quantities into the growth medium.

It is evident that, in most instances, an auxotroph will not grow unless its particular metabolite requirement is provided. This consideration allows the use of the "penicillin technique" (Davis, 1948; and Lederberg and Zinder, 1948) for selecting particular auxotrophs, because penicillin, by interfering with cell-wall synthesis, kills only those cells that can grow and divide in a particular medium; the auxotroph, which does not grow in a medium lacking in its required nutrient, is unaffected by the penicillin. A suspension of microbial cells subjected to a predetermined dosage of a mutagenic agent is inoculated into a complete broth medium to allow growth and expression of mutation for all of the surviving cells. The cells then are washed, starved in a nitrogen-free medium (Hayes, 1964), and placed in a broth medium containing penicillin but lacking one to several critical nutrients, such as particular amino acids; the choice and number of the deleted nutrients depends on the numbers of types of auxotrophs which are desired. On incubation of the cells in this medium the wild-type cells, being able to grow, are killed, and the auxotrophs remain. A variation of the penicillin treatment step includes 20 percent sucrose in the broth medium so as to prevent the bursting of the protoplasts which are induced by penicillin (Gorini and Kaufman, 1960). If only one critical nutrient was deleted from the penicillin broth, then all of the surviving cells should have the same growth requirement. In contrast, if several critical nutrients were deleted (for example, a synthetic medium without incorporating amino acids), then the surviving cells will be a mixture of auxotrophs. In this instance, the technique of "replica plating" (Lederberg and Lederberg, 1952) can be used to determine the actual growth requirements of the individual auxotrophs. The auxotrophs are allowed to grow on the surface of a complete agar medium, and then all of the resulting colonies are replica plated onto the surface of various other agar media, each of which includes only one of the possible critical nutrients; using a sterile velveteen pad (Figure 10.1), the imprint of the original plate is transferred or inoculated onto the agar surfaces of all of the test plates (Figure 10.2), and the plates are incubated. Comparison of the replica plates with the original (Figure 10.3) shows which colonies on replication did not grow and, hence, require the nutrient deleted from the particular test plate. The corresponding original colonies are then transferred and tested to be sure that they truly possess the desired metabolic block and that they are capable of accumulating some fermentation product in good yield behind this block.

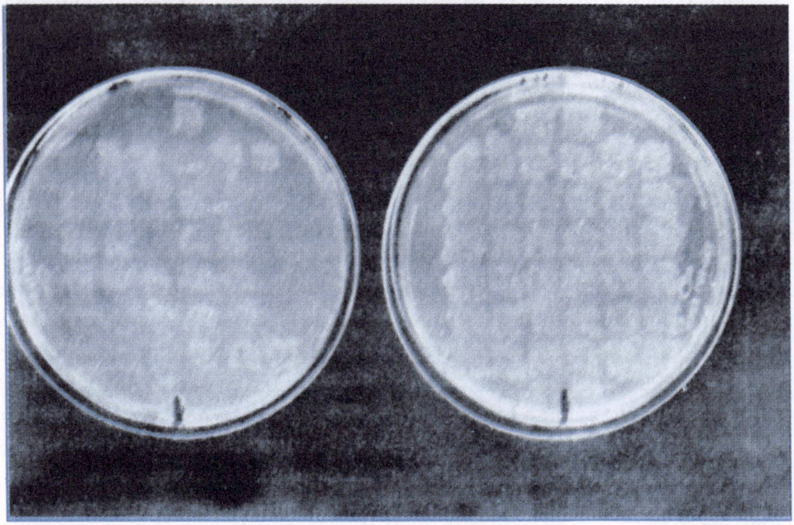

Figure 10.3 Replicated and original plates after growth. In this instance, the replica-plating technique was employed in a manner slightly different from that described in the text. The original plate at the left was inoculated as small squares with various unknown auxotrophs from a mixture resulting from the treatment of a wild-type culture with a mutagenic agent and penicillin. The auxotrophs for this particular test plate are revealed by comparing the positions of the squares without growth on the replicated plate with the corresponding positions on the original plate. Preparations courtesy of S. A. Williams.

Mutation and selection to obtain higher-yielding strains of a previously derived auxotroph or of a wild-type cell that is not an auxotroph are much more difficult, because the penicillin technique cannot be used to eliminate the lower-yielding cells; the presence or absence of the desired mutation is no longer an all-or-none phenomenon. Thus, unless an auxiliary metabolic block of value to the fermentation, that one knows about and can detect, can be introduced into the cells, all cells will grow in the presence of penicillin and be killed. In essence, then, unless a specific screening type of bioassay can be devised, all of the cells or, at least, many of the cells that have survived the mutagenic agent must be tested, preferably first on agar then in liquid medium, for their yield potential as well as for their rate of product formation. Another problem enters at this point. Media that were balanced for yields of fermentation product with the parent mutant or wild-type strain may not be properly balanced for the hoped-for higher-yielding capacity of a new mutant. Also, other fermentation conditions may no longer be the same. Thus, a richer medium or, possibly, several media may have to be tested to detect and evaluate the high-yielding mutant.

A newly derived mutant need not necessarily be a higher-yielding strain if, in the process of mutation, the genetic stability of the parent mutant or wild-type strain has been increased. However, selection of organisms surviving mutagenic agents for those possessing increased genetic stability is rather difficult and requires extensive further testing.

References

Davis, B. D., 1948. Isolation of biochemically deficient mutants of bacteria by penicillin. *J. Am. Chem. Soc.,* **70,** 4267.

Gorini, L. and H. Kaufman, 1960. Selecting bacterial mutants by the penicillin method. *Science,* **131,** 604–605.

Hayes, W., 1964. *The genetics of bacteria and their viruses.* John Wiley and Sons, Inc., New York.

Lederberg, J., and E. M. Lederberg, 1952. Replica plating and indirect selection of bacterial mutants. *J. Bacteriol.,* **63,** 399–406.

Lederberg, J., and N. Zindare.1948. Concentration of biochemical mutants of bacteria with penicillin. *J. Am. Chem. Soc.,* **70,** 4267–4268.

CHAPTER 11
Phage

Phages are viruses that attack bacteria and actinomycetes but not fungi or yeasts, at least so far as is known. They are not by themselves capable of multiplication but require a susceptible host. Phages are of great importance in industrial microbiology, because their ability to be carried by dust in the air allows them to infect microorganisms employed in industrial fermentations. Since a phage attack is an ever present possibility, it is essential that the industrial microbiologist know something about phages and the means for combating phage infections.

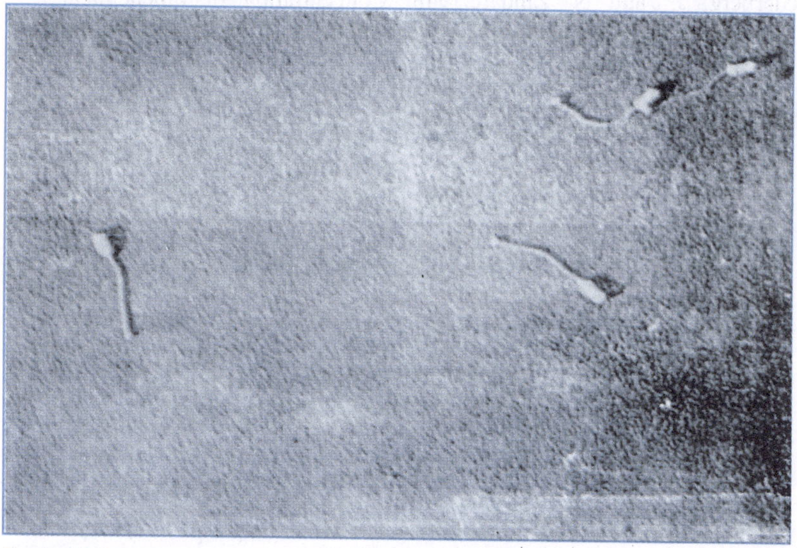

Figure 11.1 Staphylococcus phage at 40,000 magnification. (Seto, Kaesberg, and Wilson. 1956. J. Bacteriol, 72. 847–850.)

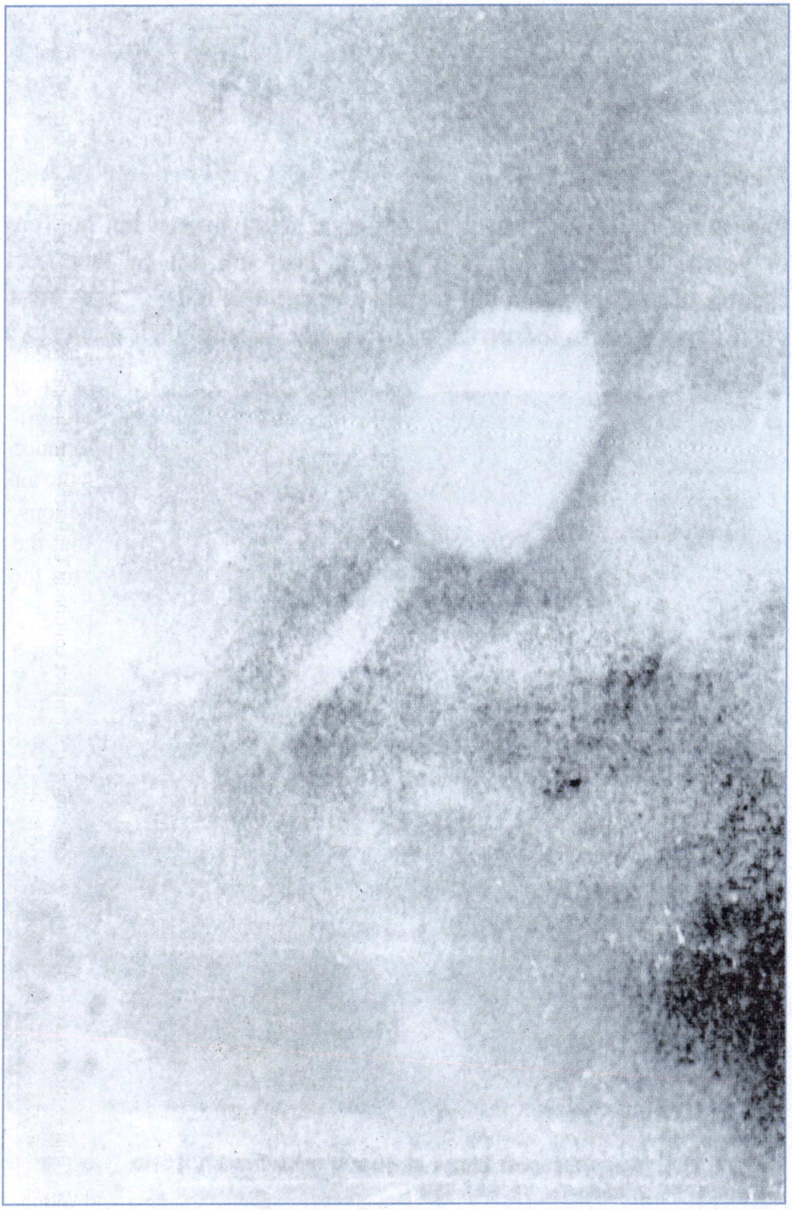

Figure 11.2 Coliphage T_2 negatively stained with phosphotungstic acid and magnified 310,000 fold. Courtesy of E. H. Cota-Robles.

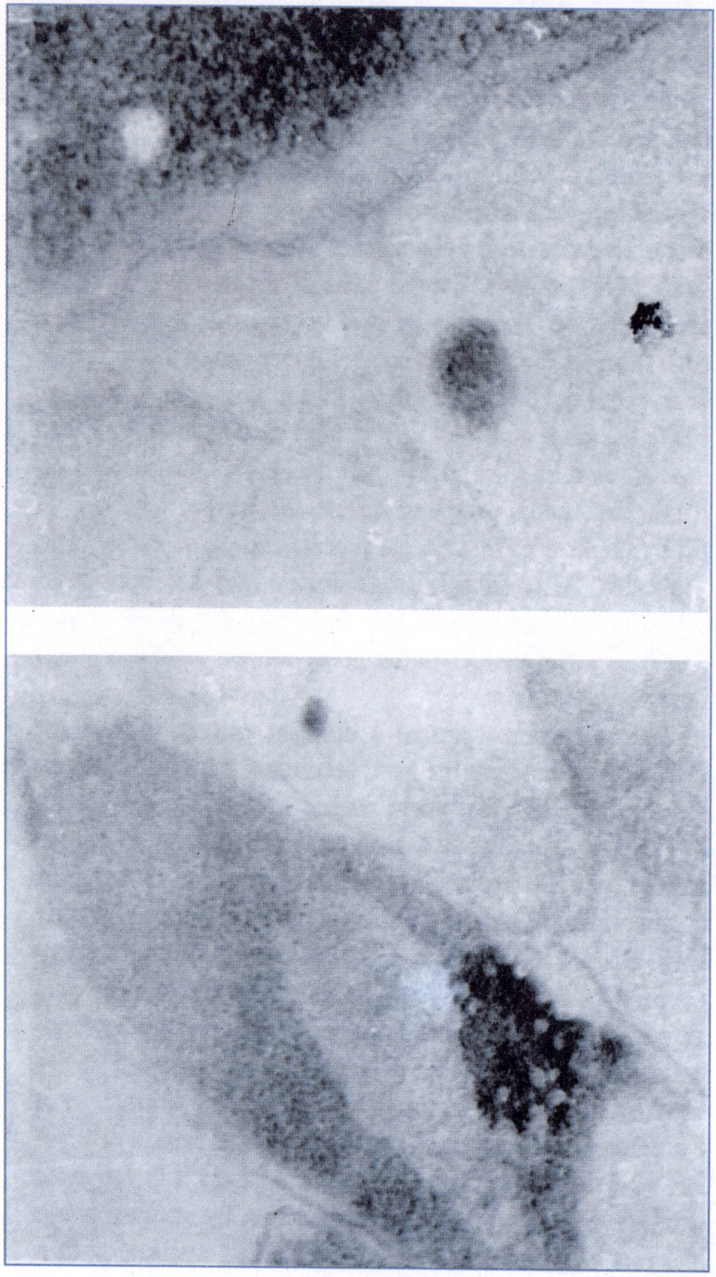

Figure 11.3 Thin section of an Escherichia coli cell showing an intact coliphage T_2 attached to the cell wall. (Cota-Robles and Coffman, 1963. J. Bacteriol., 86, 266–273.) × 52,000 (Left) and 164,000 (Right).

Phages contain a head to which a tail mayor may not be attached depending on the particular phage (Figures 11.1 and 11.2). The overall length of a phage (including the tail) is in the general range of 50 to 200 millimicrons, and the head averages 50 to 90 mμ in width. Thus, the size of these viruses is small enough to allow their passage through a bacteriological filter, such as a fritted glass, Seitz, or membrane filter, which provides pore sizes with a diameter of approximately 0.2 to 0.45 microns. Such filters do not allow the passage of bacteria and actinomycetes and, therefore, they can be used to separate a phage in a culture broth from its host. Phages contain either deoxyribonucleic or ribonucleic acid, but not both, surrounded by a protein coat. The phage first adsorbs to the surface of a sensitive host microorganism, and then injects its nucleic acid into the host (Figure 11.3). This nucleic acid, on entry into the host, takes over and directs the further synthesis of nucleic acid by the host so that, in the process, the phage nucleic acid becomes replicated. After enough phage nucleic acid has been replicated, it is surrounded by a protein coat, also synthesized by the host, and the host lyses so as to liberate the newly-formed complete phage into the surrounding medium.

Lysogenic microorganisms present a different picture in that the phage nucleic acid, on entering the host, becomes a part of the genetic make-up of the host, but the phage nucleic acid is not extensively replicated. The host continues to grow and function in a normal manner without lysing. However, in a normal population of lysogenic bacteria or actinomycetes, a minute portion of the population apparently is less stable in relation to the phage, and phage production with attendant lysis occurs for these cells. Thus, in such a population, the only evidence of phage is their presence in a filtrate prepared by bacteriological filtration of the culture. The phages in this culture filtrate are demonstrated by addition of a small amount of the filtrate to a culture of a different host which is not lysogenic and which will lyse on infection with the phage. The presence of a phage in a lysogenic microbial culture does not prevent super-infection by another phage unless the phages are extremely closely related. Thus, application of a phage to a microbial culture to make it lysogenic cannot be used to protect the culture from further phage attack.

Phages are detected and counted by use of the "phage plaque" plating procedure. The phages are separated from their host bacteria or actinomycetes by passage through a bacteriological filter, and dilutions of the filtrate are prepared which include dilutions as high as 10^{-7} to 10^{-10}. These dilutions are required because of the high "titers" of phage which occur at times in microbial cultures. Petri plates are prepared with a base layer, of agar medium containing 1.5 percent agar. Aliquots from the various phage dilutions are mixed with portions of a suspension of a sensitive host microorganism, the

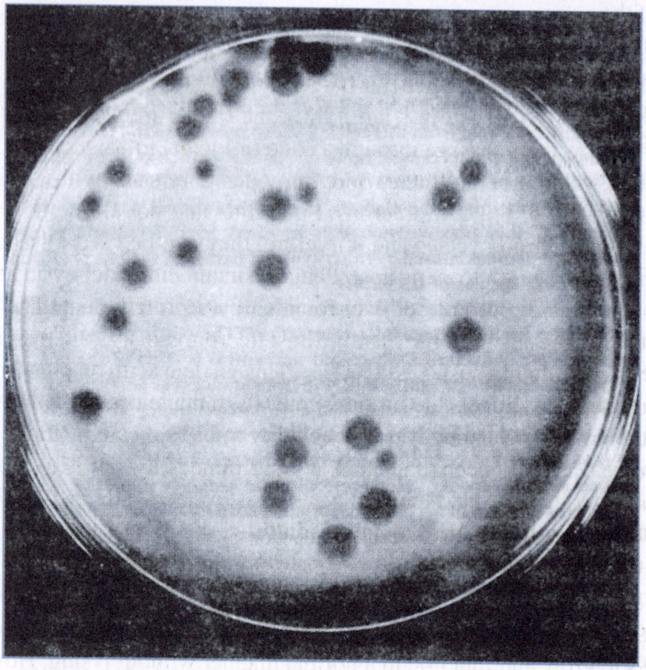

Figure 11.4 Plaques produced by a mixture of three phage strains acting on an indicator bacterial culture. The plaques produced by one of the phage are very small, being just barely visible. Courtesy of C. F. Pootjes.

indicator strain and with growth medium containing 0.6 to 0.8 percent melted agar. This mixture then is added as a thin layer to plates containing hardened basal agar, and the seeded layers are allowed to solidify before incubation. The agar of this seed layer is just concentrated enough to allow solidification, and the surface layer provided is quite soft. At those dilutions of the culture filtrate great enough to provide good separation of the individual phage particles on the plates, phage plaques occur in the growth of the indicator microorganism (Figure 11.4). These plaques are round, from less than a millimeter to 5 or 10 mm in diameter, and appear as cleared areas lacking visible microbial growth. The size of the plaque is a reproducible characteristic for the interaction of a phage and its indicator microbe. The reason for this becomes evident when we consider that phage reproduce in their indicator host only during active growth of the host organism. Therefore, during the active growth of the host, the initially infected host cell plus the cells subsequently infected by the phages released from this cell lall yse to result in plaque formation. This sequence of events ceases, however, as the growth of the host cells slows with age of the culture and, thus, after a suitable incubation period for formation of the plaques, the plaques should not increase in size. In fact, this phenomenon can be used to differentiate phage plaques from plaques caused by other types of parasites such as protozoa or *Bdellovibrio* species of bacteria.

The gross appearance of a phage plaque also is a reproducible characteristic for the phage-host interaction. The edges of the plaque may be sharply defined or diffuse, and the central portion of the plaque may be translucent or slightly milky in appearance.

The host range for a strain of phage is narrow to broad depending on the particular phage. It may attack only a single microbial strain, or it may attack a group of closely related strains within a species, or even two or more species. However, within a sensitive natural population, such as a strain of a host microorganism, there will be found a few individual cells that are resistant to infection by a particular phage. In the event of a phage attack, these organisms survive and multiply so that, given enough time, the microbial culture will recover from a phage attack and will be composed largely of organisms resistant to the phage. Obviously, there is a strong selection for the resistant organisms. A microbial culture resistant to a particular phage because of a previous attack by this phage usually, however, is not resistant to the next different phage that comes along. Assuming that the phage does not induce lysogeny in its host, the culture again will go through the same sequence of lysis of a high percentage of the cells followed by a slow recovery and growth of the few naturally resistant cells.

Just how serious is a phage attack as regards fermentation yields? In answer, the actual amount of damage to a fermentation caused by a phage attack depends on the particular fermentation and on the phase of the fermentation at the time at which the attack occurs. Thus, a phage infection of a fermentation is not a problem if the phage happens to be one that can neither lyse nor establish lysogeny in the fermentation organism. However, if the contaminating phage finds rapidly growing sensitive host microorganisms mediating an industrial fermentation, it will multiply in and lyse these organisms so that, within a relatively short time, a high percentage of the cells will have disappeared. The surviving cells are those few that were naturally resistant to the phage, and these cells will slowly multiply and repopulate the fermentation medium. Obviously, this occurrence markedly extends the incubation period for the fermentation. In contrast, an infection occurring late in the fermentation probably will be hardly noticed, since phage multiplication and cell lysis require young, actively growing cells. Therefore, the most critical time for a phage attack is during logarithmic growth of the sensitive fermentation organism.

An example of a phage attack on a bacterial fermentation occurs with *Clostridium acetobutylicum* as employed in the acetone-butanol fermentation (Chapter 18). Evolution of the fermentation gases, carbon dioxide and hydrogen, ceases as the cells are lysed by the phage, but then slowly recovers as resistant cells begin to grow. If the clostridium has produced the adaptive enzymes for converting acetic and butyric acids to acetone and butanol before the phage attack has become severe, then the fermentation will slowly recover to provide fair yields of solvents. However, a severe phage infection occurring before the adaptive enzymes have been formed will so prolong recovery of the fermentation that further incubation for product formation is not feasible.

Every precaution should be taken to prevent contamination of a fermentation with dust from the air which may be carrying phages. Also, every attempt should be made to prevent contamination of the stock cultures and inoculum. Nevertheless, if it is suspected that a phage attack has occurred, the presence of the phage should be demonstrated by filtration of a sample of the culture broth followed by plating of the culture filtrate for plaque formation with the uninfected host fermentation organism. If this procedure reveals the presence of phage, a sample of the culture filtrate is frozen as a source of the phage for later testing, or the phage is recovered by inoculation from the plaques into an actively growing culture of the host. Also, the fermentation microorganism is reisolated from the fermentation broth after regrowth of resistant cells has occurred, and the isolates thus obtained are purified and tested against the phage to be sure of resistance. The fermentation microorganism can also be mutated, using the phage filtrate to select the phage-resistant mutants, but this procedure is more involved. Regardless of which procedure is utilized, the resulting phage-resistant strains must also be retested for production capacity for the fermentation product. Thus, it is possible that, in the process of obtaining a phage-resistant strain, we may have selected a normally poor-yielding strain from the natural population, or that phage resistance, for some mutants, may be genetically tied to low-yield capacity.

A fermentation microorganism selected as above for resistance to a phage will not be resistant to subsequent attacks by other phages. Should another phage attack occur, we must start over again to obtain resistance to the new phage. By mutation and selection during process development, we cannot incorporate phage resistance into fermentation microorganisms, since there are too many different phage-strain possibilities to be able to make the fermentation culture resistant to all the possible phages that conceivably could attack it during industrial production. Thus, we must be constantly on the watch for a phage attack and be ready to recover a high-yielding, phage-resistant strain of the fermentation organism.

Recent reports indicate that some media possibly may allow increased protection for a fermentation organism against phages. Also, the incorporation of low concentrations of antibiotics into fermentation media has been reported to have this effect. These points definitely are worth further experimental study.

A phage that establishes lysogeny in a fermentation microorganism presents a different type of problem for industrial fermentations. Cell lysis is negligible and, thus, the presence of the phage is not detected unless culture filtrates are plated for plaque formation with a sensitive indicator organism. This procedure usually is not followed, however, because these phages usually are considered to have little influence on an industrial fermentation and are not determined in the routine observations of the progress of an industrial fermentation. This is a faulty assumption. The nucleic acids of the phages carry genetic material that is incorporated into the genetic material of the host microorganism and, as a result, new enzymes may be formed or old enzymes deleted from the normal enzymatic complement of the cell. Obviously, this can have a profound effect on the growth and yield potential of the fermentation organism.

The genetic changes induced by a phage during lysogeny resemble a mutation of the host organism, but as regards an industrial fermentation, they differ in one important aspect. The frequency of a particular mutation in a normal population of microorganisms is very low, and rigorous selection is required for the mutant to gain ascendancy in the population. In fact, in an inoculum or production tank, the selection forces often are not great enough to allow excessive multiplication of the mutant and, hence, little if any effect on growth and yields is observed. A phage that established lysogeny in the fermentation organism in an inoculum or production tank presents a different picture, however. The phage multiplies rapidly in the few sensitive organisms present, liberating further phages so that most of the microbial population becomes lysogenic. The genetic changes attributable to phage in the host organism, therefore, are incorporated rapidly into the entire microbial population, and selection for the genetic variant is not required. Thus, if the genetic change affects growth or yields, it will become apparent relatively quickly.

There is little that can be done about a phage attack that induces lysogeny in a fermentation microorganism. All fermentation equipment should be carefully cleaned and sterilized, but this may have little effect if the phage is still present in high numbers in the air of the plant. Obviously, we should be extremely careful that such a phage does not get into stock cultures. However, from a different viewpoint this type of phage attack on a fermentation could be a boon, for example, when the genetic changes associated with lysogeny cause increased yields instead of the more likely decreased yields. In this case, it would be advantageous to reisolate and purify the fermentation organism from this rare high-yielding tank.

Fermentations utilizing enzymatic reactions to accomplish oxidative transformations of a substrate (Chapter 21) sometimes require that the enzyme or enzymes be liberated from the microbial cells. For example, toluene is used to lyse *Aerobacter aerogenes* cells to obtain α,ε-diaminopimelic acid decarboxylase enzyme (Chapter 20). Lysis by phage also has been proposed at one time or another for liberating such enzymes. However, it is felt that the potential is far too great for the particular phage to get loose in the production plant so that it cannot be controlled.

References

Adams, M. H., 1959. *Bacteriophages.* Interscience, New York.

Luria, S. E. and J. E. Darnell., 1967. *General Virology,* 2nd ed. John Wiley and Sons, Inc., New York.

Stent, G. S. 1963. *Molecular Biology of Bacterial Viruses.* W. H. Freeman and Co., San Francisco.

Chapter 12

Dual or Multiple Fermentations

Dual or multiple fermentations are those fermentations in which more than one microorganism is employed. The organisms may be inoculated simultaneously into the growth medium, or one organism may be grown first in the medium, followed by the inoculation and growth of a second microorganism. Alternatively, after growth has occurred in the original media, two separate fermentations may be combined for further fermentation activity. The basic concept is that two or more microorganisms accomplish something that neither organism can do alone. Admittedly, in the state of present-day fermentation technology, this concept is more of a dream than a reality. The most obvious use of dual or multiple fermentations is to utilize one microorganism to produce a fermentation product that is then converted or changed by a second microorganism or further microorganisms into a different fermentation product possessing greater economic value. Thus, a yeast first produces ethyl alcohol, and then an *Acetobacter* species converts the alcohol to vinegar. Another approach is to use one microorganism to change or prepare the medium so that it becomes suitable for the growth of a second microorganism. For example, the first microorganism may provide amylase or protease activity for the second microorganism, which lacks these abilities. Further uses of dual or multiple fermentations are the use of an organism to remove the toxic metabolic by-products of another organism, an organism to provide growth factors for another organism, an organism to remove oxygen or depress oxidation-reduction potential for an anaerobic organism, or an organism to maintain a pH range critical for a second organism. In addition, one organism may produce a metabolic product, such as lactic acid, which both is beneficial to the growth of a second organism, such as a yeast, and at the same time helps to control contamination.

Simultaneous growth of two fermentation microorganisms in a single medium presents a problem in microbial ecology. Each organism must contend with the physiological, growth and nutrient utilization activities of the other, and it is likely that their growth rates will differ so that one organism will outgrow the other. Thus, extensive studies of media and other fermentation conditions are required to balance the growth of the two or more organisms. This problem becomes either simplified or magnified if some form of symbiosis exists between the organisms, so that they are dependent on each other for growth. A possible fermentation utilizing the symbiosis phenomenon would be the commercial growth of lichens, which are composed of algae plus fungi or actinomycetes. An example of a dual simultaneous fermentation not involving symbiosis might be one in which one microorganism utilizes glucose to produce α-ketoglutaric acid while the second organism, also utilizing glucose for growth, aminates the α-ketoglutaric acid to glutamic acid. An example of a dual simultaneous fermentation which has been worked out and which has industrial potential is that for producing β-carotene, the carotenoid pigment related to vitamin A and used as a coloring matter in foods (see Chapter 24). Two phycomycetes, *Choanephora cucurbitarum and Blakeslea trispora*, individually have the ability to produce this compound in aerated, submerged fermentation. However, the dual fermentation employs one or the other of these organisms, but not both. The fermentation is dual in that two different mating types, plus and minus, of the organism are grown Simultaneously. The two mating types are inoculated into the other so that the resulting yield of β-carotene are 15 to 20 times greater than the yields obtained when either mating type is grown by itself. Obviously, this fermentation is a simplified form of a dual simultaneous fermentation, because the two organisms employed are really the same organism but differing only in mating types.

Dual or multiple fermentations in which one organism is grown in a medium followed by the inoculation and growth of a second organism are easier to control from a fermentation standpoint. This is particularly true if it is feasible to kill the first organism by heat or other form of sterilization before inoculation with the second organism. The basic achievements of this approach are similar, however, to those of simultaneous-inoculation dual fermentations. Examples of this approach are the initial growth of a proteolytic or amylolytic organism in the medium to prepare it for succeeding growth of an organism not possessing these activities, the growth of lactic acid bacteria for succeeding yeasts, and the production of ethanol by a yeast followed by oxidation of the ethanol to acetic acid by an *Acetobacter* species.

The combining of separate fermentations to yield further fermentation activity already has found industrial application. In this fermentation approach, usually one fermentation yields a product that must be enzymatically changed to a second product of greater economic value, and the second fermentation provides the microorganisms containing the pertinent enzymes for carrying out this enzyme-mediated change. For example, such a dual fermentation has been used in production of L-lysine (Chapter 20). An *Escherichia coli* auxotroph in one fermentation produces, α, ∈-diaminopimelic acid; in a second fermentation, *Aerobacter aerogenes* cells are grown which contain diaminopimelic acid decarboxylase. These two fermentations are then combined so that the *Aerobacter aerogenes* diaminopimelic acid decarboxylase can decarboxylate the α, ∈-diaminopimelic acid from the Escherichia coli auxotroph fermentation to provide L-lysine. Toluene also is added at the time of combining the fermentations so that the diaminopimelic acid decarboxylase becomes liberated from the Aerobacter aerogenes cells, and so that the cells of both species will be killed and not carry out further metabolic utilization of medium components or fermentation products.

Dual or multiple fermentations, as described above, present intriguing possibilities for the industrial utilization of microorganisms. However, much study still is needed in this area, particularly in those instances in which microorganisms are to be grown simultaneously in the same medium. Thus, a greater understanding a microbial ecology would contribute greatly to the industrial potential for various of these fermentations.

CHAPTER 13

Continuous Fermentations and Late Nutrient Additions

Continuous fermentations are those in which fresh nutrient medium is added either continuously or intermittently to the fermentation vessel, accompanied by a corresponding continuous or intermittent withdrawal of a portion of the medium for recovery of cells or fermentation products. This is in contrast to a batch fermentation process in which a large volume of nutrient medium is inoculated, and growth and biochemical synthesis are allowed to proceed only until maximum yields have been obtained. At this point, the batch fermentation is stopped for product recovery, the fermentor is cleaned and resterilized, and a new fermentation is started up. At first glance, the continuous fermentation would appear to be the better of the two procedures, because the fermentation equipment is in constant usage with little shutdown time and, theoretically at least, after the initial inoculation, further production of inoculum is not required. However, as we shall see, the inherent problems associated with a continuous fermentation process often do not allow the achievement of this goal.

A continuous fermentation can be conducted in various ways. It can be carried out as a "single stage" in which a single fermentor is inoculated, then kept in continuous operation by balancing the input and output of nutrient solution and harvested culture, respectively. In a "recycle" continuous fermentation, a portion of the withdrawn culture, or of the residual unused substrate plus the withdrawn culture, is recycled to the fermentation vessel. Thus, the immiscible hydrocarbon substrate of a hydrocarbon fermentation can be recycled for further microbial attack. A portion of the organisms being produced during a continuous fermentation also can be recycled in certain instances in which the actual available substrate level in the nutrient solution for microbial growth is quite low. An example of this type of substrate is sulfite waste liquor with its low available carbohydrate content; in this instance, the recycling of cells provides a higher population of cells in the fermentor and, hence, a greater productivity.

A third type of continuous fermentation, the "multiple-stage" continuous fermentation, involves two or more stages with the fermentors being operated in sequence. To accomplish this approach, the fermentation is divided into phases, so that a growth phase occurs in the first-stage fermentor, followed by a synthetic stage in the second or succeeding fermentors. The multiple-stage continuous fermentation is particularly applicable to those fermentations in which the growth and synthetic activities of the cells are not simultaneous; that is, synthesis is not growth-related but occurs after the cell-multiplication rate has slowed (see Table 13.1).

Table 13.1 Representative Chemical Products from Continuous Fermentation

Growth-Associated	Not Growth-Associated
Acetic acid	Acetone
Butanediol	Butanol
Ethanol	Glycogen
Gluconic acid	Subtilin
Hydrogen sulfide	Chloramphenicol
Lactic acid	Penicillin
	Streptomycin
	Vitamin B_{12}

Source. W. D. Maxon., 1960. *Adv. Appl. Microbiol.*, 2, 335–349.

There are several possible means by which microbial activity in continuous culture can be controlled, although only two of these approaches, the "turbidostat" and the "chemostat," have gained general acceptance. It must be pointed out, however, that all of these approaches are easily applied only for the relatively more simple growth-related fermentation processes (Table 13.1), and for the production of microbial cells as fermentation products. In the turbidostat, the total cell population is held constant by employing a device that measures the culture turbidity so as to regulate both the nutrient feed rate to the fermentor and the culture withdrawal rate from the fermentor. If the population numbers rise above a predetermined level, a greater amount of fresh medium is added to the fermentor so as to dilute the cell concentration. Thus, there is no limiting nutrient consciously imposed with this process so that the cell growth rate should always be maximal. However, the growth must be maintained in the logarithmic growth phase or very close to it. This factor is a disadvantage in that the fermentation must be operated at a lower maximum cell population than is possible with a chemostat, and this causes a greater residual of unused nutrient to be lost from the fermentation with the withdrawn harvested culture.

In contrast to the turbidostat, a chemostat maintains the nutrient feed and harvest culture withdrawal rates at constant values, but always less than that which allows a maximum growth rate. The growth rate is controlled by supplying only a limiting amount of a critical growth nutrient in the feed solution. Thus, cell multiplication cannot proceed at a rate greater than that allowed by the availability of this critical nutrient. The controlling factor for growth, however, does not necessarily have to be a limiting nutrient; it can also be a relatively high concentration of a toxic product of the fermentation, the pH value, or even temperature. The chemostat concept of continuous fermentation is employed more often than the turbidostat, because fewer mechanical problems are encountered, and because of the occurrence of less residual unused nutrient in the harvested culture.

With either approach, it is necessary to maintain a constant cell population in the fermentor or fermentors. In this regard, the feed of fresh nutrients to the fermentor is critical as it relates to the generation time of the organism. Too low a flow rate can allow the culture to go into maximum stationary phase growth so that the continuous aspect of the fermentation cannot be maintained. In contrast, too high a flow rate in relation to the generation time can dilute out the cell population in a fermentor by removing the cells in the culture discharge faster than they can be replenished by growth. Obviously, the mathematical considerations of determining nutrient supply rates and culture withdrawal rates are complicated, and the reader is referred to excellent treatments of the appropriate mathematical considerations as published by Aiba, Humphrey, and Millis (1965), Maxon (1960), and Deindoerfer and Humphrey (1959).

Many fermentation processes have been investigated, at least on the pilot plant scale, for their possible conversion to a continuous fermentation process. Table 13.2 presents a list of representative microorganisms investigated for their possible use in continuous fermentations, and Table 13.1 presents representative chemical products investigated for their possible continuous fermentation application. In addition, Table 13.3 presents possible experimental applications of the continuous fermentation approach. From among these potential continuous fermentation processes, only the production of beer, fodder yeast (from sulfite papermill waste), vinegar, and baker's yeast (from molasses) have found commercial application. However, the activated sludge system for the processing of waste waters also may be considered as a commercialized continuous fermentation, differing from the more conventional fermentations only in that it deals with a mixed microbial population acting on a heterogeneous substrate.

Table 13.2 Representative Genera of Organisms Grown in Continuous Culture

Organisms	Genera
Actinomycetes	*Streptomyces*
Algae	*Chorella*
	Euglena
	Scenedesmus
Bacteria	*Aerobacter*
	Azotobacter
	Bacillus
	Brucella
	Clostridium
	Salmonella
Fungi	*Ophiostoma*
	Penicillium
Protozoa	*Tetrahymena*
Yeast	*Saccharomyces*
	Torula
Mammalian Cells	Embryo rabbit kidney

Source. W. D. Maxon., 1960. *Adv. App. Microbiol,* **2,** 335—349.

There have been several reports that the productivity of a continuous fermentation is greater than that for a batch fermentation. Assuming that this is a true statement, then why have so few batch fermentations been successfully converted to a continuous fermentation process? There are several answers. A successful continuous fermentation requires a thorough knowledge of the dynamic aspects of microbial behavior and growth, knowledge that is lacking or deficient for most industrial fermentation processes because of the complexities of the growth and synthetic patterns of the organisms. Also, contamination and mutation present a distinct problem for the development of a successful continuous fermentation process. The prolonged incubation periods associated with continuous fermentations can allow contaminating microorganisms the time that they require for gaining ascendency in the culture, although certain fermentations, such as that for Torula yeast on sulfite waste liquor, provide built-in contamination control, in this instance, the presence of sulfite and a low pH. As regards the contamination problem, suggestions have been made that antibiotics or other chemicals be added to continuous fermentations to hold down the level of contaminant growth. Mutation of the fermentation organism becomes a problem only if the resulting mutant cells have a selective growth advantage during prolonged incubation and, at the same time, produce less of the desired fermentation product. It has been proposed that the answer to the question of mutation is to use multistage continuous fermentations, with the first fermentor of the sequence being periodically reinoculated. Nevertheless, the real overall solution to both contamination and mutation is to reduce their rates of occurrence, so that the offending cells will be flushed from the fermentors before they have a chance to multiply.

Table 13.3 Experimental Applications of Continuous Culture

Independent Variables	Dependent Variables
Time	Metabolic rates
Growth rate	Metabolic patterns
Nutrient concentration	Cell composition
Product concentration	Cell morphology
pH	Enzyme induction
Inhibitors	Mutation rate
Enzyme inducers	Mutant expression time
Mutagenic agents	Virulence
Aeration-agitation	
Temperature	

Source. W.D. Maxon., 1960. *Adv. Appl. Microbiol.*, **2**, 335—349.

Continuous fermentations often waste nutrient substrate. Thus, the fermentation broth as it is continuously withdrawn for product recovery contains a certain amount of the residual unused nutrients of the medium as well as a portion of the fresh nutrient constituents being continuously added to the fermentation. However, in a few instances, it is possible to separate the residual nutrient substrate from the harvested culture so that it can be recycled through the fermentor. A specific instance occurs with certain hydrocarbon fermentations, such as that yielding feed yeast, in which the harvested culture is deemulsified, and the residual hydrocarbon is channeled back to the fermentation.

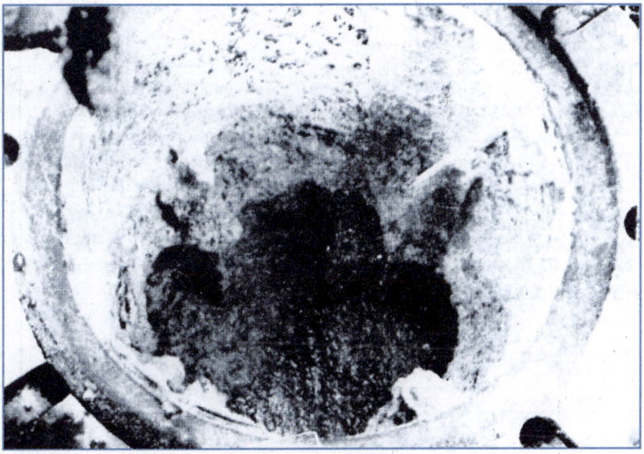

Figure 13.1 Mycelium accumulation on the walls of a fermentor during a continuous penicillin fermentation. (Bartlett and Gerhardt.,1959. *J. Biochem. Microbiol. Technol. and Eng.*, 1, 359–377.)

Certain fermentation media are rather viscous and require that strong mixing activity be employed in the fermentor to equally distribute the incoming fresh medium to all parts of the broth already in the fermentor. Obtaining adequate mixing also is a problem when slow feed rates of fresh nutrient are employed, regardless of the viscosity of the medium. From another standpoint as regards mixing, the mathematical considerations and process regimes for continuous fermentations assume that the microbial cells grow freely in the aqueous medium and do not become attached to the walls of the fermentor. However, the latter phenomenon occurs often with filamentous microorganisms such as streptomycetes and fungi (Figure 13.1) and, in fact, this surface growth can also occur in piping and valves to the point that a shutdown is required. The occurrence of this type of growth means that the cells are immobile and, hence, are not exposed uniformly to the fresh nutrients being fed to the fermentation. In addition, the level of cells or hyphae freely suspended in the aqueous nutrient can be quite erratic, because the growth sloughs from the walls of the fermentor, and because the organisms may sporulate above the liquid line with the spores falling back into the medium to supply an internal inoculum source for the fermentation. Obviously, this condition makes difficult a proper adjustment of the input and output flow rates for the fermentation.

Continuous fermentations become more complex and difficult to accomplish when a chemical product and not a microbial cell is the desired product (see Table 13.1). Thus, the conditions that are optimal for growth of

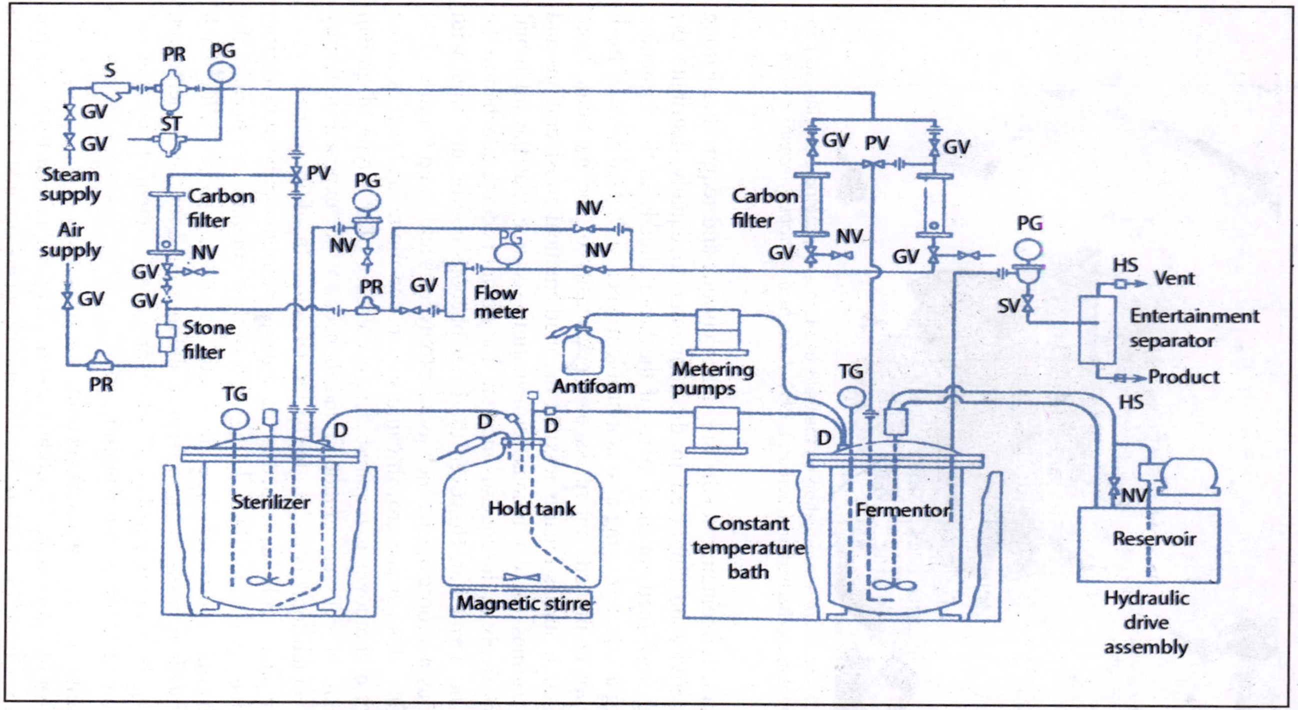

Figure 13.2 Schematic diagram of a pilot plant for single-stage continuous-fermentation antibiotic production. GV, Gate valve. NV, Needle valve. SV, Saunders-type valve. PV, Plug valve. PR, Pressure regulator. PG, Pressure gauge. ST. Steam trap. S. Strainer. HS, Heat seal. D, Diaphragm. (Bartlett and Gerhardt., 1959. J. Biochem. Microbiol. Technol. and Eng., 1, 359–377.)

the cells often are not optimal for the formation of a chemical fermentation product. This picture becomes yet more complicated if we observe, in a corresponding batch fermentation, a sequence in which formation of intermediate products in the cells or in the broth is followed by a reuse of these compounds by the cells during further growth and product formation. Obviously, if a single-stage continuous fermentation is to be carried out for these fermentations, then a compromise must be reached on the nutrient and physical conditions applied to the fermentation. The alternative would appear to be a multistage continuous fermentation that can allow growth in the first stage and product formation in the second or succeeding stages.

Antibiotic fermentations are included in this group of complex fermentation processes for which a continuous fermentation would seem

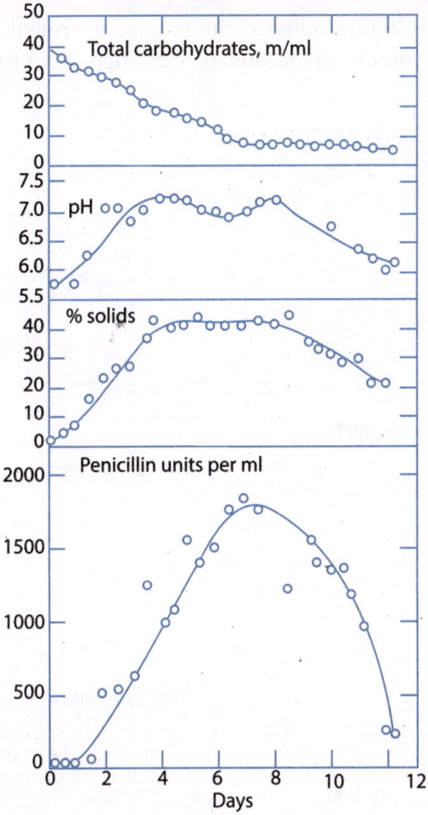

Figure 13.3 Batch penicillin fermentation. (Bartlett and Gerhardt., 1959. J. Biochem. Vlicrobiol. Technol. and Eng., 1, 359–377.)

difficult to accomplish. In this regard, the feasibility of a single-stage continuous fermentation for chloramphenicol and penicillin was investigated by Bartlett and Gerhardt (1959) (Figure 13.2). These workers reported that, at dilution rates of 1 and 0.5 volume changes per day, respectively, they were able to obtain yields from 1/4 to 1/2 of the maximum observed in batch fermentations, and that these rates were maintained in a steady state for more than two weeks. A comparison is made in Figures 13.3 and 13.4, respectively, of the results that they observed with the batch penicillin fermentation and with the continuous penicillin fermentation operated at 0.5 volume changes per day. It will be noted from this figure that, after eight days, the primary carbon source was changed from lactose to glucose (see Chapter 16 on the penicillin fermentation).

Sikyta, et al (1959) studied the streptomycin fermentation as a continuous process, but, in contrast to the studies of Bartlett and Gerhardt, employed a

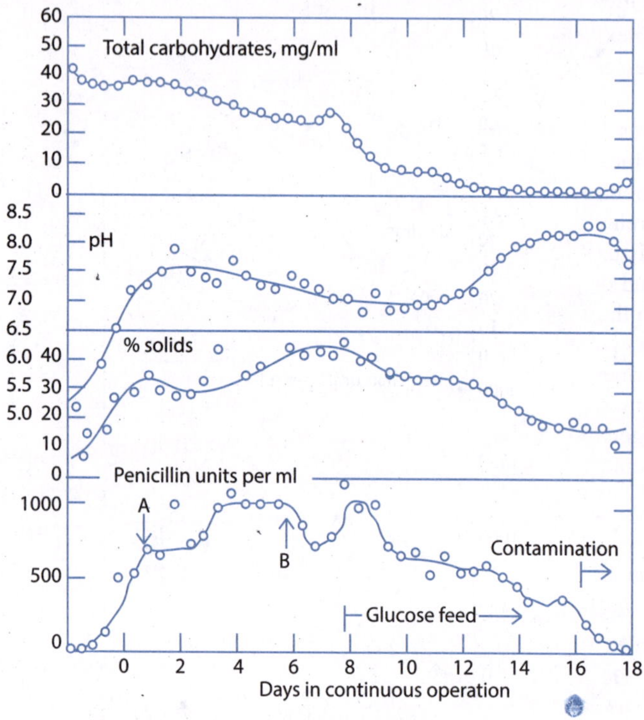

Figure 13.4 Penicillin fermentation at 0.5 volume changes per day, initially with lactose and then with glucose as the carbohydrate source. (Bartlett and Gerhardt,. 1959. *J. Biochem. Microbiol. Technol. and Eng.*, 1, 359–377.)

three-stage fermentation plus an overpressure of air in the whole system to maintain aseptic conditions. They applied uniform flow velocities through the three fermentors, but the flow velocity differ for each of the three stages of the fermentation to correspond with the growth and synthetic processes of the microorganisms occurring in the particular fermentors. Thus, they attempted to match the three stages of the continuous fermentation to the three phases of the fermentation as commonly observed in batch production. The first stage allowed logarithmic mycelial growth which was accompanied by a rapid consumption of amino nitrogen and phosphorous from the medium, and by a sharp increase and subsequent sharp decrease in the levels of the keto acids of the medium. In the second stage, a rapid consumption of reducing substances and ammonium nitrogen occurred. Also, in this stage there was a decrease in pH and an increased rate of antibiotic formation. The third stage allowed a rapid synthesis of antibiotic accompanied by a rapid increase in pH. Obviously, these antibiotic fermentations and other fermentations of like complexity will require considerable further study if continuous fermentation processes are to be commercialized.

A somewhat similar, although not continuous, fermentation approach utilizes late nutrient additions to a batch fermentation. Thus, if a substrate is somewhat toxic to the microorganism, it can be added at the time of compounding of the medium and at intervals during the fermentation so that relatively low total levels are maintained. Also, if the organism utilizes the diauxie phenomenon, the first substrate can be added initially, and the second or alternate substrate can be added during the fermentation at a time when the first substrate has almost disappeared. A late nutrient addition also occurs when ammonia is added during a fermentation to counteract decreases in fermentation pH values. This ammonia supplies additional nitrogen for the microorganism, and it can cause variable fermentation results if the nitrogen level of the medium should happen to be a controlling factor in the fermentation.

References

Aiba, S., A. E. Humphrey, and N. F. Millis. 1965. *Biochemical Engineering.* Academic Press, N.Y., Pp. 107–132.

Bartlett, M.C. and P. Gerhardt. 1959. Continuous antibiotic fermentation—Design of a 20 litre, single-stage pilot plant and trials with two contrasting processes. *J. Biochem. Microbiol. Tech. and Eng,* **1,** 359–377.

Deindoerfer, F.H. and A.E. Humphrey, 1959. A logical approach to—Design of multistage systems for simple fermentation processes. *Ind. Eng. Chem.,* **51,** 809–812.

Gerhardt, P. and M.C. Bartlett, 1959. Continuous Industrial Fermentations. *Adv. Appl. Microbiol.,* **1,** 215–260.

Hastings, J.J. H., 1958. Present trends and future developments, pp. 299–318 in Biochemical Engineering (ed. R. Steel). The Macmillan Co., N.Y.

Maxon, W.D., 1960. Continuous fermentation. *Adv. Appl. Microbiol.,* **2,** 335–349.

Sikyta, B., J. Doskocil, and J. Kasparova. 1959. Continuous streptomycin fermentation. *J. Biochem. Microbiol. Tech. and Eng.,* **1,** 379–392.

Chapter 14

Biological Waste Treatment

Most industrial processes produce waste waters that contain varying amounts of salts and organic matter. Thus, the waste waters associated with the industrial fermentation industries contain spent media, wash waters, and waters accumulating in various steps of product recovery. Organic solvent wastes also accumulate during the recovery of industrial fermentation products, but these wastes present entirely different problems and are not considered here. The waste waters resulting from industrial fermentation processes contain water-soluble, colloidal, and suspended wastes, and in this respect, they somewhat resemble municipal sewage wastes in their treatment requirements. In fact, these wastes without additional treatment at times are added to sewerage for processing by municipal sewage-treatment facilities. In any event, these wastes should not be discarded directly into streams, lakes, or rivers because of their high content of undecomposed organic matter.

Certain fermentation wastes require special handling before initiation of treatment. Thus, if a plant or animal pathogen has been employed in the fermentation, the fermentation wastes may require sterilization before undergoing waste treatment. In fact, at times it may be advantageous to sterilize fermentation wastes regardless of whether a pathogen was used so that the particular fermentation microorganism cannot be reisolated with ease from the waste waters by a competing industrial concern. The spent media or media residues also may require preliminary filtration before further treatment to remove the larger solids and masses of microbial cells. Finally, strongly acidic or alkaline waste waters may require neutralization before further biological waste treatment.

A fermentation company, depending on its size and on the type of waste waters that it produces, either may process its own waste waters or arrange with the local municipality for adding the waste waters to municipal sewerage for treatment at the local sewage treatment plant. The latter arrangement is not always feasible, because it may require the installation of extensive additional treatment facilities at the treatment plant. Also, the discharge of fermentation wastes to sewage waters may be sporadic, which results in a high but intermittent loading of the treatment facilities. In addition, the fermentation wastes may require the development of a special natural microbial flora for its decomposition, a microflora that cannot be maintained if the delivery of fermentation wastes to the treatment plant is sporadic. Finally, the municipality may require some form of pretreatment of the fermentation wastes before discharge to municipal sewerage.

Because of the similarity in biological waste-treatment systems required for fermentation wastes and for municipal sewage, municipal sewage, in the present instance, will serve as an example of the biological treatment of waste waters. However, it must be pointed out that a fermentation company treating its own waste waters does not necessarily employ all of the treatment procedures to be discussed, but may may use only those that are applicable to its own particular types of wastes.

The goal of biological treatment of waste waters is to employ microorganisms to completely oxidize to carbon dioxide and water all of the organic components of the waters. However, depending on the particular treatment techniques employed, inorganic salts present initially in the waste waters or released during waste treatment also undergo oxidation, if oxidation is possible. Thus, as a result of these various oxidations, the effluent waters from the treatment plant should contain only small amounts of incompletely decomposed organic matter, but they might contain considerable amounts of inorganic sulfates, phosphates, and nitrates or ammonia. Regardless of their composition, however, these waters should no longer be able to support extensive growth of heterotrophic or autotrophic microorganisms, including algae, so that the water can be added to natural bodies of water without causing more than a minimal growth of a balanced ecology of autotrophic and heterotrophic microorganisms. Thus, incompletely treated waste waters, on disposal in streams or other bodies of water, are subject to further microbial oxidation of organic matter with a consequent decrease in the level of dissolved oxygen in the water. This lack of dissolved oxygen favors the less desirable types of fish, in extreme cases killing fish and other forms of higher water life, and yields anaerobic conditions with consequent foul odors. Residual solids in incompletely treated waste waters also settle to the bottom of a stream or lake to cause undesirable changes in the types of microorganisms that inhabit the bottom. With municipal sewage treatment, there is the additional possibility that disease-producing microorganisms may survive in incompletely treated waters, particularly if chlorination has not been practiced.

The oxidized inorganic salts present in both completely and incompletely treated waste waters also present additional problems for the natural bodies of water receiving these waters. The phosphate, nitrate, and to some extent, sulfate, ammonia, and other salts are good fertilizers that promote the growth of algae and aquatic weeds, a condition not particularly beneficial to the appearance or odor of a body of water. These plants use up dissolved oxygen at night when photosynthesis is not occurring, and their cellular tissue also, at some time, must undergo decomposition, which makes further demands on the dissolved oxygen content of the waters.

The level of decomposable organic matter present in industrial or municipal waste waters is measured in terms of "biochemical oxygen demand" (BOD) or "chemical oxygen demand" (COD). BOD measures the milligrams of oxygen consumed during the biological decomposition of organic matter occurring in a liter of waste water during a specified period of time, usually five days. In making this determination, the waste water may be first seeded with sewage, activated sludge, pure or mixed cultures, or any other source of microorganisms in which the organisms are known to be well acclimated to the particular substrate or waste. COD determines the milligrams of oxygen per liter of waste water which are consumed during the oxidation of the organic matter by hot acidified dichromate. This procedure, being nonbiological, may not present a true picture of the ease of organic matter decomposition for biological waste treatment and, hence, it must be compared with BOD results for particular types of waste waters. Both BOD and COD determinations can be employed at any stage in the treatment of industrial or municipal wastes so as to ascertain the efficiency of the treatment or the load of decomposable organic matter still present.

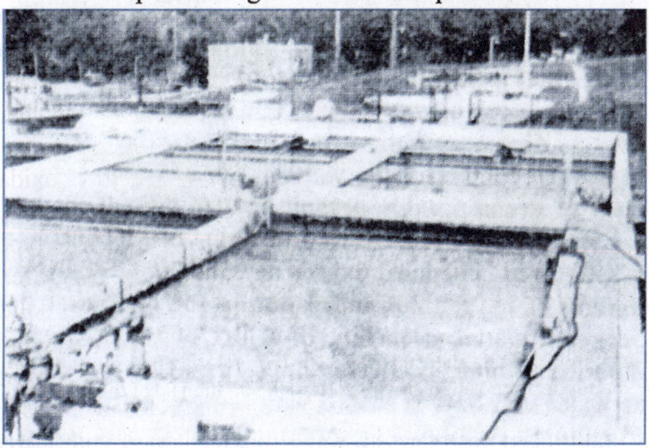

Figure 14.1 Initial aeration tank followed by a primary settling tank.

As is evident from the foregoing considerations, the treatment of industrial and municipal wastes is really a fermentation process, although pure cultures of microorganisms usually are not employed for inoculation. The natural microbial flora of the waste waters is allowed to become enriched with those components of the natural microbial population which are most active in the decomposition of the types of organic matter that must undergo decomposition. These organisms include heterotrophic bacteria and, to a certain extent, actinomycetes and fungi. Protozoa also are very active in organic matter decomposition. The autotrophic bacteria, although incapable of organic matter decomposition, nevertheless are active and, thus, ammonia and reduced sulfur compounds liberated from proteinaceous and other wastes are quickly oxidized to nitrate and sulfate by these microorganisms. Anaerobic bacteria in anaerobic digestion tanks are active in the decomposition of organic matter, particularly the more resistant organic matter. Their activities yield simple organic molecules, such as acids, alcohols, glycerol, amines, and other products of anaerobic metabolism, as well as gaseous products such as carbon dioxide, ammonia, hydrogen, methane and hydrogen sulfide. However, under ideal conditions, methane-producing bacteria utilize most of the simpler organic molecules resulting from the metabolic activities of the other anaerobes, in the process yielding carbon dioxide and methane so that these gases become the main gaseous products of anaerobic organic matter decomposition.

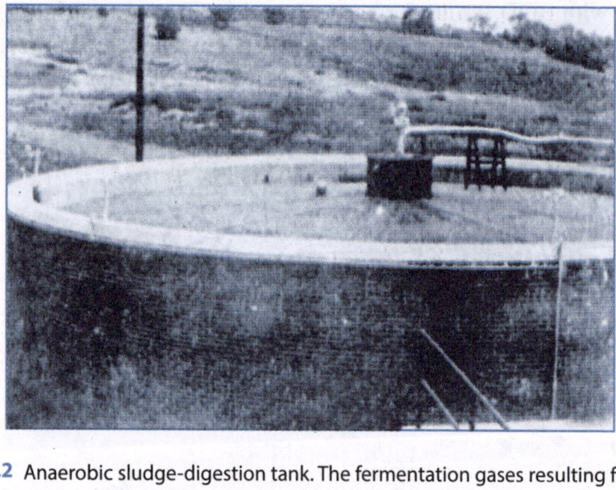

Figure 14.2 Anaerobic sludge-digestion tank. The fermentation gases resulting from anaerobic organic-matter decomposition are piped from the floating lid of the tank.

The actual procedures of waste-water treatment vary with the type and amount of waste water to be treated and may consist of only a single treatment or of a combination of treatments. Some treatment systems utilize an initial or "primary settling tank" (with or without a preceding aeration tank) with the waters moving at a slow rate to allow sedimentation of the larger suspended solids and flotation of fatty materials (Figure 14.1). The sediments and fatty materials accumulating in this tank are separated for treatment in an anaerobic digestion tank (Figure 14.2). However, the more efficient aerobic treatment systems, such as the complete mixing activated sludge process, require only that gritty material be sedimented from the waters before further treatment.

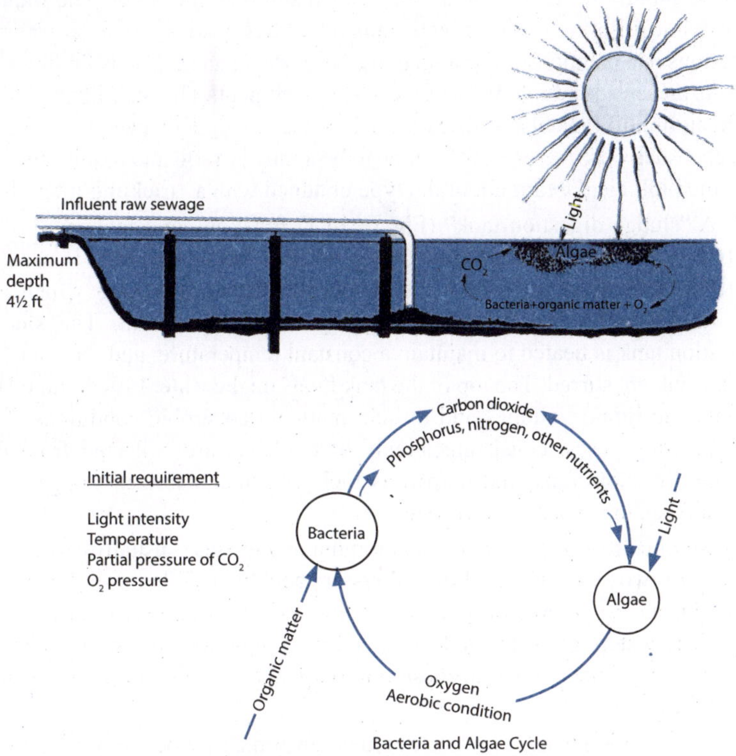

Figure 14.3 Sewage disposal by the waste-stabilization pond method. (Sidio, Hartman, and Fugazzotto, 1961. Public Health Reports, 76, 201–208.)

Septic and Imhoff tanks are anaerobic digestion chambers used for bringing about the decomposition of simple or complex organic materials to simple organic molecules and fermentation gases. They may be used with or without an initial primary settling tank treatment of the waste water. The septic tank is a relatively small closed tank vented for the escape of fermentation gases, and it finds little present-day industrial use. The more resistant organic matter, which through fermentation becomes stabilized and somewhat resistant to further anaerobic microbial degradation, accumulates as a sludge in the bottom of this tank and may be dried, ground, and spread on soil as a fertilizer. The effluent waters from a septic tank still contain both dissolved and suspended organic compounds capable of supporting the growth of aerobic heterotrophic organisms and, hence, they cannot be added to a body of water. This effluent must receive further aerobic microbial oxidation and is often spread on soil or sand, although the porosity of sand may be rapidly decreased by the suspended solids in the water. The Imhoff tank, while differing from the septic tank in its physical design and larger size, functions in a manner similar to that of a septic tank, and it also is finding less use in present-day biological waste-water treatment. The stabilized sludge from an Imhoff tank also is dried for use as a fertilizer. However, the effluent waters usually are too great in volume to be applied to soil and require further aerobic biological treatment of the type obtained with a "trickling filter."

A "sludge digestion tank" (Figure 14.1) functions in a manner similar to but much more efficient than that of the Imhoff tank, and it is used to anaerobically degrade or digest sedimented or floating wastes which are separated from waste waters undergoing aerobic treatment. The sludge digestion tank is heated to maintain a constant temperature, and the contents of the tank are stirred. The top of the tank floats on the water to accommodate changes in liquid volumes and to help maintain anaerobic conditions. The fermentation gases, consisting largely of methane, are collected from the sludge digestion tanks and burned as fuel. The final stablized sludge from this tank again is used as a fertilizer.

Aerobic treatment of industrial or municipal wastes is usually carried out by one of two systems—trickling filters or "activated sludge"—although, in some instances, "oxidation ponds" are finding increased use. In any event, the waste waters are subjected to moderate to high aeration to maintain an active aerobic metabolism of those microorganisms decomposing the waste organic matter.

An oxidation pond (or waste stabilization pond, as shown in Figure 14.3) is a large shallow body of water, two to four feet in depth, into which waste waters are discharged at a single point such as at one edge or in the middle. Wind action brings about the little mixing that occurs. Oxygen is available to the microorganisms by diffusion from the air into the shallow waters, and as a result of algal photosynthesis. The effluent waters from these ponds are discharged into a stream or into another oxidation pond in series with the first pond, and the ponds must be cleaned at intervals to remove solids that accumulate on the bottom. To date, these ponds have been used mainly for the small-scale treatment of sewage and industrial wastes in areas where much cheap land is available.

A trickling filter (Figure 14.4) employs a bed of coarse rock, with the individual rocks being two to four inches in diameter and the depth of the

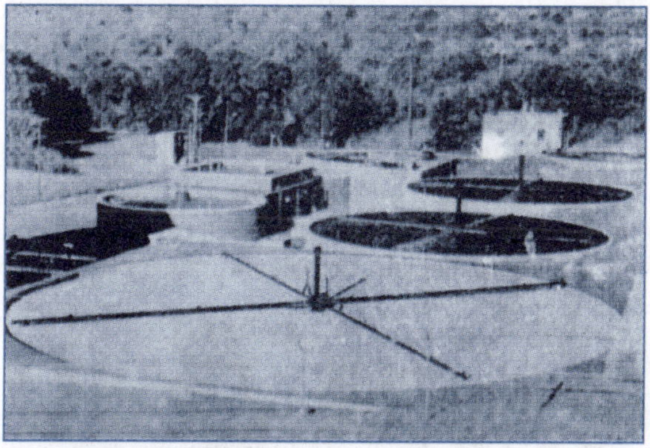

Figure 14.4 Trickling filters. The trickling filter in the foreground is not in use and, hence, does not have microbial growth coating the rocks; see Figure 14.6.

bed being approximately six to ten feet. Waste waters are sprayed over the rock bed intermittently or continuously, respectively, from fixed nozzles or from nozzles located on a horizontal rotating arm (Figure 14.5). These waters may be preaerated before spraying, although some aeration occurs during

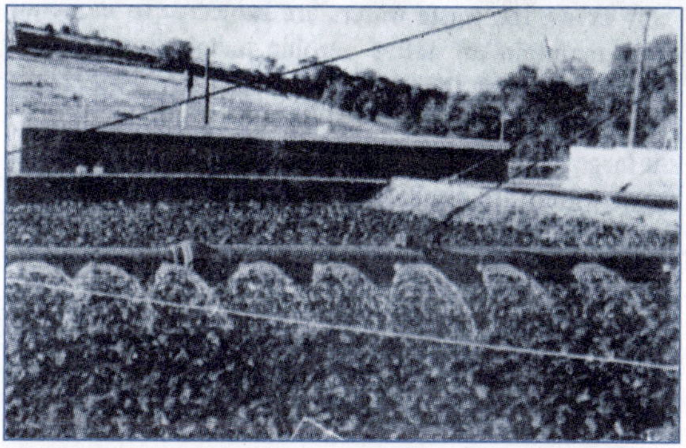

Figure 14.5 Waste waters being sprayed from a rotating arm onto the surface of a trickling filter.

the spraying. Microorganisms become attached to and grow on the surfaces of the rocks to produce a slimy layer of microbial cells (Figures 14.6 and 14.7). This growth is composed largely of heterotrophic and autotrophic bacteria and of protozoa, and the colloidal and dissolved organic matter in the waste waters is attacked and degraded by these microorganisms as the waters percolate down through the rock bed. Conditions within the trickling filter must be maintained aerobic, even at the bottom of the filter, and the application of waste water to the filter is adjusted to accomplish this end. Thus, a trickling filter continuously saturated with water quickly becomes anaerobic because of the high oxygen requirements of the microorganisms. At times, much of the microbial growth sloughs from the rocks and appears suspended in the effluent waters from the bottom of the filter, although there also is a continuous sloughing of small amounts of microbial growth from the filter. The effluent waters are passed slowly through a final settling tank (Figure 14.8) to remove the sloughed microbial cells and other debris before the waters are chlorinated and discharged into a stream or other body of water.

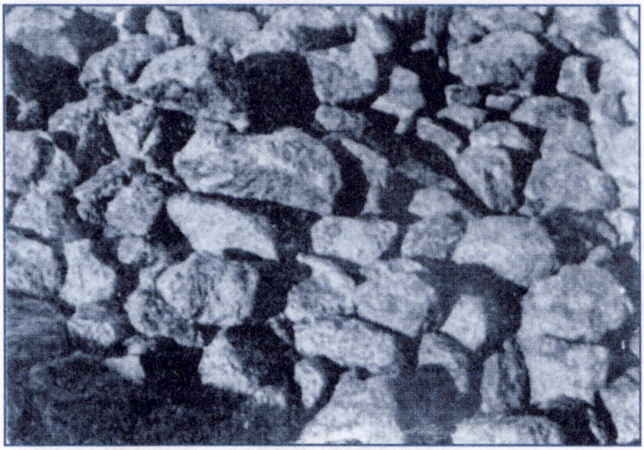

Figure 14.6 Trickling-filter rocks coated with microbial growth.

The activated sludge process is a highly efficient system for the aerobic biological treatment of industrial or municipal wastes. The waste waters are passed in succession through coarse screens to remove the larger debris, a grit chamber to sediment the heavier gritty materials, and a primary settling tank. Effluent waters from the primary settling tank are then mixed or inoculated with somewhere in the range of 20 percent of activated sludge that has been recovered from the final settling tank of the activated sludge system. These inoculated waste waters are introduced into one end of an oblong, deep, activated sludge aeration tank (Figure 14.9) in which air, introduced under pressure as small bubbles along one or both long side walls of the tank, aerates the waters and provides vigorous agitation. Smaller tanks, however, may utilize stirring without air incorporation, with the waters being aerated by contact with the atmosphere. The microbial population that degrades

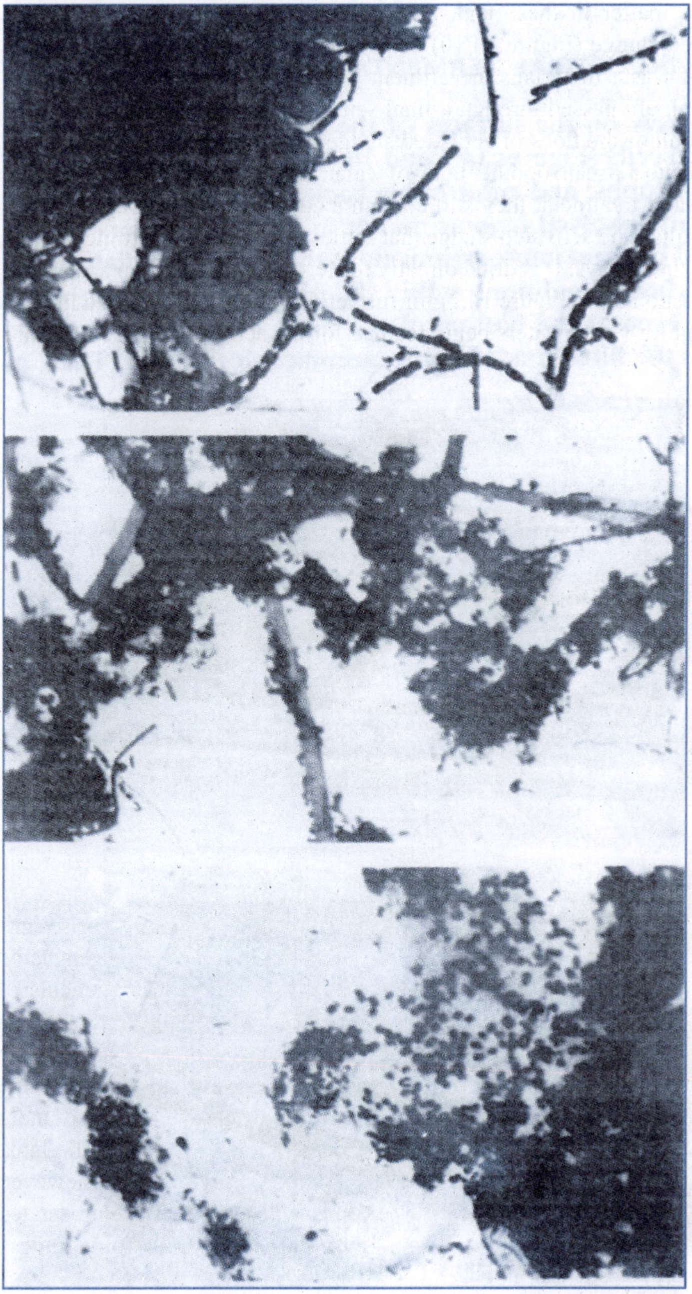

Figure 14.7 Microorganisms on trickling filter rocks as observed at 1300-fold magnification.

the organic matter in these tanks occurs as dispersed gelatinous masses, the activated sludge (Figure 14.10) consisting of an admixture of cells and particles of waste material. The effluent waters from the activated sludge aeration tank are passed through a final settling tank (Figure 14.8) to allow sedimentation of the flocs of activated sludge, then they are chlorinated and discharged into a stream or other body of water, although, as for other methods of waste-water treatment, they still contain a considerable level of oxidized inorganic salts. The activated sludge that settles from the final settling tank is handled in three ways. It is dried directly for fertilizer, added to an anaerobic sludge digestion tank (Figure 14.2) for further decomposition, or used in part as inoculum for waste waters being readied for the activated sludge aeration tank.

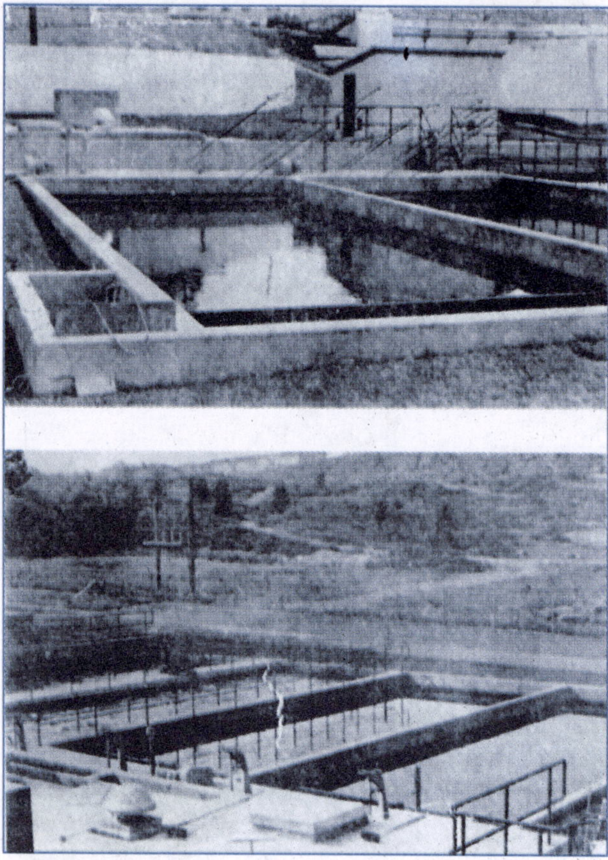

Figure 14.8 Final settling tank.

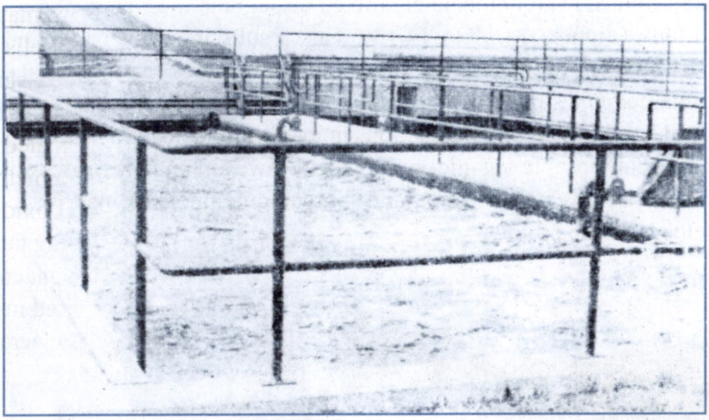

Figure 14.9 Activated-sludge aeration tank. All is being of the water along both long walls of the tank.

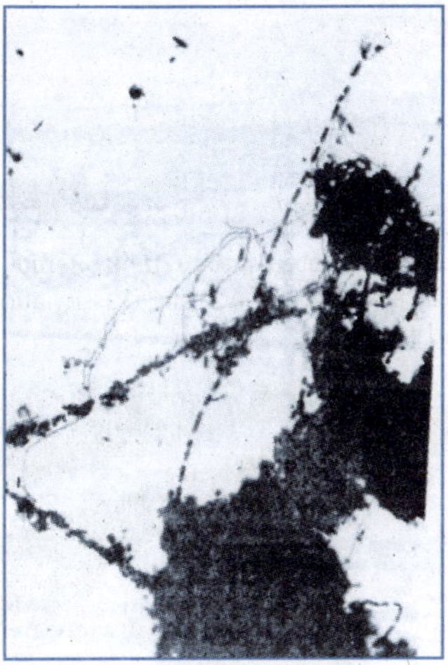

Figure 14.10 Activated-sludge microorganisms as magnification.

The aeration tank described for the activated sludge system receives a heavy load of decomposable organic matter at the input end, and this organic matter is largely degraded by the time it reaches the effluent end of the tank. As a result, the demand for dissolved oxygen is much greater at the input end of the tank, and the organisms at the effluent end are metabolically less active. This situation is corrected in a "complete mixing" activated sludge system. This system differs from the activated sludge system previously described in that the waste water, without passing through a primary settling tank, is introduced and immediately mixed throughout the waters of a round, aerated tank (Figures 14.11 to 14.13). This results in an even demand for dissolved oxygen throughout the waters so that most of the microbial cells are maintained in a similar physiological state. Such a system is more stable, capable of handling greater fluctuations in loading, and better able to degrade toxic but decomposable organic compounds. However, more activated sludge accumulates in this type of tank, and inorganic compounds may not be as completely oxidized.

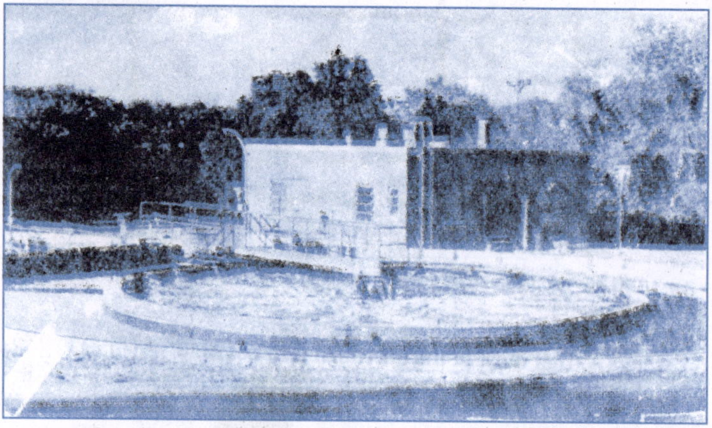

Figure 14.11 Complete mixing activated-sludge tank. Rapid and complete mixing is achieved by air incorporation all along the inner walls in association with the circular form of the tank; see Figures 14.12 and 14.13.

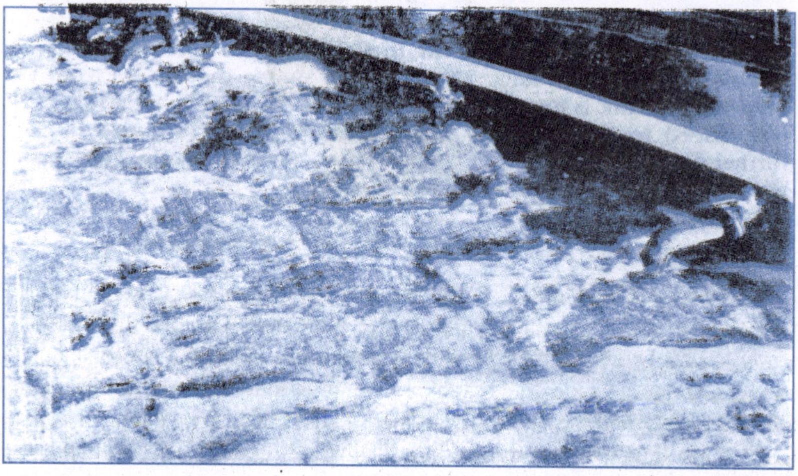

Figure 14.12 Agitation and mixing of waters in a complete mixing activated-sludge tank.

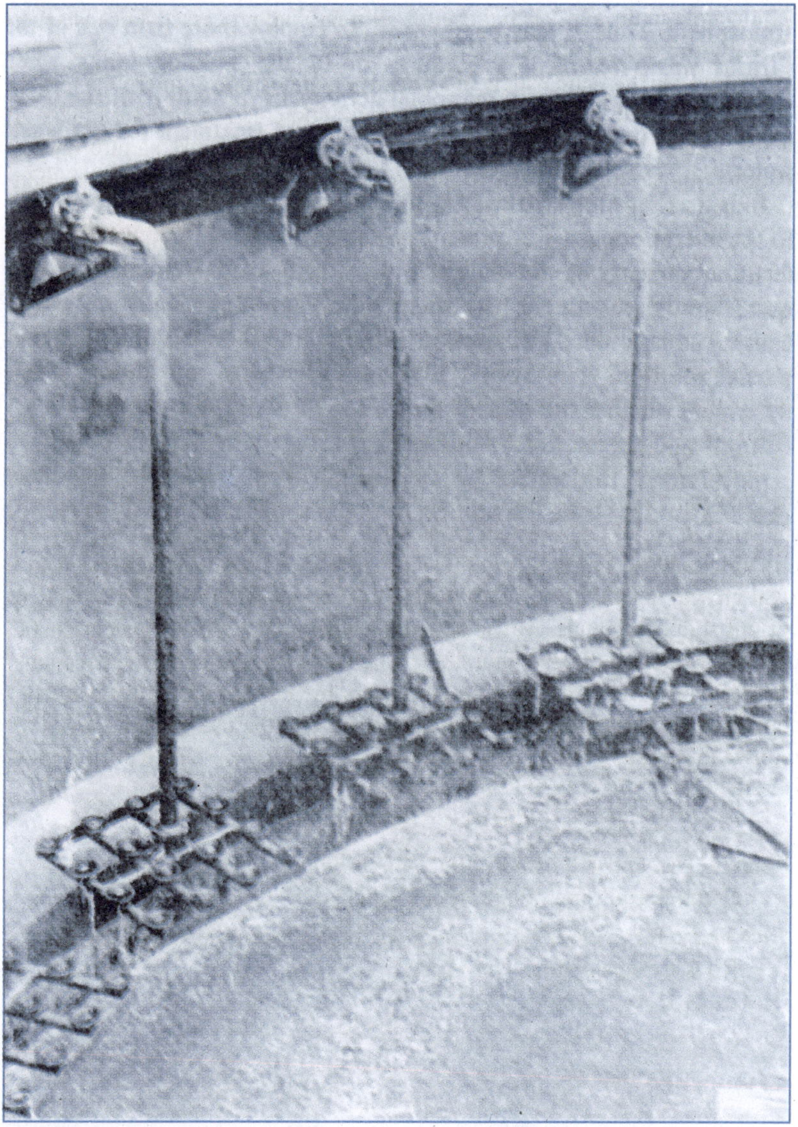

Figure 14.13 Banks of aeration spargers as observed along the inside wall of an empty complete-mixing activated-sludge tank.

The techniques for treatment of industrial and municipal wastes still leave leave much to be desired. They must be carefully controlled, because they demonstrate faults similar to those for all microbial processes. For instance, the active microorganisms comprise a natural population and, hence, this population can fluctuate widely in its relative composition of microbial forms. Obviously, certain microorganisms are much more active than are others in the decomposition of waste materials. In this vein, the pH picture during treatment must be watched as it influences the types of microorganisms and their activities in organic matter decomposition. Also, except for sludge digestion tanks, the incubation temperature cannot be controlled as in industrial fermentation, because waste-water treatment facilities are usually large and exposed to the atmosphere. Thus, it may be necessary to employ more than one of the various waste-treatment procedures or to use holding tanks when changes in the weather, in microbial activity, or in loading of the treatment system cause a slowing or inefficiency of treatment for the waste waters.

Industrial or municipal wastes that are poorly biodegradable or toxic to the microflora are ever-present problems and need further study. The fertilizer capacity of the effluent waters from waste treatment also requires study in order to use these waters more efficiently instead of causing aquatic weed and algal growth in natural bodies of water. As a partial solution, it is known that various studies are under way to determine whether the effluent waters can be used for irrigation of agricultural and forest soils. Additional investigations involve phosphate removal from the waters by tertiary chemical treatment, combined chemical and biological treatment, and the use of algal ponds to remove these salts.

References

Gainey, P.L. and T.H. Lord, 1952. *Microbiology of Water and sewage.* Prentice-Hall, Inc., Englewood Cliffs, N.J.

McKinney, R.E., 1962. *Microbiology for sanitary engineers.* McGraw-Hill Book Company, Inc., New York.

Chapter 15

Patents and Secret Processes

The economic and competitive position of a fermentation process depends on several factors, some of which are recoverable yields, research costs, size of the market, profit potential, and patent or secret process position of the fermentation process or product. The latter consideration is particularly important, because patents and secret processes provide a degree of protection to the competitive position of a commercial fermentation. But which approach should be taken by an industrial concern? Should a fermentation process or product be patented, assuming that they are patentable, to provide 17 years of monopoly, or should the fermentation process and know-how be kept a secret so as to possibly allow many additional years of protection for the process? A yet more basic question, however, concerns what can and cannot be patented. The answers to these and other questions relating to the patenting of inventions will become more clear if the basic concepts behind the granting of patents by the Patent Office of the Federal Government are examined.

Patents are granted to inventors in return for a public disclosure of their inventions. These disclosures add to the knowledge of the respective art and help to advance the state of that art. The patent, in turn, gives the inventor the right to exclude others from making, using, or selling his particular invention as disclosed in the "claims" of the patent. Most inventors will settle for the 17 years of protection rendered to them by a patent and will apply for a patent on their invention instead of attempting to maintain secrecy during the use of their invention. Obviously, secrecy about a fermentation process is difficult to maintain. Special contracts must be negotiated with trusted employees so that they will not reveal their knowledge of the process and, in addition, other problems arise which will not be discussed here. Regardless of these considerations, however, in a few instances, secrecy concerning a fermentation process has allowed the maintenance of a good competitive position for a commercial fermentation for many years in excess of the 17-year monopoly of a patent. A notable example is the commercial production of citric acid by *Aspergillus* niger as the fermentation process is conducted by the Charles Pfizer Company, Incorporated.

A fermentation process or product protected by a patent, however, also may have secrets associated with it. Special fermentation and recovery techniques associated with obtaining high yields and good product recoveries are often secret information known only to the inventor and his associates and not disclosed in the patent itself, since such data are generally developed after the application for the patent has been filed. Also, the patent describes a workable process and a product without necessarily describing minor variations in process technique and product recovery, considerations that may be, however, of extreme importance in maintaining the competitive position of the fermentation. There is some protection available form state or federal courts for this type of information. Thus, an individual or individuals can be prosecuted for stealing microbial cultures and technical data such as secret process information.

The individual working in an industrial research laboratory or any laboratory in which fermentation process of potential economic value are under study should know how to read a patent in order to be able to determine the points of the invention which are actually protected by the patent. This knowledge should prevent his infringing on the rights of other inventors. He should also understand the types of information that are required for filing a patent application so that research can be directed towards obtaining this information. He should be able to decide the extent of process variations or ranges in variations in chemical structure of a product which should be claimed in a patent application. As we shall see, claiming too little or too much about the process or product can be disastrous. Guidance in these problem areas frequently can be obtained by consulting a qualified patent attorney.

HISTORY OF THE PATENT CONCEPT

It will be easier to understand patents of we first consider how the concept of patents has developed during the past few hundred years. Patents in one form or another have been in existence at least since 1332, when Bartolomeo Verde of Venice received a revocable 12-year patent on a windmill. A patent statute enacted in Venice in 1474 allowed the granting of exclusive rights for 10 years to "inventors of new arts and machines." In 1501, Aldus in Venice obtained a patent on *italic* type. Galileo, in 1594, received a patent for a machine to be used for raising water and irrigating land. This patent was for a 20-year term, and within one year of granting of the patent, he had to construct his new form of machine. This patent also provided for the punishment of infringers, and it was based on the assumption that the machine had not previously been invented or thought of by others, and that it had never been the subject of a previous patent or grant. Thus, Galileo's patent included several principles found in modern patent law. It provided a reward to the inventor and to the first inventor only, it provided a requirement for compulsory working of the invention, and it provided the right to exclude others from practicing the invention.

Monopolies of a different sort were commonplace in England during the reign of Queen Elizabeth. These monopolies were granted by the Crown on a favoritism basis to various individuals, although this practice was illegal, based on English common law. Such products as salt, starch, glass, and paper were included in these monopolies. The power to enforce the monopoly was also granted to the holders of the monopolies and, obviously, this led to high prices and poor quality. Regardless of these monopolies, however, a patent was granted by the Crown in 1565 for a furnace, and this probably was the first example in England of a reward to an inventor. In contrast to monopolies, the granting of a patent such as this was legal under English common law. This question of the legality of patents versus monopolies was decided when the Statute of Monopolies was enacted in 1623 during the reign of King James, since this statute protected inventions by the granting to inventors of monopolies (patents) by the Crown, but it prohibited the Crown from granting other forms of monopolies. These early English patents did not include a written description of the invention, nor were drawings included. In fact, it was not until the middle of the eighteenth century that these became a part of a patent.

The early American colonists were well aware of the injustices that had occurred in England through the granting of monopolies. Therefore, a Massachusetts statute of 1641 stated that monopolies should not be granted or allowed, although such new inventions that might be profitable to the colony might receive a monopoly for a short period of time. In succeeding years, patents were granted by the various states and, in fact, an inventor had to obtain a separate patent from each state. The constitution of the United States, however, provided for patents, and the first Federal patent act enacted in 1970 allowed the patenting of "any useful art, manufacture, engine, machine, or device or improvement therein not before known or used." There have been many changes in the patent laws of the United States since this first Federal patent act, and further changes are under consideration at the present time.

United States Patent Office

2,771,396
Patented Nov. 20, 1956

2,771,396
PREPARATION OF DIAMINOPIMELIC ACID AND LYSINE

Lester Earl Casida, Jr., Baldwin, N.Y., assignor to Chas. Pfizer & Co., Inc., New York, N.Y., a corporation of Delaware

No Drawing, Application December 9, 1955
Serial No. 551, 987
11 Claims. (Cl. 195—30)

This invention is concerned with an improved method for the preparation of lysine which is an essential amino acid of commercial importance. In particular, it is concerned with a method for preparing lysine from the compound diaminopimelic acid and with the method for preparing diaminopimelic acid itself.

Although the work in this field was begun rather recently, because of the importance of lysine, there has been considerable work reported in the literature. Davis reported in Nature, volume 169, page 534 (1952), that certain lysine-requiring auxotrophs of Escherichia coli produce relatively large amounts of diaminopimelic acid. An enzyme that decarboxylates diaminopimelic acid to yield lysine has been reported to occur in many bacteria, (A Symposium on Amino Acid Metabolism, 1955, E. Work), but to be absent from *E. coli* auxotrophs that require lysine. (Dewey, Hoare and Work, Biochemical Journal, volume 58, page 523 (1954). See also Wright and Cresson, Proceedings of the Society for Experimental Biology and Medicine, volume 82, page 354 (1953).)

It has now been found that diaminopimelic acid may be produced in high yield and subsequently converted to lysine in high yield by the use of certain novel controlled conditions of the reactions. Thus, a method of preparing lysine, at a price substantially below that at which the compound is currently sold in commerce, has been developed.

The first step in this novel synthesis of lysine is the production of diaminopimelic acid. This is accomplished by means of an aerated deep tank, i.e., submerged, fermentation, using a mutant of *E. Coli* which is unable to decarboxylate diaminopimelic acid to lysine. Such mutants may be obtained by the penicillin method of Davis, (op. cit.). It has been found that several strains of *E. coli* which are not able to convert diaminopimelic acid to lysine and which require lysine for their growth, are useful for carrying out this reaction. In particular, one strain, selected from numerous other mutant strains, has been found to carry out this reaction in the best yield although the other strains of *E. coli* requiring lysine also work. A growing culture of this preferred *E. coli* strain which requires lysine for its growth and which carries out the production of diaminopimelic acid in high yield has been deposited with the American Type Culture Collection in Washington, D.C. and added to their permanent collection where it has been given the number ATCC 12,408. In order that this reaction producing diaminopimelic acid be carried out in high yield, conditions must be carefully controlled. It has been discovered that during the fermentation, the pH should be maintained near neutrality. During the fermentation, the pH tends to drop and neutrality is maintained by the addition of alkali, for example NaOH, KOH, and preferably ammonium hydroxide. Urea may also be used for this purpose, as it is converted to ammonia. Toward the end of the fermentation the pH tends to rise, and neutrality

is held by adding sulfuric acid. It has also been discovered that the addition of glycerol to the medium is extremely helpful. It has been found that mannitol may be used in place of glycerol; however, glycerol has been found to be the most effective and economical. In addition, it has been found that cornsteep liquor is a particularly good constituent of the fermentation medium. This cornsteep liquor supplies the lysine required for the growth of the *E. coli* auxotrophs and also possibly acts as an economical source of precursors such as aspartic acid and lactic acid. Thus, by means of these three newly discovered controls of the fermentation, that is (1) the careful control of pH at or near neutrality, (2) the addition of glycerol in from 1 to 10% by volume, and (3) the use of cornsteep liquor, it has been found possible to produce diaminopimelic acid in economical large scale industrial quantities.Diaminopimelic acid is, of course, an extremely valuable compound. It is useful in itself and it is also useful as an intermediate for the synthesis of lysine, as will be shown below. We have also obtained some evidence to show that diaminopimelic acid may be used as a supplement in the feeding of poultry where it may take the place of lysine.

This fermentation is conducted at about 28°C, and in general approximately three days are required to obtain optimum yield. It is, of course, understood that conditions for obtaining the best yield vary somewhat with the particular strain of organism employed.

The final step in the synthesis of lysine is the conversion of the diaminopimelic acid to lysine. This is accomplished by treatment of the diaminopimelic acid, preferably in the original broth containing the cells, with the enzyme diaminopimelic acid decarboxylase obtained from organisms of the species Aerobacter aerogenes and also from ordinary members of the species *E. coli*, that is, members of the species *E. coli* which do not require lysine for their growth. The enzyme is liberated from the cells of these organisms by any of the standard methods used to liberate enzymes. These include treatment with a solvent such as butanol, treatment with ultrasonic energy, and the preparation of acetone-dried powder. We have found that the preferred method for liberating the enzyme diaminopimelic acid decarboxylase from organisms of the genus *A. aerogenes* and organisms of the genus E. coli which do not require lysine for their growth, is treatment with the solvent toluene, which has the additional advantage of maintaining sterility during the latter stages of the reaction in which the enzyme is used. The cells may be treated with toluene either before or after the addition to the original diaminopimelic acid broth, but in either case it is preferred that the toluene be present in the conversion mixture and not separate off. One particular strain of *A. aerogenes*, which gives very high yields because it lacks the enzyme lysine decarboxylase, has been deposited with the ATCC and given the number 12,409.

For maximum conversion of the diaminopimelic acid to lysine, it is desirable that certain conditions be used. It has been discovered that the addition of chelating agents such as citrate ions and ethylenediaminetetraacetic acid tetrasodium salt is very helpful to carrying out this reaction. The addition of vitamin B6 is helpful also. The chelating agent and the B6 are especially helpful when high concentrations of diaminopimelic acid are being reacted. It has also been discovered that carrying out this reaction in the absence of light also increases the yield, but is not essential.

Figure 15.1 An example of a United States Patent. Included are the specifications and Claims, with the latter starting with the statement, "What is claimed is:"

This conversion of diaminopimelic acid to lysine is carried out in approximately 24 hours. A temperature of approximately 28°C, has been found to give good results.

Following this reaction, the lysine is then purified by filtration of the enzyme reaction mixture, absorption of the lysine on a strong cation exchange resin, such as the sulfonic acid resin Amberlite IR–120 (TM of Rohm and Haas Co.), elution of the lysine from the cation exchange resins by dilute alkali, such as potassium hydroxide or sodium hydroxide, passage of this eluate through a weak cation exchange resin such as the carboxylic resin Amberlite IRC–50 (TM of Rohm and Haas Co.), which will not absorb the lysine, and drying of the effluent. Additional purification is then carried out by standard method of recrystallization.

The following examples are given solely for the purpose of illustration and are not to be construed as limitations of this invention, many variations of which are possible without departing from the spirit or scope thereof.

EXAMPLE I

Production of diaminopimelic acid

E. coli, ATCC 12,408, was grown for 20 hours at 28°C, with shaking on the following medium which had previously been sterilized by autoclaving for 30 minutes at 20 pounds/square inch pressure:

$(NH_4)_2HPO_4$	percent	0.5
Cornsteep liquor	do	0.5
Glycerol	do	0.5

pH adjusted to 7.5 with potassium hydroxide

Another medium was prepared for actual preparation of the diaminopimelic acid. This medium had the following composition:

$(NH4)_2HPO_4$	percent	4
Cornsteep liquor	percent by volume	4
Glycerol	do	6
$CaCO_3$	percent	0.5

pH adjusted to 7.5 with potassium hydroxide

Two liters of this medium were autoclaved for one hour at 20 pounds/square inch pressure.

100 cc. of the original inoculum was added to 2.1. of the production medium. The reaction was carried out at 28°C with stirring at the rate of 1750 revolutions/minute and aeration at the rate of one volume of air/volume of reaction mixture/minute. A trace of soybean oil was added as an antifoam agent. After 72 hours, the mixture assayed as having a diaminopimelic acid content of 9.0 mg/ml.

EXAMPLE II

Alternate production of diaminopimelic acid

E. coli, ATCC 12,408, was grown on the nutrient medium described in Example I to obtain an inoculum. One liter of this inoculum was added to 25 gallons of the following sterilized production medium:

$(NH_4)_2HPO_4$	percent	2
Cornsteep liquor	percent by volume	4
Glycerol	do	7
$CaCO_3$	percent	0.5

pH adjusted to 7.5 with potassium hydroxide

The reaction was carried out at 28°C, with stirring at the rate of 1750 revolutions/minute and aeration at the rate of one volume of air/volume of reaction mixture/minute. A trace of Dow Corning Antifoam A (brand of silicon defoamer) was added as an anti-foam agent. During the reaction, the pH was maintained near neutrality by adding ammonium hydroxide gradually, beginning at the end of approximately 24 hours of reaction time. The pH tends to drop and it is preferred to add ammonium hydroxide gradually so as to keep the pH very slightly (between 7 and about 7.5) above neutrality and thereby prevent the development of a low pH. After the reaction had proceeded for 64 hours, it was necessary to add sulfuric acid in order to maintain neutrality, since at this stage of the reaction the pH tended to rise. After 68 hours, the reaction mixture was assayed as having a diaminopimelic acid content of 6.5 mg/ml.

EXAMPLE III

Conversion of diaminopimelic acid to lysine

One hundred ml. of a broth in which diaminopimelic acid had been produced in a manner similar to that described in Example I above and assaying at 2.5 mg. of diaminopimelic acid/ml. was adjusted to a pH of 7.2. It should be noted that the cells of *E. coli* used toproduce the diaminopimelic acid were not removed from this broth but were allowed to remain in it. This broth was contained in a 300 cc. Erlenmeyer flask and 5 cc. of toluene were added.

A. aerogenes, ATCC Number 12,409, was grown for 20 hours in two liter batches of the following medium:

Glycerol	percent	0.5
$(NH_4)_2HPO_4$	do	0.5
Cornsteep liquor	do	0.5

pH adjusted to 7.5 by potassium hydroxide

The conditions for growth were a temperature of 28°C., agitation at the rate of 1750 revolutions/minute, aeration at the rate of one volume of air/volume of mixture/minute, with a trace of soy bean oil added as an anti-foam agent. After 20 hours, 25 cc of the broth containing suspended cells were centrifuged and the supernatant liquid discarded. These cells were then added to the Erlenmeyer flask containing the diaminopimelic acid broth and toluene. This flask was then shaken for 16 hours at 28°C at the end of which time the diaminopimelic acid was converted to lysine in 100% yield. The lysine was recovered by ion exchange treatment.

EXAMPLE IV

Alternate method of converting diaminopimelic acid to lysine

100 cc of diaminopimelic acid broth was added to a 300 cc Erlenmeyer. The pH was adjusted to 7.2 and 5 cc of toluene were added.

A. aerogenes, ATCC Number 12,409, was grown as in Example III and at the end of 20 hours, 7 ml of the cell broth suspension was centrifuged and the supernatant discarded. The cells were freeze-dried to yield 75 mg of solids which was added to the above Erlenmeyer flask containing diaminopimelic acid broth and toluene. This Erlenmeyer flask was shaken for 16 hours at 28°C following which time the diaminopimelic acid was found to be converted to lysine in 100% yield.

EXAMPLE V

Use of chelating compounds

In other experiments concerning the conversion of diaminopimelic acid to lysine conducted in a manner similar to that described in Examples III and IV above, it was found that in cases where the diaminopimelic acid containing broth contained a high concentration of this acid, the conversion to lysine could be made to take place more completely and more rapidly than would otherwise be the case with broths contain-

5

ing these high concentrations by adding a chrelating agent to the mixture Citric acid and ethylenediaminetetraacetic acid tetrasodium salt were found helpful when added in concentrations of from about 0.004 molar to about 0.032 molar. Use of higher concentrations is not recommended.

The addition of vitamin B6 during the conversion of diaminopimelic acid to lysine is also helpful in carrying out the reaction. Only trace amounts of the vitamin are required.

What claimed is:

1. A process for the preparation of lysine which comprises the steps: (a) fermenting on a nutrient medium comprising glycerol and cornsteep liquor under submerged, aerobic conditions with a mutant of E. coli which requires lysine for its growth and lacks the enzyme diaminopimelic acid decarboxylase, while maintaining the pH of the medium near neutrality, and (*b*) treating di-aminopimelic acid with the enzymes produced by an organism selected from the group consisting of *A. aerogenes*, and those strains of E. *coli* which do not require lysine for their growth.

2. A process for the preparation of diaminopimelic acid which comprisesfermenting on a nutrient medium comprising glycerol and cernsteep liquor under sub-mdrged, aerobic conditions with a mutant of *E. coli* which requires lysine for its growth and lacks the enzyme diaminopimelic acid decarboxylase, while maintaining the pH of the medium near neutrality.

3. A process for the preparation of lysine which comprises treating diaminopimelic acid with the enzymes produced by an organism selected from the group consisting of *A. aerogenes* and those strains of *E. coli* which do not require lysine for their growth.

4. In a process for the preparation of diaminopimelic acid

6

by a submerged, aerobic fermentation with a mutant of *E. coli* which requires lysine for its growth and lacks the enzyme diaminopimelic acid decarboxylase, the improvement of maintaining the pH of the medium near neutrality.

5. In a process for the preparation of diaminopimelic acid by a submerged, aerobic fermentation with a mutant of *E. coli* which requires lysine for its growth and lacks the enzyme diaminopimelic acid decarboxylase, the improvement of adding glycerol to the nutrient medium.

6. In a process for the preparation of diaminopimelic acid by a submerged, aerobic fermentation with a mutant of *E. coli* which requires lysine for its growth and lacks the enzyme diaminopimelic acid decarboxylase, the improvement of adding cornsteep liquor to the nutrient medium.

7. In a process for the preparation of lysine by the treatment of diaminopimelic acid with the enzymes produced by an organism selected from the group consisting of *A. aerogenes* and those strains of *E. coli* which do not require lysine for their growth, the improvement of adding a chelating agent to the-reaction mixture.

8. A process as in claim 7 wherein the chelating agent is the citrate ion.

9. A process as claimed in claim 7 wherein the chelating agent is ethylenediaminetetraacetate tetrasodium salt.

10. A process as claimed in claim 2 wherein the organism employed is *E.coli* ATCC 12, 408.

11. A process as claimed in claim 3 wherein the organism employed ia *A. aerogenes* ATCC 12,409.

References Cited in the file of this patent

Advances in Enzymology, vol. 16, 1955, pages 297–299.

COMPOSITION OF A PATENT

A patent consists of three parts: the grant, specifications, and claims. The grant is filed at the patent office and is not published. It is a signed document and is the agreement that grants patent rights to the inventor. The specifications and claims are published as a single document (Figure 15.1) which is available to the public at a minimal charge from the Patent Office. Thus, this the part of a patent that one normally sees. The specifications section is a narrative description of the subject matter of the invention and of how the invention is carried out. Therefore, anyone skilled in the particular branch of learning relating to the patent should be able to reproduce the invention on reading the specifications section. The claims section specifically defines the scope of the invention to be protected by the patent. That which others may not practice is defined here and, if the patent relates to industrial fermentations, it should be clearly understood from the claims just how the invention differs from known products and processes. The inventor may claim a part or all of that which is described in the specifications. In fact, the exact wording of the claims is important, because it states exactly what is to be protected and what is not. Thus, a patent stands or falls depending on the statements included in the claims section. It is obvious, then, that the inventor must decide as best he can that which he should and should not claim. If he does not claim certain variations in the process or product, it may be possible for others utilizing these variations to carry out the process or make the product without infringing on the rights of the inventor. In contrast, if in the claims the inventor attempts to protect all possible variations in the process or product without experimentally establishing the validity of each of these variables, he may find that the patent is in jeopardy because of nonworkability of some of the claims. Thus, the inventor should claim those variables of which he is sure and, if possible, he should experimentally test all other variables which, if not claimed, might allow others to circumvent the patent.

SUBJECT MATTER AND CHARACTERISTICS OF A PATENT

Inventions are divided into various categories or "classes" of subject matter. Several of these classes do not apply to microbial processes or products, however, and therefore are not considered in the present discussion. Microbial processes or products usually fall under one of two classes: an "art or process" or a "composition of matter." The second class pertains to new chemical compounds or novel compositions or mixtures, and a microorganism or its enzymes may be used to aid the accomplishment of a chemical synthesis or in producing such compositions. The art or process class of patents pertains to methods, including microbial fermentations, for bringing about useful chemical or physical results.

Implicit in the patentability of a microbial process is the concept that man has adjusted the environment of the microorganism to such an extent that the organism will carry out, in the laboratory or commercial production plant, a process that it could not carry out, to any extent, under the conditions occurring in nature. Thus, *Clostridium acetobutylicum* (Chapter 18), in nature, possibly might produce small amounts of acetic and butyric acid, but it is considered to be highly unlikely that natural environmental and nutritional conditions would be favorable for the further formation of acetone and butanol. Likewise, many investigations designed to demonstrate antibiotic production by microorganisms in soil, for the most part, have yielded negative results. If this phenomenon does occur in nonsterilized soil, it is probably on a microscale in the immediate vicinity of the individual microorganism or on the surface of a particle of readily decomposable organic matter.

The microorganism utilized in a microbial process cannot be patented, and this statement also is true for mutants. However, the utilization of a microorganism not previously described or of a newly derived mutant does lend "novelty" or newness to an invention. This consideration has caused considerable difficulty for the classification of industrial microorganisms, because a large number of supposedly new microorganisms have been given species names in patent applications, although these organisms often differed only slightly from recognized species. In fact, extensive studies of certain groups of these organisms are underway to establish their taxonomic relationships so as to reduce the numbers of species described in the patent literature to those that really differ taxonomically.

It is possible that the inventor of a microbial process may have the alternatives of patenting either the process or the product, or of patenting both. Obviously, if the product is a compound already well known (for example, the amino acid L-lysine), a product patent cannot be obtained, and the patent application must cover only the process for manufacture. In contrast, a newly discovered product not previously described, such as certain new antibiotics, may allow application for a product patent. This product patent has distinct advantages over a process patent in that there may be more than one microbiological route or even a chemical route to formation of the product. A specific example is the Pfizer product patent, U.S. 2,699,054 on the antibiotic tetracycline, since there are at least two processes involving microorganisms yielding this antibiotic. Thus, tetracycline can be produced by a direct fermentation, or chlorotetracycline can be first accumulated through fermentation followed by its chemical conversion to tetracycline.

The United States has an "examination" patent system in contrast to the "registration" system in use in some other countries. The examination system requires that a patent application be studied for "novelty" in the light of "prior art" and for usefulness or "utility." The prior art consists of all printed material, including patents, that was available previous to the time of patent application. This material may be from any country and in any language. The invention must be new in respect to use in this country, so that any unpatented process, even if secret, already in use cannot be patented. For example, Pfizer's secret citric acid process cannot now be patented. Prior experimental use, an abandoned experiment, or lost art does not affect novelty. Based on this, a research worker should not abandon experiments in his research book, and he should not state in writing that he has given up on the experimental approach. A research worker also must be careful that his own scientific publications do not constitute a bar to obtaining a patent. Thus, the Patent Office considers that a patent for which the application was filed within one year after a pertinent publication or public use by the inventor still may be granted, but that longer time periods forfeit novelty. Publication or prior uses by others than the inventor can be antedated.

Too many patent applications are presented to the U.S. Patent Office for a rapid determination of novelty. This backlog rersults in a prolonged period between the time of patent application and patent issue—as much as three years or more.

The requirement for usefulness or utility means that the invention must perform some beneficial function. Thus, it is considered that utility is absent for inventions that are inoperative, frivolous, or injurious to the health, morals, and good order of society. No particular degree of utility is required, however, and there need not be a presently existing practical usefulness. For example, a compound may be useful under the patent statutes if it can be employed for research purposes, as in the case of intermediates that may be used in the synthesis of other compounds of a useful class.

The basic criteria for patentability are set forth in the patent statutes. For example, Section 101 of Title 35 U.S.C. states:

> Whoever invents or discovers any new and useful process, machine, manufacture, or composition of matter, or any new and useful improvement thereof, may obtain a patent therefore, subject to the conditions and requirements of this title.

Thus, apart from utility, the basic requirements for patentability are new and nonobvious subject matter and adequacy of disclosure. In regard to the latter point, in microbiological applications, the drafting of a proper disclosure is quite complex and involves problems that require competent professional assistance. Also, where a new organism is involved, in addition to a proper description in the specification, a culture should be deposited with a recognized depository culture collection prior to filing, although public access to the culture may be restricted until the patent issues.

Based on novelty and utility, the Patent Office decides whether a patent should be granted for a particular invention. If this decision should be unfavorable as it relates to a particular patent application, an appeal can be made to a Board of Appeals within the Patent Office, and one can even appeal to various federal courts. Also, amendments can be made to the original patent application in order to make the invention more acceptable in the eyes of the Patent Office.

There is no requirement that a patent granted in the United States must be put to actual use. In fact, there are many "defensive" patents and patents on small improvements that are never sold or used commercially. Despite such nonuse, these patents seldom impede economic development, since they provide valuable information and encourage invention of modifications or alternatives. Also, in many cases, a patent of this type may be licensed to "unblock" another invention. A study by the Patent, Trademark, and Copyright Foundation of George Washington University (Washington, D.C.) showed that 55 to 65 percent of assigned United States patents and 40 to 50 percent of unassigned United States patents were actually produced for sale or used for making commercial articles at some time during the life of the patent, which indicates a rather high rate of commercial utilization of patents.

The patent concepts discussed thus far apply not only to "basic" patents but also to "improvement" patents that follow and are closely related to the basic invention. Thus, if an inventor obtains a basic patent for an invention, but later finds an improved way of carrying out the invention, he may obtain an improvement patent. The situation is more complex, however, if an inventor other than the original inventor obtains the improvement patent, since it is likely that the second inventor cannot utilize the improvement without permission or license from the holder of the basic patent. Thus, the solution usually calls for negotiation and sale of rights so as to allow utilization of the improvement patent. A specific example of basic and improvement patents is associated with a fermentation process for the manufacture of L-lysine (see Chapter 20). The basic patent (U.S. 2,771,396) pertains to a fermentation process for utilizing an *Escherichia coli* mutant to produce 2, 6-diaminopimelic acid (DAP), with this compound then being decarboxylated to L-lysine by a wild-type strain of *Aerobacter aerogenes*. This basic patent was followed two years later by an improvement patent (U.S. 2,841,532), which was secured to protect the decarboxylation of (DAP) by Escherichia coli back mutants that accumulated during inoculum growth and production, a situation in which the DAP decarboxylase of the *Aerobacter aerogenes* was not needed. In this instance, negotiations were not required, since both the basic and improvement patents were assigned to the same fermentation company.

WHO IS THE INVENTOR: WHO OWNS AN INVENTION

In the United States, a valid patent is granted only to the first inventor, regardless of filing dates for patent applications. It is not always clear, however, just who really is the first inventor and, therefore, the patent laws provide for "interference proceedings" to determine priority of invention. These interference proceedings may be initiated by the Patent Office before issue of the patent, or they may be initiated by another applicant who has a copending application or who files within one year after the patent issues. The inventor is considered to be that individual who first conceived the idea of the invention, regardless of whether the idea had at that time been reduced to practice. But, to be considered as the inventor, one also must have demonstrated reasonable diligence in carrying out the invention (reducing it to practice), or be able to prove reduction to practice prior to the other party's conception. As can be seen, it is of utmost importance for the inventor to establish the actual date on which he conceived the idea of the invention. To establish this date, the inventor should immediately get the inventive idea down in writing, sign and date the paper on which it is written, and have witnesses sign and date the document who can verify the date and content of the description of the invention. This recording of the invention is often done in a research book, and it should include what is considered to be the results and means for obtaining the results of the invention. In addition to recording the invention, every page in the research book on which further experimental work has been recorded should also be signed and dated by the inventor and by one or two witnesses who understand the invention. These witnesses possibly may be called on at a later date to identify the writing in the research book and to establish its date and content. The procedures outlined above establish both the date of conception of the invention and the progress in its reduction to practice but, to prove reduction to practice, the inventor must be able to produce corroboration that the invention was actually carried out, generally through witnesses who actually observed the experimental work. Alternatively, however, a patent application itself can serve as a "constructive" reduction to practice without further proof being required, but by so doing, the invention is placed in a less favorable position as regards considerations for patentability.

Implicit in the concept of granting of patents is the premise that a "spark of genius" or "inventive ingenuity" is involved. In other words, individuals other than the inventor, even with the knowledge at hand which was available to the inventor, could not have conceived the invention. At times, however, questions arise as to who among several individuals working in a single laboratory or for an industrial concern is the actual inventor. In other words, who actually possessed the inventive ingenuity? If a supervisor presents an idea and the experimental approach for reducing it to practice to a laboratory technician, then the invention is the property of the supervisor and not of the technician who merely carried out instructions to reduce it to practice. However, the supervisor who presents the idea without a solution may possibly not be the sole inventor. At times, the actual inventor may be difficult to decide, and the names of more than one inventor may appear on the patent application as joint inventors. Usually, however, an invention is thought to be conceived by a single individual.

Aside from determining who the inventor is, there is the question of who owns the patent. This is a particularly pertinent question, because patents can be of great economic value in addition to the monopoly that they afford, since they can be sold, licensed for a return of royalties, or assigned to an industrial concern or to the federal government. Also, patents are heritable property and can be part of an estate. Research workers employed by an industrial concern often sign contracts stating that they will assign their inventions to the concern so that the resulting patents are actually owned by the concern.

In fact, it is often a condition of employment that such agreements be signed. Problems arise at times when an individual with such a contract invents something "in basement" which may be directly related to the interests of the company, or when the individual utilizes company equipment and facilities to make an invention, whether or not the invention is directly related to the interests of the company. Although there are some ground rules applying to these situations, it still may be difficult to make a fair decision as to actual ownership of such a patent.

A published patent states at the top of its first page the type of ownership that is to be associated with the patent. There are three categories. The first category, in which most patents occur, is that in which commercial rights are retained by the inventor or the concern to which the patent has been assigned, although these rights may be further licensed, assigned, or sold (see Figure 15.1). In the second category are those patents that are assigned to the federal government, for instance, those assigned to the U.S. Department of Agriculture. The assigning of patents to the federal government allows it some control in the licensing of the use of these patents. The last category includes those patents "dedicated to the public". Such patents do not provide a monopoly for any individual or any industrial concern but make the inventions available for all. In regard to this category, the absence of exclusivity for these patents may not provide adequate incentives to invest in the development or marketing of products.

PROTECTION OF THE RIGHTS OF THE INVENTOR: INFRINGEMENT

A patent grant to an inventor confers on that inventor the right to exclude others from making, using, or selling his invention for a period of 17 years from the date of patent issue. In case of "infringement," that is, a violation of these patent rights, the inventor can call on the federal courts for help. In the courts, the inventor may sue the infringer for up to triple damages plus court costs, and the damages include profits that the infringer has accumulated in the practice of the invention. Thus, the infringer has a great deal to lose when he violates the patent rights of others. However, the potential infringer may feel that he has not infringed the subject matter specifically stated in the claims of the patent. Also, he may be able to show that certain of the claims, or all of the claims, are seriously defective so that the patent grant is no valid. If, as a result of these proceedings, certain of the patent claims are declared invalid by the courts, the patent may still be preserved by filing a "disclaimer" with the Patent Office for the faulty claims. Also a "reissue" patent may be granted to correct errors in the patent as originally granted. In certain instances, there are apparent infringements of inventor's rights in which United States courts generally do not enjoin or penalize the infringer. This occurs when someone uses information from the patent claims on an experimental basis, or for private, noncommercial, use. For example, a patent covering a new process for the manufacture of wine might be employed by an individual in his basement to make a small batch of wine for home consumption. While this is technically an infringement, it is difficult to conceive of expensive infringement proceedings being brought against such an individual.

Drugs, pharmaceuticals, and other fermentation products manufactured in a foreign country and imported for use or sale in the United States present special problems. If such products are protected in the United States by a product patent, then importation and use or sale of the product constitute infringement. A specific example can be cited for the antibiotic tetracycline as produced by fermentation in Italy where patent coverage cannot be obtained for pharmaceutical products or processes of manufacture. In this instance, importation and use or sale of tetracycline by American concerns not licensed by the holder of the tetracycline product patent are considered to constitute infringement, although the Italian companies themselves cannot be used.

COST OF A PATENT

The costs for patent application and issuance have recently been greatly increased. Formerly, a fee of $30 was paid to the Patent Office at application and an additional $30 at patent issue. At present, these fees are $65 on filing plus certain extra charges for claims, and $100 on issuance plus $10 for each printed page of specifications. Also, there are additional fees for drawings and appeals, and patent attorney fees may be considerably more. In regard to this point, in rare instances patent attorneys will accept a percentage of royalties from the monies accruing from use of the patent instead of a specific fee. Research personnel for an industrial concern do not pay fees since these are absorbed by the employer as a part of the agreement for assignment of patents. Obviously, the real expenses associated with a patent occur if an infringer is challenged. Nevertheless, usually the high potential monetary returns from a useful patent outweigh all these consideration.

POSSIBLE CHANGES IN UNITED STATES PATENT LAW

As previously stated, over a period of years, various changes have occurred in United States patent law, and further changes are still being considered. For instance, under consideration is a change to grant the patent to the first-to-file rather than to the actual first inventor, a procedure that would totally eliminate patent interferences. Another change would permit the filing of one or more preliminary patent applications prior to the filing of a complete application within one year. In addition, all applications would automatically be published 18 to 24 months from the earliest filing date. Finally, the life of the patent would be for 20 years from the date of filing of the patent application, rather than for the present 17 years from the date of granting of the patent.

PATENTS IN OTHER COUNTRIES

To protect his invention, an inventor may well wish to apply for patents in countries other than the United States. However, this is more complicated than it would seem, because the procedures for application, the structures of patents, and the protection afforded by a patent vary markedly from one country to another, so that separate and differing patent applications must be prepared for each country. Several countries use a "registration" system for filing patent applications instead of the "examination" system employed in the United States. In the registration system, the proper filing of the patent application and payment of government fees automatically result in the granting of a patent. This system is operative in France, Switzerland, Italy, Belgium, Luxemburg, and some other countries. Also, the small and less industrially developed countries utilize this system, because it is simpler and less costly. Some of the countries utilizing the registration system do not require a definite listing of claims, but merely a short resume. Other countries require that the claims be stated, but this is only to help in deciding whether more than one invention is involved. With the registration system, the scope of the patent is not limited by the exact wording of the claims and, if infringement litigation ensues, the entire disclosure is studied in light of prior art. Thus, the registration system for patents makes no decision on scope and validity before granting of the patent, so that these considerations are left to the decision of the courts.

Many countries, excluding the United States and Canada, consider the inventor to be the individual who first files a patent application, and not necessarily the one who first conceives the invention and reduces it to practice. Also, in many countries, the determination of novelty and prior art includes all publication and public use of the invention prior to the date of filing of a patent application. This is in contrast to the one-year grace period allowed to an inventor in the United States between the time of published description or use of an invention and the filing of a patent application.

At present, pharmaceuticals and the microbiological processes for making them cannot be patented in Italy. In contrast, Germany and the Netherlands provide patent grants for processes for making chemicals and pharmaceuticals, but the products themselves cannot be patented.

Most countries other than the United States require the payment of periodic maintenance fees to keep a patent in force. Also, many countries require that a patent actually be used within the country granting the patent if the patent is to stay in force. In fact, if the government feels that the public would benefit from the exploitation of a patent not being used, it may request the granting of a compulsory license to others who are willing to use the invention. In a few countries, a patent may be revoked if not used.

The many variations in patents and patent application procedures make it difficult for an inventor to know how to proceed in obtaining patents in countries other than the United States. However, a summary guide for the inventor may be found in a special report entitled "Common Patents for the Common Market" published in *Chemical and Engineering News* (June 16, 1964, pp. 96–97). In this guide, the following patent considerations are compared for 22 countries: (1) what is considered as prior art, (2) what cannot be patented, (3) language patent written in, (4) type of examination, (5) opposition, (6) life of patent, (7) maintenance fees, and (8) working requirements.

References

Biesterfield, C.H. 1949. Patent *law for lawyers, students, chemists and engineers.* Second Edition. John Wiley and Sons, Inc., New York.

Calvert, R. 1964. *The encyclopedia of patent practice and invention management.* Reinhold Publishing Corp., New York.

Special Report. 1964. Common patents for the common market. *Chem. and·Eng. News.* June 16, pp. 86–98.

U.S. Department of Agriculture. 1952. Patent manual for employees of the U.S. Department of Agriculture, U.S. Department of Agriculture, Washington.

Wise, J.K. 1955. *Patent law in the research laboratory,* Reinhold Publishing Corp., New York.

CHAPTER 16

Fermentation Economics

MARKET POTENTIAL

The ability to produce a fermentation product in high yield is only a part of the requirement for a commercially successful fermentation process. Thus, the product must be sold so as to recover costs along with an acceptable profit. However, in order to sell a fermentation product, there must be a demand, or market, for the product. Two possibilities exist. A market for the product may already exist, because the same or similar product has previously been sold by others. In contrast, a newly discovered fermentation product not previously sold commercially (such as a new antibiotic or food flavoring agent) will require that a market be established. Of course, certain of these new fermentation products also will require approval by the Food and Drug Administration or other agencies before they can be placed on the open market.

Sometimes, a fermentation product cannot be placed on the market because it appears to have relatively few uses and, thus, public demand for the product is either low or nonexistent. Obviously, for such a product, it is often difficult to obtain patent coverage because of an apparent lack of utility. Fermentation products of this type are extensively studied by the fermentation company to find uses for them, and samples may also be sent to other companies on an experimental basis for testing to find whether they might possibly discover uses for the compound. An example of this situation is when a fermentation product is a chemical possessing one to several reactive chemical groups, which might conceivably serve as an intermediate compound for chemical preparation of further commercially valuable products.

For some fermentation products a market already exists, because the product has been previously sold to the public, and the public has found it to be acceptable. This already-available commercial product may be produced either by fermentation, chemical synthesis, or extraction from a natural source. Obviously, if a market already exists, then competition also already exists for the production and sale of the product. The industrial concern newly entering the market with a fermentation product therefore must be able to produce it cheaply enough that it can be sold at or at slightly less than the going price. In other words, the fermentation process and its product must be able to compete on an economically sound basis with similar products already on the market, and this ability to meet competition must apply both at the time of entering the market and at later times when competitors increase their own yields and lower the market price.

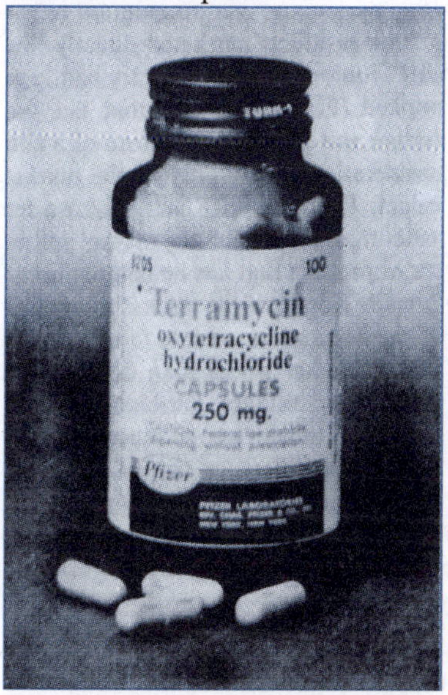

Figure 16.1 Fermentation product which has been packaged and labelled for sale to the public. In this instance, Terramycin is both the trademark and the proprietary name for the product, while oxytetracycline hydrochloride is the generic name. Photo courtesy of Charles Pfizer and Co., Inc.

A fermentation product also may be used internally by an industrial concern so that it is never sold directly to the public. For example, a company that manufactures and sells aspirin might produce salicylic acid by fermentation of naphthalene, followed by a chemical conversion of the salicylic acid to aspirin. Alternatively, a fermentation product may be sold directly to another industrial concern that chemically transforms the fermentation product before sale to the public. Fermentation products sold in this manner do not usually encounter the additional costs of advertising, packaging, and distribution to retail outlets which apply to fermentation products marketed directly to the public. Also, they do not usually require that a proprietary name, generic name, and trademark be applied (Figure 16.1) so that the general public can recognize the product and purchase it instead of a competing product.

Additional considerations also apply to the market potential for a fermentation product. Thus, the price charged for a fermentation product can be no greater than that which the market will bear. In fact, even a patented process or product that has no competition on the open market is not commercially feasible if the price is too great for public acceptance. Obviously, the demand for certain fermentation products allows the charging of much higher prices than does the demand for other fermentation products; for instance, antibiotics for medical use are expensive when compared to vinegar produced by fermentation. This example demonstrates the difference between a fermentation product produced in relatively small amounts, but which has a high sales price and high profit margin per unit sold, and a fermentation product produced in high volume but with a relatively low unit cost of production, sales price, and profit.

The life expectancy of the public demand for a fermentation product is often difficult to predict. Thus, the market for an antibiotic can be short-lived if undesirable but unforseen physiological side reactions show up during mass usage of the antibiotic. An antibiotic may also cease to possess public appeal if a subsequently discovered antibiotic is found to be more efficient in fighting disease. The life expectancy for a fermentation product market also may be short if the latter is protected only by a process patent, since discovery by others of an alternate more economical fermentation process or of an economically competitive direct total chemical synthesis will cause a decrease in demand for the fermentation product. We can see, therefore, that it is possible for what would appear to be an economically sound process to lose its market or provide such a small return from the market that costs of original research and production are not reimbursed and profits do not accrue.

Foreign sales present additional market potential for fermentation products although, obviously, it must first be determined whether a market actually exists abroad for these products. If a market does exist, then there are the alternatives of utilizing production facilities in the United States or in a foreign country. Nevertheless, regardless of where the fermentation product is to be made, there is still the requirement for distribution facilities abroad so that the product can reach its specific markets. In contrast, fermentation products produced in foreign countries may be imported into the United

States to serve as direct competition for American products in the American market. Such a situation involves questions of tariffs and potential patent infringements and, obviously, fermentation products imported from countries with low labor costs markedly affect the market potential for a similar fermentation product produced in the United States.

FERMENTATION AND PRODUCT RECOVERY COSTS

The economic position of a fermentation product is closely tied to the costs associated with its production and distribution. These costs can be placed in several categories, although all sources of costs must be considered.

Medium Constituents

The competitive position and potential profits from a fermentation product are closely tied to the costs of the various components of the production medium. Inoculum medium, while important on a cost basis, is usually less expensive, because less is required, and because it is utilized only to provide rapid cell growth and not to convert a large amount of carbon substrate into microbial cells or fermentation product. In contrast, a single high-cost medium component for the production medium can virtually dictate the selling price for the fermentation product. Obviously, all attempts should be made to find an alternate or a substitute low-cost replacement for such a medium component. Any component of the medium, however, may be subject to marked fluctuations in costs and availability. Thus, the price and availability of cane black-strap molasses because of the world political situation can have a marked effect on the commercial position of a fermentation utilizing this substrate. It is advantageous, therefore, to have at hand an equally good alternate medium for use, should such a situation occur. It must be remembered, however, that the use of an alternate medium sometimes requires the use of a different fermentation microorganism or strain of the organism.

The medium components do not constitute the only source of cost for a fermentation medium. Some media require pretreatment to make them acceptable for microbial growth or fermentation product accumulation. Thus, it may be necessary to remove certain unwanted components from the medium, such as certain metal ions removed by ion-exchange resins.A particular medium component also may require pretreatment so that it is in a form available to the microorganism. Thus, starch must be pretreated with amylase to release fermentable sugars for yeast growth. In the same way, proteins must be degraded by proteolytic enzymes to release amino acids for yeasts. The adjustment of pH values for a freshly made-up medium or at intervals during production requires acid or alkali. These reagents would appear to contribute very little cost to the expense of a medium, but we must remember that considerable reagent may be required for adjusting the pH value of a large volume of medium, particularly if the medium is well buffered by proteins, inorganic salts, or other buffering agents.

The particular composition of a microbial fermentation medium can produce costs not readily apparent from the media component schedule. A medium that has a tendency to foam during air incorporation and impeller action can provide additional cost because of the inherent lower aeration potential for a foaming medium and the markedly increased possibility for contamination. This consideration also applies to a fermentation microorganism that, during growth, produces peptides with foaming characteristics from protein constituents of the medium. A medium that makes fermentation product recovery difficult also adds measurably to the overall fermentation costs, since a high fermentation yield may be meaningless if fermentation product recovery is poor or the expense of product recovery in good yield is great. Thus, medium components should be chosen to obtain the highest possible final recovery of fermentation product and not only just to obtain a high yield of product in the fermentor.

Labor Costs

Labor costs apply to nontechnically and technically trained personnel at all levels of competence; all labor must be considered. This includes labor associated with handling of cultures, inoculum, production, product recovery and purification, maintenance of product sterility (if required), packaging, steam production, equipment maintenance and cleaning, administration, and so forth. These labor costs vary from fermentation to fermentation, and they may be greater for fermentations requiring a prolonged incubation period.

Fermentation Incubation Period

Short incubation-period fermentations usually are less costly, and this applies both to inoculum buildup and to production. Thus, short incubation-period fermentations allow a greater turnover of fermentation equipment; that is, more fermentations can be run in the same equipment during the same period of time. In this regard, it is assumed that at the termination of a fermentation, accessory storage and work-up tanks will be available so that the fermentation tank itself can be drained, since the holding of completed fermentation broth in a fermentor ties up equipment needed for further fermentation runs. As mentioned previously, fermentations requiring long incubation periods provide additional requirements and costs for labor, and they present greater potential for contamination, since contamination is an ever-present hazard.

Contamination and Sterilization

Contamination at more than a minimal level almost always presents additional costs to a fermentation, since most fermentations do not survive serious contamination, and the medium must be discarded. Moderate contamination, however, may not be serious enough to require discarding of the fermentation broth, although fermentation yields may be seriously affected. Certain fermentations are more prone to contamination than others. This applies particularly to those fermentations in which foaming is a problem, the fermentation incubation period is prolonged, the fermentation microorganisms competes only poorly with contaminants for fermentation nutrients, and the fermentation product itself is easily degraded or chemically changed by contaminating organisms. Some fermentations also are more sensitive to phage than are others, and this is particularly true for certain of the bacterial and actino mycete fermentations. Fermentations whose economics do not allow the cost of media sterilization usually provide some type of alternate method for containing contaminant growth. Such methods include low pH of the medium, a substrate poorly amenable to attack by contaminants, partial heat treatment of the medium, and inclusion of specific chemicals to retard contaminant growth. These provision for containing contamination are not foolproof, and thus contamination costs also must be considered for these fermentations.

Fermentations employing microorganisms which, because of their natural state or because of mutation, are genetically unstable may encounter costs similar to those for contaminated fermentations. Thus, a relatively high population of low-yielding cells in a genetically unstable population is analogous to contamination by outside organisms.

Yields and Product Recovery

The ability of a fermentation to produce high yields and to allow good product recovery is a prime consideration in fermentation economics and, in this regard, yields and product recovery must be considered together, since a high yield is of little value if the product cannot be properly recovered for sale. It also is this consideration that allows a fermentation to maintain its competitive position on the open market. Thus, unless a fermentation product is protected by a patent monopoly, the maintenance of a competitive market position probably will require a continuing research program in order to increase the fermentation yields and better the methods of product recovery. Further considerations of fermentation yields and product recoveries are included in Chapter 10 and elsewhere in this book.

Product Purity

Fermentation products are marketed at various levels of purity. At one end of the scale, some products, such as certain antibiotic preparations, must be sterile and free from pyrogens. In contrast, other products, such as exemplified by various other antibiotic preparations, are sold in crude form for mixture with animal feeds. Thus, obviously, the purity level required for the marketing of a fermentation product has a profound effect on the costs associated with that product. Specific fermentation products also may be marketed at more than one concentration as well as level of purity. For example, fermentation lactic acid (Chapter 18) is sold at strengths ranging from approximately 20 to 85 percent and at purity levels ranging from the relatively crude Technical grade to high purity Edible and U.S.P. grades. Each of these grades of lactic acid has a place on the market, and the fermentation lactic acid can be channeled into those forms yielding the greatest overall profits.

Complicated solvent extraction and fractionation procedures, successive recrystallizations, and other requirements for fermentation product purification contribute greatly to the overall costs. This cost is associated not only with the expense of carrying out the various steps of product purification, but also with the fact that small to considerable losses of fermentation product may occur in each step in the purification process.

Overhead

Overhead expenses refer to general expenses incurred in the running of a business. These expenses include rent, taxes, insurance, light, heat, accounting and other office expenses, depreciation, and so forth. These expenses must be considered in the total costs of a fermentation product, but they are not tied to or do not fluctuate to any extent with a particular fermentation.

Waste Disposal

Costs attributable to waste disposal range from a minimal to a major factor in fermentation product costs. A critical consideration in this cost is whether local or municipal waste-treatment facilities will accept the fermentation wastes with or without pretreatment, or whether the fermentation company must maintain its own waste-treatment system. Thus, disposal of fermentation wastes into streams, rivers, or other bodies of water is no longer permissible in many localities because of state and federal regulations. Certain fermentation wastes also require an additional expense of sterilization before discarding; included in this class are wastes from fermentations utilizing plant or animal pathogens as the fermentation organism.

Fermentation wastes include wastes from the actual fermentation, wastes from recovery processes, as well as cleaning and cooling waters. Various of these wastes, particularly cooling waters, can at times be utilized in media makeup for similar or other fermentations. Also, at times it is feasible to recover by-products from the fermentation wastes. These by-products may be either alternate fermentation products present in the harvested culture broth or cells, such as riboflavin from the acetone-butanol fermentation, or they may be spent components from the fermentation medium itself. Thus, "spent grains" from the "mashing" step in the preparation of media for beer brewing are separated by filtration, dried, and sold as cattle feed. Obviously, recovery of economically valuable by-products from a fermentation improves the overall cost and profit picture for the prime fermentation product.

Research Costs

The cost picture of a fermentation process must include those expenses incurred in the research that discovered and developed the process, as well as the research required for the maintenance of a competitive commercial position for the process. These research costs can be considerable, for instance, for those fermentations such as provide new antibiotics where the probability of success in their discovery and development is low. While the costs of research may seem high, it is often the situation that a company cannot afford not to carry out a continuing research program if it is to maintain a competitive position in the market.

There are less tangible research costs that also must be considered in the overall cost picture of a fermentation. Research of this type is more exploratory in nature, and it may not be tied to any specific fermentation product; in fact, it may not be intended to yield a marketable product. This type of research is pursued in the hope that the resulting basic information obtained on the grouth and synthetic activities of microorganisms inorganisms will be of later value in defining areas of exploration and approaches for discovering new fermentation processes and bettering old processes. The costs attributed to this type of research must be absorbed by fermentation processes already in production.

Capital Expenditure

A newly developed fermentation may require an outlay of capital before commercial production can be undertaken. In this regard, the greatest potential requirement for capital expenditure is associated with fermentation equipment and facilities. These are expensive, and they are usually in continuous use for fermentations already in production. Thus, a new fermentation can require the preempting of existing facilities or the construction of additional facilities. A similar situation also holds for product recovery and purification facilities. A newly developed fermentation also may require the installation of unusual or newly designed fermentation equipment. Obviously, installation of this equipment adds greatly to the fermentation costs, and this is especially true if some question exists about the life expectancy of the fermentation in regard to its market position.

Patent Position

A sound patent position (Chapter 15) for a fermentation process or product markedly influences the profit picture. Thus, a sound patent position allows that the price charged for a fermentation product be as high as the market will bear and that extensive commercial competition will not be encountered. This is particularly true for a product patent, although it is assumed that a process associated with a process patent is efficient enough to meet competition by other processes for the same or similar product. Thus, overall, a good patent position provides greater potential for the recovery of costs and the obtaining of an acceptable profit.

The costs associated with obtaining a patent are relatively small. However, patents become costly if infringement proceedings must be initiated. Nevertheless, if infringement is shown, the infringer may have to pay up to triple damages plus court costs.

Patents can yield revenue to the holder by means other than or in addition to the utilization of the patent in the production and marketing of the fermentation product. Thus, the patent can be licensed to other fermentation companies, even to competing companies, for a return of royalties, and the holder of the patent can still produce the fermentation product. In fact, it even is possible that the federal government might require compulsory licensing of the process for use by competitors if it is felt that the benefits of the fermentation product to mankind are great enough that high market prices attributable to the patent monopoly are not beneficial to the general public. An extreme theoretical example of this situation would occur if a patented fermentation product could, with ease, cure all forms of cancer, and the patent holder, realizing the importance of this fact, placed a price on the fermentation product which would allow profits completely out of line with all costs associated with the discovery and production of the product.

At the opposite extreme are patents that really are of little use to the holder. Obviously, nuisance patents fit this category. However, other reasons may be forthcoming. The patent holder may not have the capital or facilities to produce and market the fermentation product. Also the fermentation raw materials may be too costly to the patent holder to allow the fermentation product to compete on the open market, although there may be others who produce and market such fermentation raw materials, or who have these materials as by-products of other processes, and who thus might be in a more favorable position than the holder of the patent to utilize its potential. Thus, in these situations, it may be to the advantage of the patent holder to license the patent without producing the fermentation product, or to sell the patent outright. If there is a demand for the patent, either alternative can yield enough revenue to recover all of the costs discovering and developing the fermentation process and, in addition, to provide an acceptable profit.

PROCESS APPRAISAL

An appraisal of the economic potential for a fermentation process requires that all of the preceding considerations be evaluated both under present and future market conditions. This evaluation should be made as early as possible during process development, as well as at the time of deciding whether to enter the market with the fermentation product. Also, the process should be reevaluated at later dates during commercial production. For these evaluations, it is necessary to estimate present and future availability and price of fermentation substrates, costs of labor and overhead, public demand for the product, competition, potential for bettering yields and product recoveries, and ability and facilities to meet market demands for the product. It is also necessary to consider all present and future costs, profits desired, and a selling price for the product that the market will bear. All of these points are utilized to decide whether the fermentation product can be produced and sold at an acceptable level of profit. If this decision is negative, then the alternatives are to abandon the process, to carry out further research on the process or product recovery, or to license or sell the patent and know-how to others who can produce and market the fermentation product at an acceptable profit level. A great deal of money often is at stake in these decisions; thus, a fermentation company should carefully consider all of the alternative possibilities.

PART III

TYPICAL FERMENTATION PROCESSES

In recent years, many fermentations of potential commercial value have been studied extensively, but of these fermentations only a few actually are practiced at the present time. The existence of a better process (either chemical or microbiological), poor economics, or a lack of demand for the product has prevented the commercial usage of many of these fermentations, although they may in the future be practiced commercially when these conditions have changed. In the following chapters, examples of various types or classes of fermentations are described, and these include those practiced at the present date, as well as those that no longer find commercial application or that have never reached this stage of development. No attempt has been made to describe all of the possible microbial fermentations, since many employ similar organisms and are carried out in a similar manner in similar fermentation equipment. Also, in several instances, little process information is generally available, because of secrecy and a lack of patent disclosure associated with process details. However, several fermentations are described at length, as examples of classic fermentations that have found great commercial use, and as examples of type fermentations or somewhat complex fermentations that may or may not have been reduced to a routine production basis. Other fermentations are described, but in less detail, either because process information is not available, or because many of their basic considerations are common to most microbial fermentation processes.

Chapter 17
Antibiotic Fermentations

The industrial fermentation industry received its greatest impetus for expansion and profits with the advent and exploitation of antibiotics as chemotherapeutic agents. The demand for penicillin during World War II, and later for streptomycin and other antibiotics, brought on the undertaking of intensive research programs designed to find organisms capable of producing good antibiotics, and oriented toward the development of means for producing antibiotics on a large scale. New cultural procedures were devised, and the technique of submerged-agitated-aerated fermentation in deep-tank fermentors came into being. As a result, much of the knowledge gained during the development of anti-biotic fermentation processes then became available for the commercial development of other new nonantibiotic fermentation process not previously possible on a large-scale production basis.

The term "antibiotic" has been defined by Selman Waksman as being an organic compound, produced by one microorganism, that, at great dilution, inhibits the growth of or kills another microorganism or microorganisms. Obviously, this definition does not include materials extracted from green plants or from other nonmicrobial sources, nor does it include organic acids or amines that may inhibit microbial growth, but which are not active at high dilution. An antibiotic may inhibit the growth of or kill one species of organism, a few species, or many types of organisms. However, for any one antibiotic there is a specific group of microorganisms, comprising its "inhibition spectrum," which is sensitive to the antibiotic at therapeutically possible dosage levels. Antibiotics are produced primarily by bacteria, *Streptomyces, Nocardia*, and fungi, although several other classes of microorganisms have at least limited abilities in this area. However, antibiotics produced by *Streptomyces* species have found greatest commercial application, because the ability to produce an antibiotic of some type seems to be a rather common characteristic among these organisms. Many bacteria produce antibiotics, and this is particularly true for bacteria of the genus Bacillus. However, many of the bacterial antibiotics are polypeptides, which have proven generally to be somewhat unstable, toxic, and difficult to purify. Antibiotics produced by fungi, with a few notable exceptions, also generally have been found too toxic for medical use. One obvious exception is the penicillin group of antibiotics produced by various molds. The fact that an antibiotic possesses toxicity, which usually rules out its internal administration to the animal or human body, does not necessarily, however, prevent its medical application, since in some instances the antibiotic can still be used in topical applications, such as for the treatment of burns or skin infections.

The metabolic reactions leading to antibiotic formation usually do not seem to be components of the normal metabolic systems responsible for growth and reproduction of microorganisms. In fact, antibiotic biosynthesis might be regarded as "a series of inborn errors of metabolism" (Hockenhull, 1963) superimposed on the normal metabolism of the organism. Industrial antibiotic fermentation processes have further exaggerated these errors by subjecting the microorganisms to mutagenic agents and to highly nutritious media and growth conditions quite different from those encountered by the organism in its natural habitat. The peculiar metabolic reactions involved in antibiotic formation are reflected in the unusual chemical structures that occur in some antibiotics. For example, antibiotics are known to contain fused rings, rare sugars, and unnatural isomers of amino acids. However, in at least one instance, there seems to be a rationale for the production of an antibiotic by a microorganism, and this occurs with the antibiotic bacitracin, a polypeptide antibiotic containing both D- and L-amino acids, as produced by *Bacillus licheniformis*. This antibiotic is formed by the cells only under conditions that support spore formation and, as such, the antibiotic appears to sever a structural function as a chemical component of the spore coat. These unusual chemical structures observed in many antibiotics have been a boon to the industrial fermentation industry in that, with one exception, these antibiotics have proven difficult, expensive, or even impossible to prepare by chemical synthesis. The notable exception is the antibiotic chloramphenicol produced by *Streptomyces venezuelae*. This antibiotic was first produced commercially by a fermentation process, but later it was found that its chemical structure was relatively simple and amenable to chemical synthesis and, thus, present-day production of this antibiotic is by chemical systhesis.

Antibiotics have found use in medical and veterinary applications, treatment of plant diseases, as an aid in animal nutrition when mixed with feeds or water, and in the preservation of food and other materials. In recent years, however, relatively few new antibiotics have come into commercial production and, in fact, the search for new antibiotic products has been somewhat curtailed. This is due largely to the fact that extensive screening programs have turned up only a few commercially usable antibiotics over those discovered in the 1940's and 1950's, and because any new antibiotic must be better than those already in commercial usage. This is not to say, however, that new antibiotics of great value will not be discovered in the future, although it may be that the approach to discovering valuable new antibiotics may lie in a slightly different direction. Thus, there are many potentially good antibiotics already known which, because of moderate toxicity or some other feature, are not presently usable, and manipulation of the genetic characteristics of the organism, changes in fermentation conditions, or even the use of chemical reactions to alter the structures of the antibiotic molecules might provide a change in the antibiotic that would allow its commercial acceptibility. Such altered chemical structures conceivably could provide an additional valuable feature in that sensitive organisms might be less likely to acquire the antibiotic resistance that is characteristic of some antibiotics after long exposure of the cells.

PENICILLIN

Penicillin, because of the impetus of World War II, was the first antibiotic to be produced on a large scale, and it still is one of the best antibiotics available. It is active against many Gram positive bacteria, *Nocardia*, and *Actinomyces*, but not against most Gram negative forms except at higher dosage levels. It interferes with cell-wall synthesis of sensitive organisms and is active only against growing cells. In addition, it presents the favorable characteristic of being almost nontoxic to mammals, except for certain allergic reactions that develop with a small percentage of individuals.

There actually are several penicillins, all closely related in structure and in activity against sensitive microorganisms. These penicillins have a common chemical nucleus and differ principally in the chemical structure of a side chain attached to this nucleus. The various penicillin fermentations also are unusual in that various compounds resembling the side chains can be added as a precursors to the fermentation medium, and these compounds, through microbial action, are directly incorporated into the penicillin molecule. Also, the side chain can be enzymatically removed, liberating the penicillin nucleus so that unnatural side chains can be chemically added to the nucleus in order to create new penicillins.

Several different fungi are able to produce one or more of the penicillins, although this activity resides chiefly with the aspergilli and penicillia. Today, however, the principal organisms for commercial penicillin production are highly mutated strains of Penicillium chrysogenum (Figure 17.1).

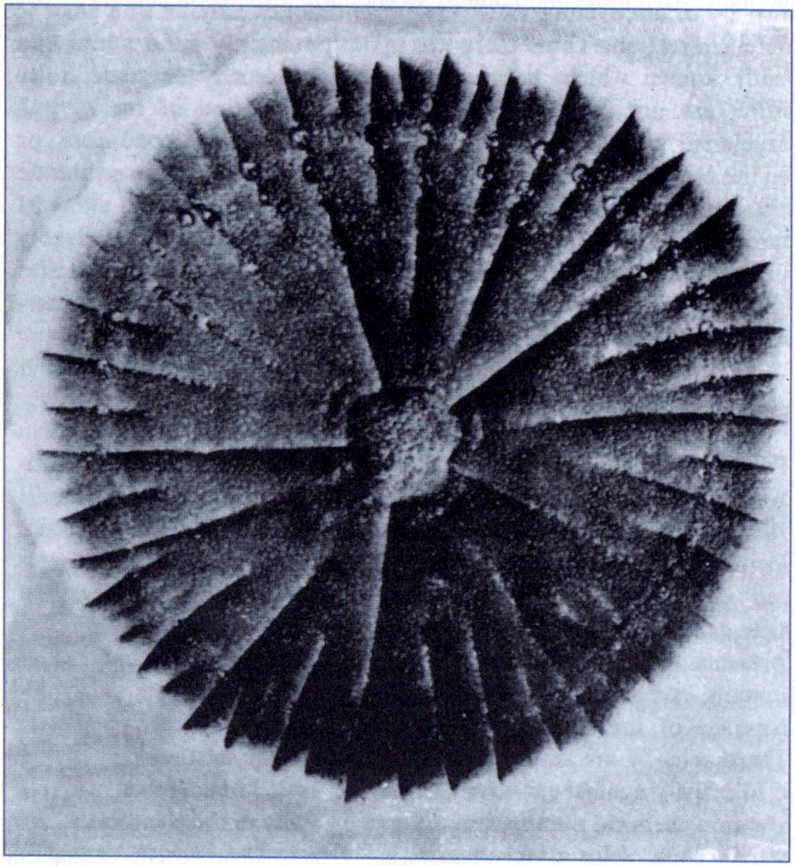

Figure 17.1 Colonial growth of Penicillium chrysogenum. Photo courtesy of Charles Pfizer and Co., Inc.

History

Sir Alexander Fleming, in 1929, first observed the antibiotic properties and possible therapeutic value of penicillin (see Chapter 2). Thus, he observed that an airborne contaminant, later shown to be *Penicillium notatum*, inhibited the growth of a culture of Staphylococcus aureus on agar medium in the area surrounding the fungal colony. Although this phenomenon of antibiosis was well known before this time, all of the microbial principles involved had proven to be toxic to the animal body. Fleming further showed that the inhibitory effect that he observed was caused by a soluble, diffusable, mold product. In addition, he demonstrated that this inhibitory activity could be obtained in concentrated form from the mold culture and that crude preparations were relatively nontoxic to animals. He called this material "penicillin" after the mold that had produced it, Penicillium notatum, and suggested that this material possibly might have therapeutic value. From what is known today, the penicillin observed by Fleming was penicillin F.

Further studies by other workers in the early 1930's showed that penicillin was an organic acid, and that at low pH values it could be extracted by organic solvents from aqueous solutions. However, penicillin was found to be easily destroyed by acidity and heat, and its activity disappeared on evaporation of a solution to dryness. The yields also were quite low, and because of these considerations further studies were abandoned. Nevertheless, penicillin was reinvestigated by the English workers Chain et al, and their studies were published in 1940. These workers grew large batches of Penicillium notatum in stationary surface mat culture to obtain enough culture broth for study. Their experiments with these culture broths showed that, at low temperatures, the antibiotic could be extracted with organic solvents from acidic aqueous solution without extensive destruction, and that an active and reasonably stable salt of penicillin could be prepared as a dry powder. Furthermore, although this preparation was impure, it did demonstrate experimental therapeutic activity. Thus, this study, as well as that of Abraham *et al* (1941), made more attractive the possible industrial production and therapeutic use of penicillin.

The advent of World War II brought a demand for an antimicrobial agent for the treatment of burns and wounds, and this demand spurred both English and American universities and the pharmaceutical industry to cooperate in the development of a penicillin fermentation. Gradually, a large-scale fermentation became operable and, although at the time not economically feasible, it did supply the needs of the military. Nevertheless, as time progressed, rapid advances in process technology, including the development of a deep-tank aerated fermetation, allowed penicillin to become generally available to the public about 1946 and at drastically lowered prices.

During World War II and for a time thereafter, penicillin-producing fungi were studied extensively in order to increase penicillin yields to commercially practicable levels. Fleming's original strain of *Penicillium notatum* as well as other early isolates provided only low yields of penicillin, and these strains responded poorly to submerged culture techniques when these became available. In contrast, an early strain of *Penicillium chrysogenum* (NRRL, 1951), isolated from moldy fruit, was found to provide greater yields of penicillin. This strain was then treated with mutagenic agents, such as X-rays, ultraviolet light, and nitrogen mustard (MBA), so as to allow selection of higher yielding mutants, and the application of these mutagenic agents in sequence, with some repeated treatments finally yielded strain Q-176, which was capable of producing much higher yields of penicillin. Thus, where the NRRL 1951 strain gave approximately 200 units per milliliter, strain Q-176 provided greater than 1000 units per milliliter. However, both the NRRL 1951 and Q-176 strains also produced the yellow, water-soluble pigment, chrysogenin, which provided a yellow tint to the penicillin, and further mutation and selection was required to yield strains that did not produce this pigment. All of these strain-development studies finally culminated with the present-day high-yielding industrial strains for penicillin production, and it should be remembered that all of these strains really are various descendants of strain Q-176.

The mutational approach with mutagenic agents as described above is simple to perform and may yet yield new and better penicillin-producing strains. However, penicillin-producing strains of *Penicillium* are asexual, so that conventional methods of genetic analysis cannot be applied to them. Nevertheless, a form of conjugation known as parasexual recombination can occur, with resultant segregation and recombination of genes. Thus, studies by Roper (1952), Sermonti (1956), and Pontecorvo (1956) have shown that when two genetically different strains of *Penicillium* are grown together, the hyphae of the two strains will fuse at several points. Cells formed from this union contain nuclei from each of the parent fungal strains and, at times, two nuclei situated in close proximity within the cell fuse to form a diploid nucleus. If this diploid nucleus happens to get into a conidium, which is uninucleate, a new strain will be perpetuated. However, diploid nuclei can also divide meiotically to form haploid nuclei possessing different genetic combinations. Using this technique, in the future it thus might be possible to derive new industrial strains of penicillin-producing fungi.

The early studies of penicillin production of penicillin-yielding fungal strains were hampered by a lack of a consistent assay unit for comparison of penicillin yields. The early assays employed an arbitrary unit of activity, the Oxford unit (Figure 17.2), which was the amount of penicillin activity required to prevent growth of *Staphylococcus aureus* over a 24 mm diameter zone using the cylinder-plate method of assay. In 1944, however, an "International Unit" of penicillin activity was established as the amount of penicillin equivalent to 0.6 micrograms of an international standard of crystalline sodium penicillin G of about 98 percent purity. Stated in another way, one milligram of current International Standard sodium penicillin G contains approximately 1665 units of activity. Thus, penicillin activity units can easily be converted to a weight basis.

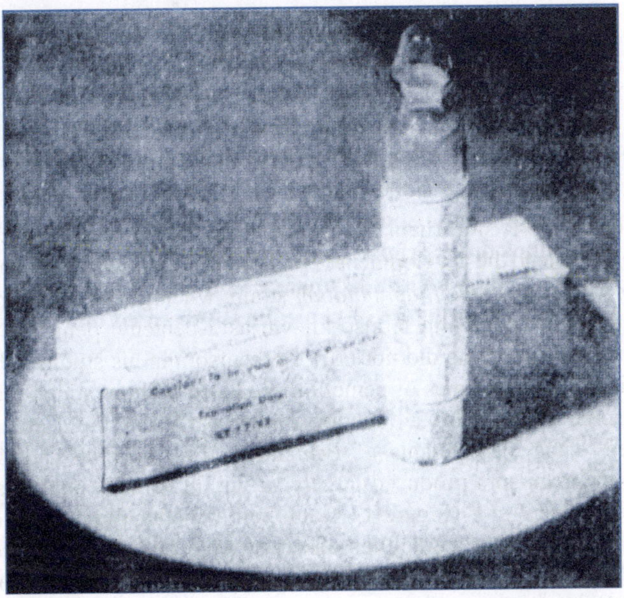

Figure 17.2 Penicillin as produced in 1943; notice the activity as stated in Oxford Units. Photo courtesy of the Upjohn Co.

As the use of penicillin for the therapeutic treatment of disease increased, it became apparent that certain pathogenic microorganisms, particularly *Staphylococcus aureus*, could develop resistance to the antibiotic. Thus, this dilemma spurred research efforts to find ways of producing new and different penicillins that would be active against penicillin-resistant microorganisms. As a result of these studies, 6-amino-penicillanic acid, the chemical nucleus of penicillin, was discovered, followed by the development of procedures for synthesizing new penicillins by adding other side chains to the penicillin nucleus.

Penicillin Molecule and Precursors

Whereas in present-day commercial terms penicillin is regarded as penicillin G, penicillin also is a generic name applied to a group of compounds having the same nucleus and approximately similar anti-biotic activity characteristics against sensitive microorganisms. The various penicillins differ primarily in the nature of their "R" side chains, which are attached by an amino linkage to the chemical nucleus of the molecule. The basic structure of penicillin is presented in Figure 17.3.

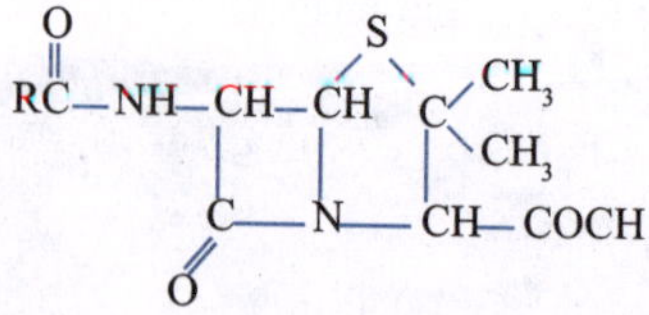

Figure 17.3 Basic structure of the penicillin molecule. The various penicillins differ as to the nature of their "R" sidechains.

Study of the R side chain in relation to the use of precursors has been highly profitable to the development of high-yielding penicillin fermentations. Fleming's original *Penicillium notatum* strain, when grown on his medium, produced largely penicillin F, also known as 2-pentenyl penicillin (Figure 17.4), in part because he did not utilize precursors in his studies. However, the particular type or types of penicillin produced without added precursors are, to some extent, also a function of the particular mold strain being employed. Thus, descendants of *Penicillium chrysogenum* Q-176 in the absence of precursors produced largely penicillin K with smaller amounts of dihydro penicillin F (Figure 17.4) and, on a chemically defined medium lacking precursors, the penicillins observed were mainly F, dihydro F and K. This overall picture was markedly changed, however, when Moyer and Coghill (1946) discovered that the addition of cornsteep liquor to the medium increased the total yields of penicillin and changed the relative amounts of various types of penicillin present. Thus, the use of cornsteep liquor made penicillin G the predominant penicillin as produced by *Penicillium chrysogenum.* This finding had considerable commercial significance, since penicillin G was the desired penicillin, because its pharmacological properties and stability were more acceptable than those of penicillins K, F, and dihydro F. On further study, the cornsteep liquor was found to contain phenylalanine and its breakdown products phenethyl amine and phenylacetic acid. When this was known, it became apparent that phenylacetic acid or other closely related precursors could be added to the medium to direct the mold synthesis toward penicillin G, at the same time minimizing the recovery problem of separating the unwanted penicillins. However, it also was observed that phenylacetic acid was toxic to the mold at low pH values, and that it was readily oxidized (or destroyed) by the mold so that it had to be added slowly or intermittently to the fermentation if it was to be incorporated as the R side

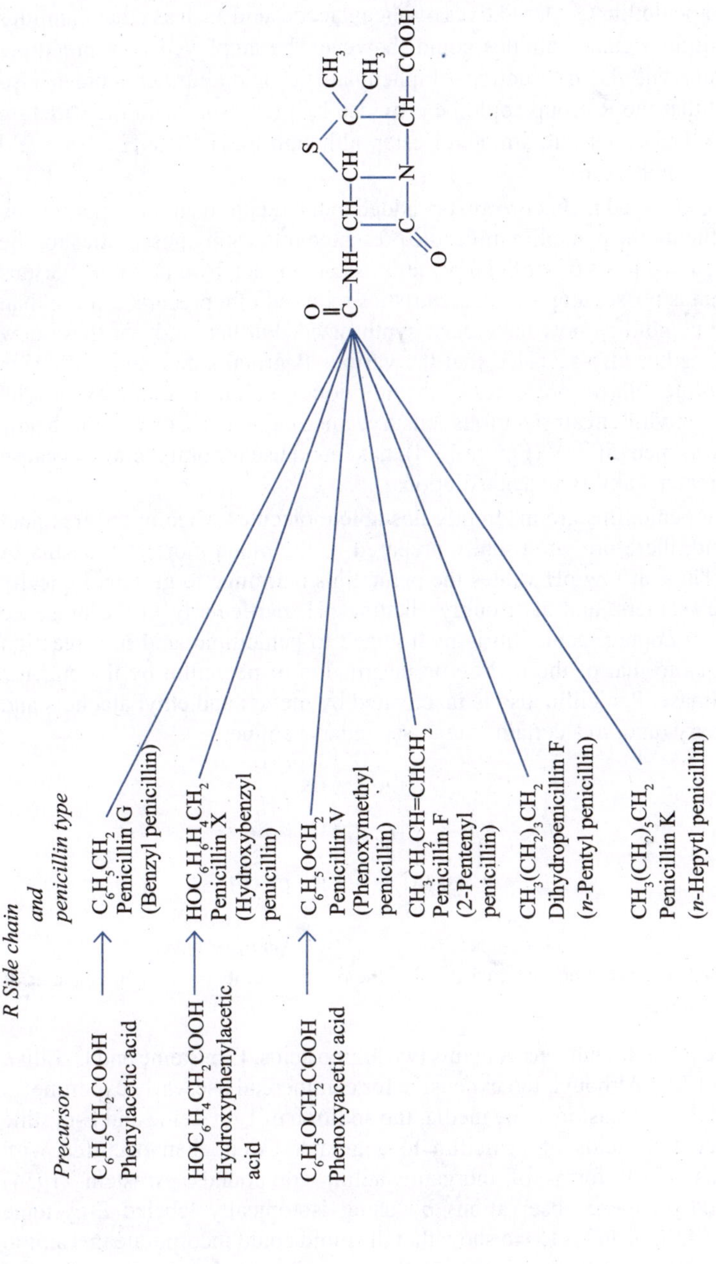

Figure 17.4 Comparison of various penicillins as to precursors and "R" side-chains.

chain of penicillin G. Derivatives of phenylacetic acid such as ethanolamides or substituted ethanolamides could, however, be employed as a precursor to circumvent the destruction of phenylacetic acid. Further studies also showed that the R group could be provided by precursors with the structure RCH_2COOH or its salt, amide, or ester, although $RCH_2CH_2NH_2$ also could serve as a precursor.

The knowledge that precursors added to the medium are incorporated by the mold into the penicillin molecule presented interesting possiblities for the fungal biosynthesis of artificial penicillins and, in fact, by employing various compounds possessing the characteristics required of a precursor, more than 50 new penicillins now have been synthesized. Further study of these new penicillins has also revealed that the various R-group side chains influence the absolute relative potencies of the antibiotics and, to a certain extent, the relative activities against various sensitive microorganisms. One of these new penicillins, penicillin V (Figure 17.4), has found use for oral therapy because of its greater stability in acid solutions.

The penicillins are inherently unstable molecules when in the free acid form and, therefore, are usually prepared as the much more stable salts or esters. Thus, at low pH values the penicillins rearrange to give biologically inactive isomers, and at strongly alkaline pH, particularly in the presence of zinc or copper, penicillin is hydrolyzed to penicilloic acid in a reaction analogous to that of the hydrolytic destruction of penicillin by the enzyme penicillinase. Penicillin also is inactivated by methyl and ethyl alcohols and by primary (and, to a certain extent, secondary) amines.

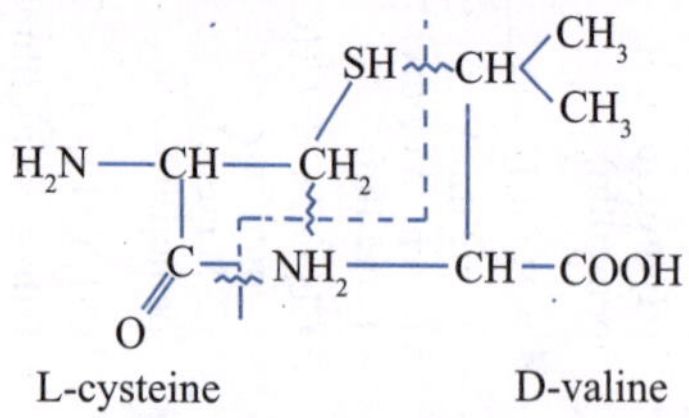

Figure 17.5 The penicillin molecule showing the positions of its component amino acids L-cysteine and D-valine.

The penicilln nucleus contains two amino acids, L-cysteine and D-valine (Figure 17.5). Although too expensive for commercial use, early experiments showed that, at least in some media, the addition of L-cysteine and L-cystine increased the yields of penicillin to a greater extent than occurred with additions of all forms of inorganic sulfur compounds. Arnstein (1954) expanded on these observations by using isotopically labeled L-cysteine (beta-C14, S35, and N15) to show that the mold could incorporate this amino acid directly into the penicillin nucleus. Similar studies by Arnstein and other workers, using isotopically labeled D- and L-valine as well as inhibitor studies, also showed that the carbon skeleton of L-valine is incorporated into the penicillin nucleus, although it may first be deaminated; there is as yet no good explanation for the inversion of the amino group of L-valine during in corporation. Although, as we have seen, Penicillium chrysogenum can incorporate L-cysteine and L-valine directly into the penicillin nucleus, it is considered, nevertheless, that these amino acids as they occur in the penicillin nucleus probably are not utilized as precursors from the medium, but are synthesized by the mold.

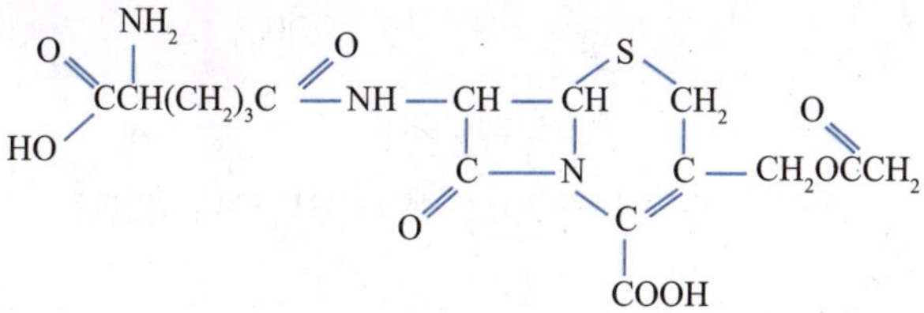

Cephalosporin C

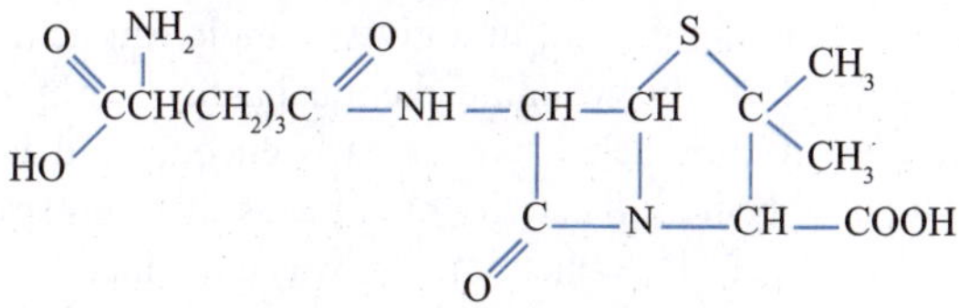

R Cephalosporin N

Figure 17.6 The cephalosporins.

The cephalosporins are antibiotics closely related to the penicillins in chemical structure and antibiotic activity, but they are produced by species of the mold Cephalosporium. Two cephalosporins have been described and studied : Cephalosporin N, also known as Synnematin, and Cephalosporin C (Figure 17.6). Of these, Cephalosporin N is of particular interest, because it is more active than penicillin against various species of *Salmonella*.

Penicillinase

Penicillinase is an extracellular enzyme adaptively produced by members of the coliform group of bacteria, by most *Bacillus* species, and by some strains of *Staphylococcus*. This enzyme hydrolyzes penicillin to penicilloic acid, as shown in Figure 17.7. Most penicillin-resistant pathogenic strains of *Staphylococcus aureus* contain this enzyme and, as such, it is a major factor of penicillin resistance during infection. Also, this enzyme rapidly degrades penicillin in penicillin fermentations if a contaminant that produces the enzyme should gain access to and be able to grow in the fermentation broth.

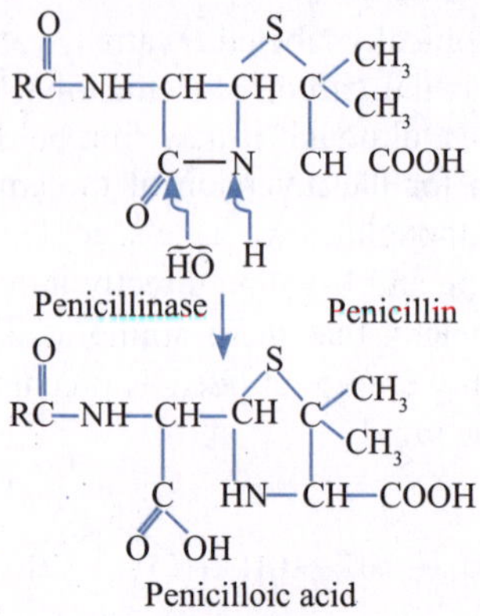

Figure 17.7 The hydrolysis of penicillin to penicilloic acid by the action of penicillinase.

6-Aminopenicillanic Acid

The quantity of penicillin present in a given sample can be determined either by the iodometric or hydroxylamine chemical assays, or by biological assay. The chemical assay approach, however, early encountered difficulty in that the apparent titers of penicillin activity by these assays were greater than those by biological methods. This phenomenon was explained in part when Kato in 1953 reported that something in addition to penicillin in the culture broth was being measured during the chemical assay. He further observed that this substance was produced in penicillin fermentations conducted in the absence of precursor and, since these chemical assays involved only the ring portion of the molecule, he postulated that this material might be the biologically inactive penicillin nucleus without its biologically active R side chain. After this initial discovery, Batchelor etal (1959) were then able to identify this material as actually being the penicillin nucleus, 6-aminopenicillanic acid (Figure 17.8), and to show that this compound was sensitive to the penicillinase enzyme, and that it could be converted to penicillin G by treatment with phenylacetyl chloride. These discoveries were of distinct interest, because they demonstrated that the primary penicillin nucleus, 6-aminopenicillanic acid, was a stable entity present in the culture broth, even though its presence had long gone undetected. Also, these findings allowed a postulation that this compound could be recovered from the fermentation broth and chemically converted to new penicillins by the chemical addition of various R side chains. However, this proved to be more difficult than anticipated, since 6-aminopenicillanic acid, because of its hydrophilic nature, was found to be difficult to isolate from the culture broths. Also, the yields of this material in fermentation broths proved to be relatively low, and it was only with the discovery of the penicillin acylase enzyme, which cleaves the side chain from penicillin, that commercial production of 6-aminopenicillanic acid and the related chemical conversion to new penicillins were accomplished.

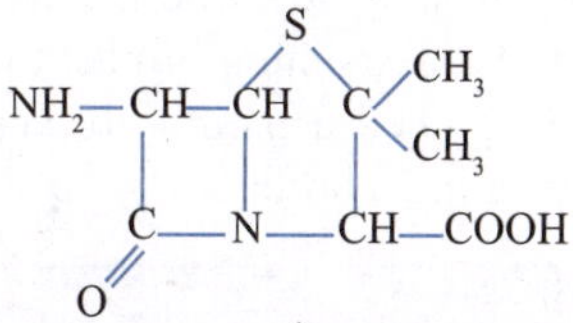

Figure 17.8 6-Aminopenicillanic acid.

Various species of bacteria, *Nocardia, Streptomyces*, and fungi were found to produce extracellular penicillin acylase and, later, it was discovered that *Penicillium chrysogenum* itself produces this enzyme. To prepare new penicillins by this method, partially purified penicillin G is first treated with acylase prepared as a culture filtrate of one of the acylase-producing organisms, and the resulting 6-aminopenicillanic acid is then acylated by chemical means. Of these new penicillins, phenoxyethyl penicillin, phenylglycyl penicillin, 2, 6-dimethoxyphenyl penicillin, and others have found therapeutic use. These semisynthetic penicillins in several instances have proven less sensitive *in vivo* than penicillin G to the penicillinase activity of penicillin-resistant staphylococci, and this consideration has aided in the treatment of infections caused by these organisms.

It is assumed that the 6-aminopenicillanic acid is synthesized by *Penicillium chrysogenum* before addition of the R side chain to the molecule and, in fact, most of the available evidence would tend to support this concept. However, it is also possible that the 6-aminopenicillanic acid present in penicillin fermentations may be attributed, at least in part, to the penicillin acylase activity of *Penicillium chrysogenum* during the fermentation splitting the R side chain from the normal penicillin product of the fermentation.

Penicillin Production

Penicillin was first produced commercially in stationary mat culture. However, with this technique, the penicillin yields suffered from the problems commonly associated with this type of culture: oxygen penetrates only poorly into the mycelial mat; that portion of the mycelium submerged in liquid is deficient in oxygen; and the aerial hyphae have only poor access to nutrients. The medium was sterilized in shallow layers in bottles, flasks and trays or pans made of metal or glass. Large numbers of wet or dry spores were added as inoculum to this medium or blown onto its surface, and the cultures were incubated at 24 to 28°C for six or seven days (Figures 17.9 and 17.10). Obviously, penicillin production by this procedure required large amounts of equipment and labor. At harvest, the broths from these stationary cultures were pooled for recovery of the penicillin, but any broths contaminated by penicillinase-producing organisms had to be first separated and discarded. Thus, if not separated from the remaining broths, the penicillinase in these cultures destroyed all of the pooled penicillin, because the enzyme activity survived in the pooled or combined broths.

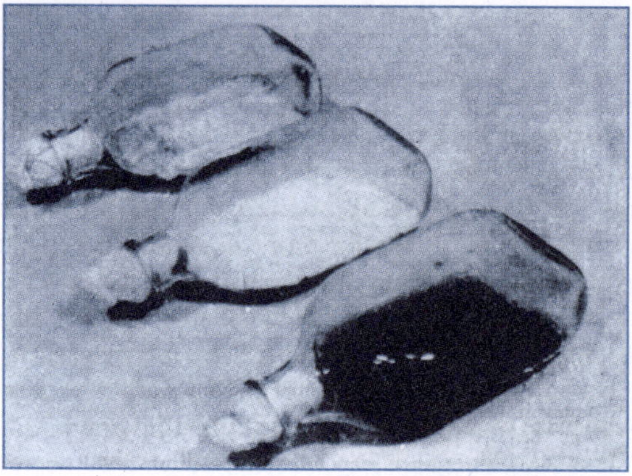

Figure 17.9 Mat-culture production of penicillin in bottles during World War II. Photo courtesy of the Upjohn Co.

At this time, there also was some commercial use of stationary mat replacement culture for penicillin production. This procedure was attractive, because the yields in the replacement medium attained maximum levels several days earlier than in the growth medium.

Deep-tank aerated fermetations for penicillin production were developed during World War II and, although both the surface and deep-tank processes were employed simultaneously for a while, it soon became apparent that the deep-tank process was the most promising from a commercial viewpoint. However, many problems were encountered in the design of fermentors, sterilization of air, and so forth and, in addition, the shift to submerged-aerated fermentations required strains of *Penicillium* with characteristics different from those employed in stationary mat culture. These problems, nevertheless, were successfully solved for penicillin production, and the methods developed proved to be applicable for later fermentations of other types.

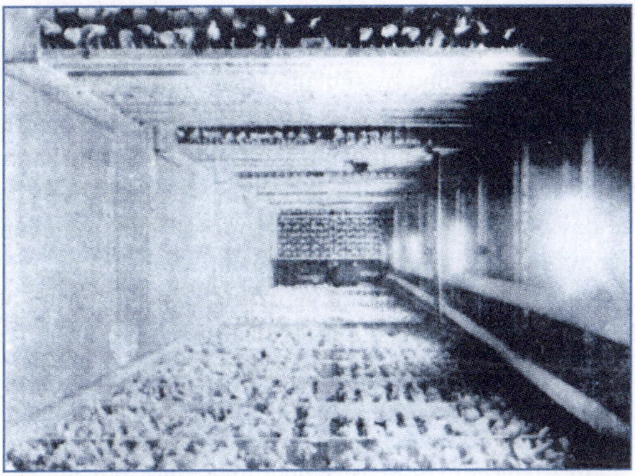

Figure 17.10 Incubation room for mat-culture penicillin production in bottles, as in Figure 17.9. Photo courtesy of the Upjohn Co.

Stock culture maintenance procedures for high-yielding strains of *Penicillium chrysogenum* required serious study, because these high-yielding strains proved to be genetically unstable and, in fact, the higher the yield capacity, the more unstable is the strain. As a result of these investigations, it has been found that frequent transfers of the mold on agar medium tend to select for those portions of the natural population which sporulate profusely, although heavy sporulation is not necessarily associated with high penicillin yields. Therefore, agar media are chosen to allow minimum vegetative growth with rapid sporulation of the entire culture, and these media are inoculated with high levels of spores. In addition, cultures maintained on agar slants are transferred as infrequently as possible. The primary stocks for these organisms are maintained by one of three methods: a well-sporulated agar slant is frozen, soil stocks are prepared and stored at 2 to 4°C, or the spores are lyophilized.

For inoculum production, spores from heavily sporulated working stocks (special agar sporulation media) are suspended in water or in a dilute solution of a nontoxic wetting agent, such as 1:10,000 sodium lauryl sulfonate. These spores then are added to flasks or bottles of wheat bran plus nutrient solution, and these are incubated five to seven days at 24°C so as to provide heavy sporulation. The resulting spores are used directly to inoculate inoculum tanks or, in some instances, they are pregerminated in a separate medium to provide a mycelial inoculum. The inoculum tanks are incubated 24 to 48 hours with agitation and aeration in order to provide heavy mycelial growth, and the resulting inoculum is used for a production tank, or it is added to a second- or even a third-stage inoculum tank to produce inoculum for larger-scale fermentations. Contamination in the inoculum tanks is tested both by microscopic observations and by subcultures to broth medium.

The production tanks are inoculated by employing air pressure to force 10 percent by volume of inoculum into the tank. The actual penicillin fermentation is incubated at approximately 25 to 26°C for approximately three to five days, although the exact duration of the fermentation depends on various factors, such as the particular fungal strain employed, the type of production medium, the aeration and agitation conditions, and other factors peculiar to the particular production facility carrying out the fermentation. However, within any one production plant, considerable effort is made to provide repeatable production times so that efficient scheduling of production facilities and labor can be maintained. During production, periodic samples are removed for determinations of penicillin yields and for contamination checks. This contamination test is particularly important, because penicillin fermentations are quite sensitive to contamination by penicillinase-producing organisms.

The exact compositions of those penicillin production media actually used in industry are difficult to determine, because these media are considered to be trade secrets. However, most of these media probably are somewhat similar. A typical medium described by Jackson (1958) contains cornsteep liquor solids, 3.5 percent; lactose, 3.5 percent; glucose, 1 percent; calcium carbonate, 1 percent; potassium dihydrogen phosphate, 0.4 percent; edible oil, 0.25 percent, and penicillin precursor. However, under high aeration and agitation conditions, the lactose content of this medium can be increased to 4 or 5 percent. The pH of this medium after sterilization is 5.5 to 6. A typical production medium, as described by Sylvester and Coghill (1954), is composed, per liter, of cornsteep liquor solids, 30 g; lactose, 30 g; glucose, 5 g; sodium nitrate, 3 g; magnesium sulfate, 0.25 g; zinc sulfate, 0.044 g; calcium carbonate, 3 g; and phenyl acetamide precursor, 0.05 g. As noted later, these media probably have undergone considerable change to increase yields and meet economic changes.

Inoculum media are similar to production media, except that lactose and precursor are not included. Glucose or sucrose serve as the carbon source because, during the development of the inoculum, growth and not penicillin production is desired.

The course of a typical penicillin fermentation is presented in Figure 17.11. As may be seen, in general, the pH remains constant at the start of the fermentation while the glucose, cornsteep liquor carbon compounds, and ammonia are being utilized. As these carbon compounds become depleted, and as some of the lactic acid of the cornsteep liquor is being used, ammonia is liberated by deamination of the amino acids of the cornsteep liquor, and the pH rises to 7 to 7.5, the optimum pH range for penicillin production. Beyond this point the pH remains constant, the mold uses the lactose to produce penicillin, and very little further growth occurs, because the mold actually is being starved at this point. At the end of the fermentation, the pH rises to 8 or higher, because depletion of the lactose brings on autolysis of the mycelium. However, usually the penicillin fermentation is harvested before this phase.

During the initial stage of carbohydrate and cornsteep liquor utilization (that is, during the first 20 to 30 hours), the fungal growth becomes very thick and heavy. This growth occurs as disperse strands or clumps of mycelium or as definite pellets of mycelium, 0.5 to 2 mm in diameter.

Penicillin yields with time are linear from approximately 48 to 96 hours, although the yields depicted in Figure 17.11 have occurred more quickly. The final penicillin yield is in the approximate range of 3 to 5 percent based on carbohydrate consumed and is probably in excess of 1500 units per milliliter. Sylvester and Coghill (1954) have estimated that "to produce 1000 gallons of fermented culture (5 to 6 lbs of penicillin) by the submerged-culture process requires approximately 500 lbs of nutrients, 7500 lbs of steam, 10,000 gallons of water, 1000 kwh of electricity, and 250,000 cu ft of air."

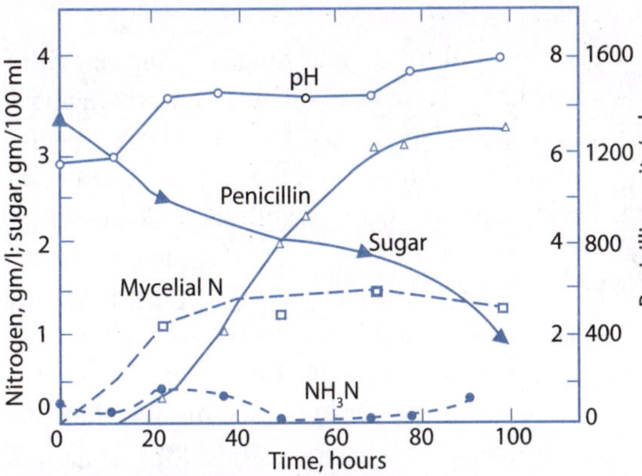

Figure 17.11 Chemical changes in a typical penicillin fermentation with added phenylacetic acid. (Brown and Peterson. 1950. Ind. Eng. Chem., 42, 1773. Copyright 1950 by the American Chemical Society and reprinted by permission of the copyright owner).

The pH picture during the penicillin fermentation is critical since, as previously noted, penicillin is sensitive to low pH values. However, penicillin also is sensitive to pH values above 7.5, especially in the presence of ammonium ion. Because of these considerations, during the stage of actual penicillin production, the pH is maintained near neutrality by calcium and magnesium carbonates in the medium and by the phosphate buffer. A rise in pH value is less of a problem since, during this period, little ammonia is being liberated to raise the pH values. However, in addition, the pH may be controlled by adding either sodium hydroxide or sulfuric acid.

As in evident to this point, the medium constituents have a profound effect on penicillin yields. The cornsteep liquor provides peptides, amino acids, and amines which are deaminated to provide the ammonia required in the early stages of the fermentation, as well as some of the carbon nutrients. The glucose is rapidly utilized to provide mycelial growth but allows very little penicillin production. The lactose, however, is only slowly degraded to glucose plus galactose, and it is this slow glucose availability from the lactose that allows the starvation conditions required for penicillin production. In fact, a series of publications by Johnson and his coworkers (Hosler and Johnson, 1953; Soltero and Johnson, 1953; and Davey and Johnson, 1953) has shown that penicillin yields equivalent to those with lactose can be obtained from glucose alone, if the glucose is added only slowly to the fermentation as required by the mold. In this regard, it is probable that with the relatively lower cost of commercial glucose today, a carbohydrate regimen somewhat similar to that described above, in fact, may be commercially employed in penicillin production.

Lipid nutrients also are utilized by the fungus during penicillin production, and fatty oils, such as lard oil, soybean oil, and linseed oil, and fatty acids of greater than 14 carbon chain lengths and their esters are especially effective. Some of the oil is added as antifoam, and the rest is purposely added directly to the medium. These nutrients increase both the amounts of mycelium and yields, but high levels can be deleterious in both early and late stages of the fermentation. Also, these nutrients can provide too great an acidity, but this is usually neutralized by the calcium carbonate of the medium. These oils probably are degraded by the fungus to the two-carbon acetate or similar compound level before being used in formation of mycelium and penicillin.

Various synthetic media have been developed for penicillin production, and it has been claimed that these media provide penicillin yields equivalent to those form a medium containing cornsteep liquor (Jarvis and Johnson, 1947; and Calam and Hockenhull, 1949). Obviously, such media are far too expensive for their industrial use in the production of penicillin, but they have been of value in studies on the mechanisms and factors involved in penicillin production.

Penicillin Harvest and Recovery

Penicillin in the acid (anion) form is solvent extractable, and the antibiotic, as dissolved in an organic solvent, can be back-extracted as a salt into aqueous solution. These considerations, in general, are made use of for the

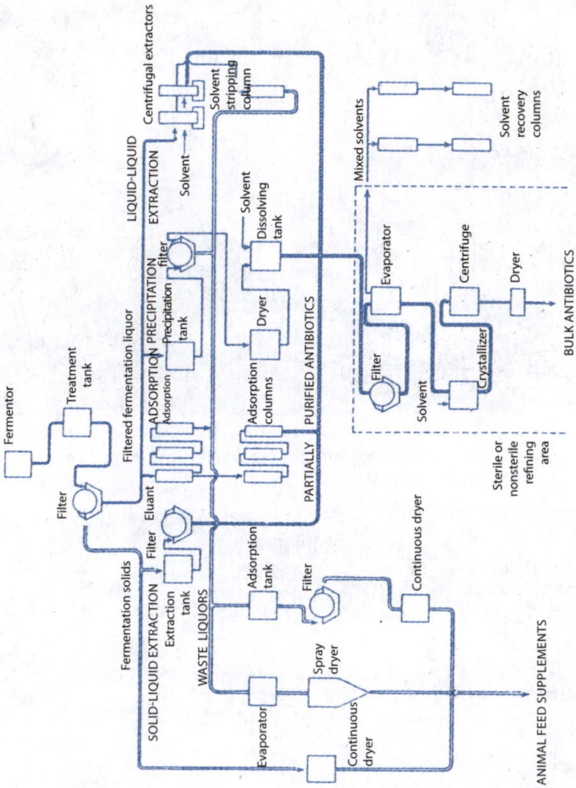

Figure 17.12 Basic flowsheet for the commercial recovery and purification of antibiotics. Photo courtesy of Charles Pfizer and Co., Inc.

recovery and purification of penicillin from harvested culture broths, although the exact procedures to be used depend somewhat on the particular production medium employed and on the final penicillin yields in this medium. Obviously, high yields in conjunction with a medium that does not interfere with recovery and purification greatly simplify the procedures required to obtain a pure product. A general flowsheet for the commercial recovery of antibiotics is presented in Figure 17.12 although, as will become apparent, the recovery of penicillin does not require all of the steps presented. Figure 17.13 is an overall view of a commercial antibiotic recovery plant.

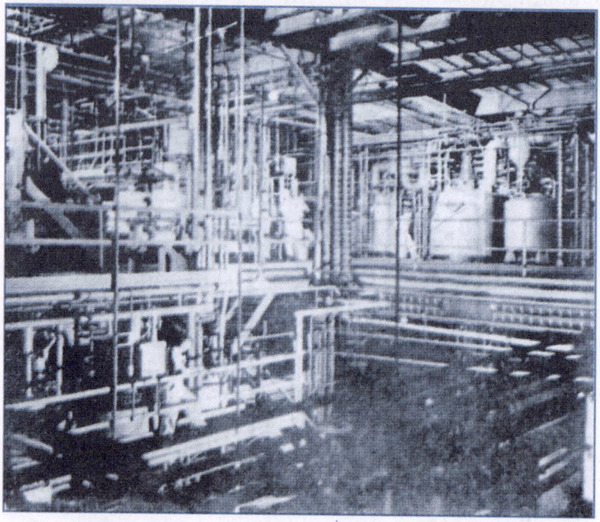

Figure 17.13 Overall view of the interior of a commercial antibiotic recovery plant. Photo courtesy of Charles Pfizer and Co., Inc.

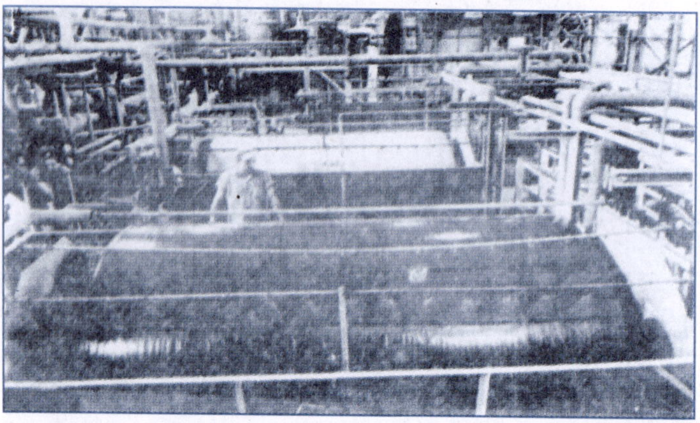

Figure 17.14 Rotary vacuum filter for the filtration separation of mycelium from antibiotic culture broths. The mycelium collects on the outside of the drum as the broth is sucked through the filter; see Figure 17.15. Photo courtesy of Charles Pfizer and Co., Inc.

To be more specific, at harvest, the completed penicillin fermentation culture is filtered on a rotary vacuum filter (Figures 17.14 and 17.15) to remove the mycelium and other solids although, under the right conditions,

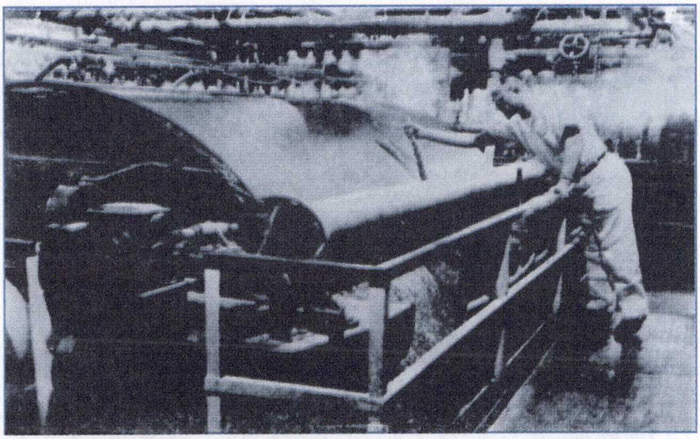

Figure 17.15 Rotary vacuum filter with caked mycelium and other solids being scraped from the filter. Photo courtesy of Charles Pfizer and Co., Inc.

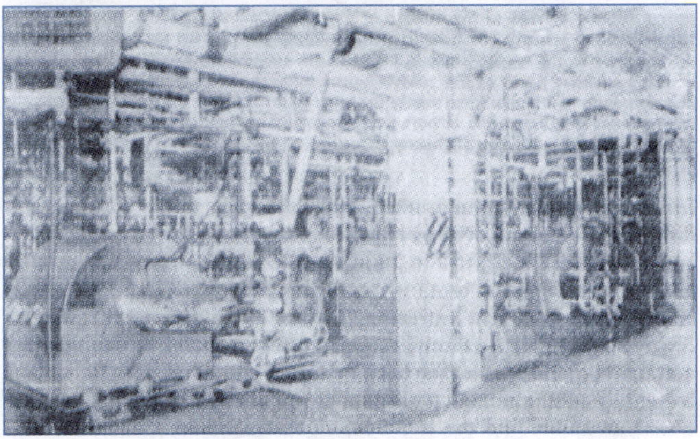

Figure 17.16 Podbielniak counter-current extractors. Photo courtesy of the Podbielniak Division of Dresser Industries.

this may not even be required. Phosphoric or sulfuric acids are added to lower the pH to 2 to 2.5 in order to convert the penicillin to the anionic form, and the broth is immediately extracted in a Podbielniak countercurrent solvent extractor (Figures 17.16 and 17.17), with an organic solvent such as amyl acetate, methyl isobutyl ketone, or butyl acetate. The penicillin is then back-extracted into water from the organic solvent by adding enough potassium or sodium hydroxide to form a salt of the penicillin, and the resulting aqueous solution is again acidified and reextracted with methyl isobutyl ketone. These shifts between water and solvent aid in purification of the penicillin. The solvent extract finally is carefully back-extracted with aqueous potassium or sodium hydroxide, but more often with sodium hydroxide, and from this aqueous solution various procedures are utilized to cause the penicillin to crystallize as sodium or potassium penicillin (Figure 17.18). The resulting crystalline penicillin salt then is washed and dried, and the final product must pass rigorous government standards. Spent solvents resulting from the above procedures are recovered for reuse (Figure 17.19).

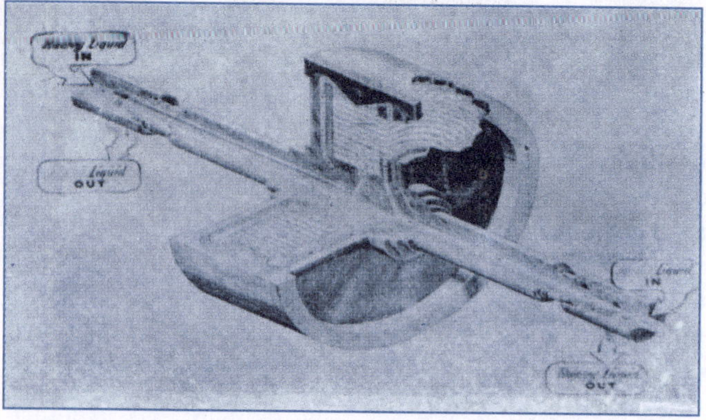

Figure 17.17 Diagram illustrating the flow of fluids through a Podbielniak counter-current extractor. The antibiotic broth is admitted near the center of the spinning rotor and the lighter solvent to the outside of the rotor. Centrifugal force then moves the antibiotic broth towards the outside of the rotor, in the process displacing the lighter solvent towards the center. Thus, in the rotor the antibiotic is extracted by the solvent from the aqueous phase as the solvent moves through the aqueous phase. Also, each phase through centrifugal force rejects the other as it exits from the rotor. This apparatus will function even when one or both phases contains suspended solids. Photo courtesy of the Podbielniak Division of Dresser Industries.

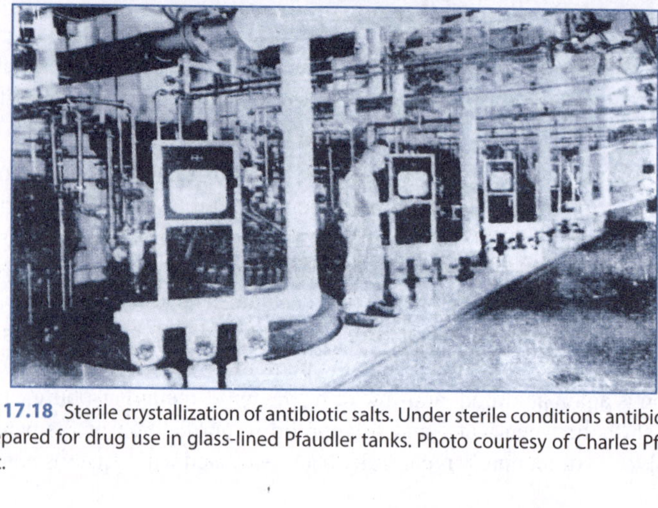

Figure 17.18 Sterile crystallization of antibiotic salts. Under sterile conditions antibiotic salts are prepared for drug use in glass-lined Pfaudler tanks. Photo courtesy of Charles Pfizer and Co., Inc.

Continuous Fermentation

At first glance, the penicillin fermentation might seem ideal for application of continuous fermentation techniques. However, a major problem is encountered because, during active penicillin production on lactose, there is very little accompanying mycelial growth with the result that culture withdrawn for harvest rapidly depletes the mycelium levels in the fermentation, because the mycelium does not grow rapidly enough to replenish the mycelium that has been removed. As a solution, Jackson (1958) has suggested the use of two fermentors in series for a continuous fermentation. The first fermentor would be used for the growth of mycelium and would utilize glucose and a higher incubation temperature. Mycelium withdrawn from this fermentor would then be added to a second fermentor containing a lactose medium, and penicillin would be produced in this fermentor. Actual trials of this continuous fermentation procedure, however, have provided lower yields than might have been expected. Other studies on continuous antibiotic fermentations are presented in Chapter 13.

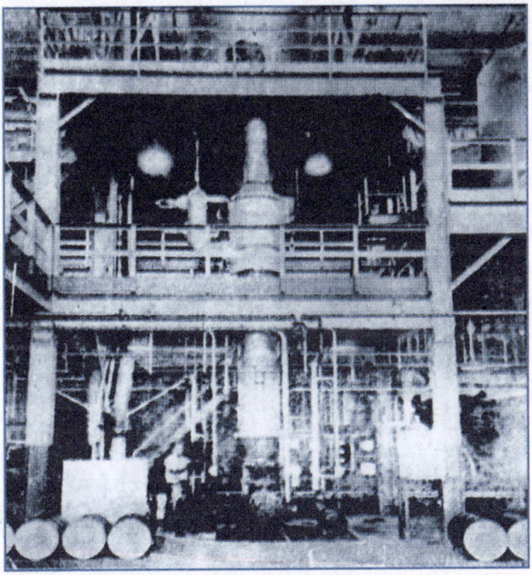

Figure 17.19 Evaporators for recovery of solvents. Photo courtesy of Charles Pfizer and Co., Inc.

Waste Disposal

Wastes from penicillin production provide high BOD and can present serious problems in their disposal as well as expense to the industry. These wastes include spent mycelium, extracted broth, wash waters, and residual organic solvents in the fermentation broths and waters. The possibilities for the handling of these wastes depend on the geographical location of the production plant, and among the various possibilities are the following. Aqueous fractions can be discharged to sanitary sewage systems, if the municipal treatment plant can handle these wastes. The mycelium can be dried for use as a feed supplement, and the extracted broth can be combined with the mycelium before drying. Alternatively, the mycelium may be buried in the ground. Liquid wastes also can be evaporated and buried or they can be treated by special sewage disposal plants maintained by the fermentation company.

References

Penicillin

Abraham, E.P., E. Chain, C.M. Fletcher, A.D. Gardner, N.G. Heatley, M.A. Jennings, and H.W. Florey. 1941. Further observations on penicillin. *Lancet,* **2,** 177–188, 189.

Arnstein, H.R.V., and P.T. Grant. 1954. The incorporation of cystine into penicillin. *Biochem. J.*, **57,** 360–368.

Batchelor, F.R., F.P. Doyle, J.H.C. Nayler, and G.N. Rolinson. 1959. Synthesis of penicillin: 6-aminopenicillanic acid in penicillin fermentations. *Nature*, **183,** 257–258.

Brown, W.E., and W.H. Peterson. 1950. Factors affecting production of penicillin in semi-pilot plant equipment. *Ind. Eng. Chem.,* **42,** 1769–1774.

Calam, C.T., and D.J.D. Hockenhull. 1949. The production of penicillin in surface culture, using chemically defined media. *J. Gen. Microbiol.,* **3,** 19–31.

Chain, E., H.W. Florey, A.D. Gardner, N.G. Heatley, M.A. Jennings, J. Orr-Ewing, and A.G. Sanders. 1940. Penicillin as a chemotherapeutic agent. *Lacet,* **2,** 226–228.

Clarke, H.T., J.R. Johnson, and R. Robinson. 1949. *The chemistry of penicillin.* Princeton University Press, Princeton.

Davey, V.G., and M.J. Johnson. 1953. Penicillin production in cornsteep media with continuous carbohydrate addition. *Appl. Microbiol.,* **1,** 208–211.

Demain, A.L. 1959. The mechanism of penicillin biosynthesis. Adv. Appl. *Microbiol.,* **1,** 23–47.

Erickson, **R.** C., and R.E. Bennett. 1965. Penicillin acylase activity of *Penicillinum chrysogenum. Appl. Microbiol.,* **13,** 738–742.

Fleming, A. 1929. On the antibacterial action of cultures of a penicillium, with special reference to their use in the isolation of *B. influenzae. Brit. J. Pathol.,* **10,** 226–236.

Hockenhull, D.J.D. 1959. The influence of medium constituents on the biosynthesis of penicillin. Pp. 1–27 in *Progress in industrial microbiology,* vol. 1 (ed. D.J.D. Hockenhull). Interscience Publishers, Inc., New York.

Hockenhull, D.J.D. 1963. Antibiotics. Pp. 227–299 in Biochemistry of industrial micro-organisms (ed. C. Rainbow and A.H. Rose). Academic Press, New York.

Hosler, P., and M.J. Johnson. 1953. Penicillin from chemically defined media. *Ind. Eng. Chem.,* **45,** 871.

Jackson, T. 1958. Development of aerobic fermentation processes. Pp. 183–221 in *Biochemical engineering* (ed. R. Steel). Heywood & Co., Ltd., London.

Jarvis, F.G., and M.J. Johnson. 1947. The role of the constituents of synthetic media for penicillin production. *J. Am. Chem. Soc.,* **69,** 3010–3017.

Kato, K. 1953. J. *Antibiotics, Japan, Ser. A.,* **6,** 130, 184.

Moyer, A.J., and R.D. Coghill. 1946. Penicillin. VIII. Production of penicillin in surface culturers. *J. Bacteriol.,* **51,** 57–58.

Moyer, A.J., and R.D. Coghill. 1946. Penicillin. IX. The laboratory scale production of penicillin in submerged culture by *Penicillium notatum* Westling (NRRL 832). J. Bacteriol., **51,** 79–93.

Pontecorvo, G. 1956. The parasexual cycle in fungi. *Ann. Rev. Microbiol.,* **10,** 393–400.

Prescott, S.C. and C.G. Dunn 1959. *Industrial microbiology.* 3rd Ed. pp. 770–784. McGraw-Hill Book Co., Inc., New York.

Roper, J.A. 1952. Production of heterozygous diploids in filamentous fungi. *Experientia,* 8, 14–15.

Rose, A.H. 1961. *Industrial microbiology.* Pp. 204–208. Butterworths, Washington.

Sermonti, **G.** 1956. Complementary genes with affect penicillin yields. *J. Gen. Microbiol.,* **15,** 599–608.

Soltero, F.V., and M.J. Johnson. 1953. The effect of the carbohydrate nutrition on penicillin production by *Penicillium chrysogenum* Q-176. *Appl. Micrbiol.,* 1, 52–57.

Sylvester, J.C., and R.D. Coghill. 1954. The penicillin fermentation. pp. 219–263 in *Industrial fermentations,* vol. II (ed. L.A. Underkofler and R.J. Hickey). Chemical publishing Co., Inc., New York.

STREPTOMYCIN

Streptomycin (Figure 17.20) is produced by *Streptomyces griseus*. It is particularly active against Gram-negative bacteria and against the tuberculosis organism *Mycobacterium tuberculosis*, although it also has some activity against other Gram-positive bacteria and has been used therapeutically in the treatment of infections caused by organisms resistant to penicillin. Streptomycin, in addition, finds use in the treatment of plant diseases caused by bacteria, because the antibiotic is active systemically in plants. In man, prolonged streptomycin treatment at high dosage can produce neurotoxic reactions, and particularly problems in balance maintenance and partial hearing loss. Chemical reduction of streptomycin to dihydrostreptomycin (Figure 17.20) decreases this neurotoxicity, and for this reason much of the streptomycin produced today is as the latter form. Some microorganisms gain resistance relatively easily to streptomycin, and streptomycin therapy, therefore, is often carried out in conjunction with para-aminosalicylic acid or isoniazid (isonicotinic acid hydrazide) to decrease this resistance buildup in sensitive microorganisms.

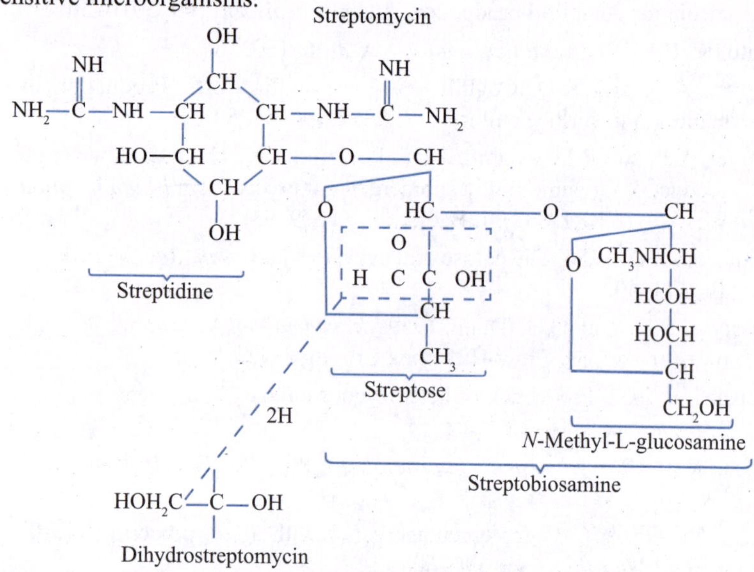

Figure 17.20 The streptomycin molecule. Dihydrostreptomycin is prepared, as shown, by the chemical reduction of the carboxyl group on the streptose moiety.

Streptomycin was discovered by Schatz, Bugie, and Waksman (1944), and one of their original soil *Streptomyces griseus* isolates (No. 18–16) was a parent of most of the industrial strains used today. Thus, mutation and selection and selection were employed to increase yields to the present-day levels. So far as is known, streptomycin is produced only by *Streptomyces griseus*, and only a few strains of this organism have the ability to produce reasonable yields of the antibiotic.

Chemical Structure

Streptomycin and dihydrostreptomycin are basic compounds (Figure 17.20) and, therefore, they are usually prepared as salts. Thus, streptomycin is available as the hydrochloride $C_{12}H_{39}O_{12}\cdot 3HCL$, as a crystalline hydrochloride double salt with calcium chloride, or as the phosphate or sulfate, and dihydrostreptomycin as the hydrochloride or sulfate. One unit of streptomycin activity, however, is equivalent to one microgram of the free base. In addition to the streptomycin of commerce, other forms also occur as fermentation products of *Streptomyces griseus*. Thus, depending on the strain of this organism being used or on the production medium, small amounts of mannosidostreptomycin or hydroxystreptomycin are accumulated in addition to the streptomycin. Also, in a normal streptomycin fermentation, some mannosidostreptomycin is produced early in the fermentation, but this antibiotic is largely enzymatically degraded by *Streptomyces griseus* to streptomycin by the time of harvest. The mannosidostreptomycin is not desired because of its low antibiotic activity.

The use of precursors does not increase yields of streptomycin. Thus, most of the carbon of the streptomycin molecule has been shown to originate from glucose and not from the more complex carbon compounds of the medium, although some of the carbon of the molecule does originate from carbon dioxide. The carbonyl function on the streptose moiety is somehow involved in the antibiotic activity of streptomycin. This is concluded from the fact that most chemical additions to this carbonyl group destroy the antibiotic activity.

Production

Most of the media for the commercial production of streptomycin are somewhat similar. Woodruff and McDaniel (1954) described a medium containing 1 percent soybean meal, 1 percent glucose, and 0.5 percent sodium chloride. Hockenhull (1963) considered a typical industrial medium to contain 2.5 percent glucose, 4 percent extracted soybean meal, 0.5 pecent distillers dried solubles, 0.25 percent sodium chloride, and a pH of 7.3 to 7.5 before sterilization.

High-yielding, mutated strains of *Streptomyces griseus* are genetically unstable, a fact to be considered in maintenance of stock cultures. Because of this consideration, spores of the organism usually are maintained as soil stocks, or are lyophilized in a carrier such as sterile skim milk. The spores from these stock cultures are then transferred to a sporulation medium to provide enough sporulated growth to initiate liquid culture buildup of mycelial inoculum in flasks or inoculum tanks.

Streptomycin yields in production fermentors respond strongly to high aeration and agitation. The optimum fermentation temperature is in the range of 25 to 30°C, probably closer to 28°C and the optimum pH range for streptomycin production occurs between pH 7 and 8, with the highest rate of production in the range of pH 7.6 to 8. The fermentation lasts approximately 5 to 7 days and provides streptomycin yields probably in excess of 1200 micrograms per milliliter. The antibiotic is not destroyed by contaminating microorganisms as occurs with penicillin, although contaminants do decrease yields. Actinophage infections, however, can be serious, whether they occur in the inoculum or production tanks, since the streptomycete quickly lyses so that yields are reduced. However, strains of *Streptomyces griseus* resistant to the more common phages have been developed and are in use today.

A commercial streptomycin fermentation passes through three phases. The first phase lasts approximately 24 hours, with rapid growth during this period producing most of the mycelium for the fermentation. The strong proteolytic activity of *Streptomyces griseus* releases ammonia to the medium from the soybean meal, and the carbon nutrients of the soybean meal are utilized for growth. However, the glucose of the medium is utilized only slowly during this period, and only slight streptomycin production occurs. Also, during this period, the pH of the medium rises from approximately 6.7 or 6.8 to 7.5 or slightly higher. Phase 2, during which streptomycin is produced at a rapid rate, lasts from approximately 24 hours to 6 or 7 days of incubation. Almost no mycelial growth occurs and, thus, the weight of mycelium remains fairly constant. Ammonia is utilized, and the glucose is rapidly withdrawn from the medium so that little is left by the end of this phase. The pH remains fairly constant in a range of approximately 7.6 to 8. In the last phase, phase 3, the sugar has been depleted from the medium, and streptomycin production ceases. The cells lyse, releasing ammonia, and the pH rises. The fermentation, however, usually is harvested before the start of this phase of senescence.

Harvest and Recovery of Streptomycin

At completion of the fermentation, the mycelium is separated from the broth by filtration, and the streptomycin is recovered by one of several procedures, the choice of procedure depending on the particular industrial concern. In one procedure, the streptomycin is adsorbed from the broth onto activated carbon and then eluted from the carbon with dilute acid. The eluted streptomycin then is precipitated by solvents, filtered, and dried before further purification. In an alternate procedure, the fermentation broth is acidified, filtered, and neutralized. It then is passed through a column containing a cation exchange resin to adsorb the streptomycin from the broth. Following this adsorption, the column is washed with water and the streptomycin eluted with hydrochloric acid before concentration *in vacuo* almost to dryness. The streptomycin then is dissolved in methanol and filtered, and acetone is added to the filtrate to precipitate the antibiotic. Finally, the precipitate is washed with acetone and dried *in vacuo* before being dissolved in methanol for preparation as the pure streptomycin calcium chloride complex. The final product must meet standards set by the Food and Drug Administration.

Vitamin B as a By-Product

Normal streptomycin fermentations by *Streptomyces griseus* produce small amounts of vitamin B_{12} in addition to streptomycin. However, the level of vitamin B_{12} is markedly increased without affecting streptomycin yields if a soluble cobalt salt is added as a precursor (Chapter 7) to the medium at concentrations just under that toxic to streptomycin production. The vitamin B_{12} may be recovered in pure form from the culture broth, or dried fermentation residues or partially purified concentrates of the vitamin can be added as a supplement to animal feeds. However, regardless of this by-product possibility for the streptomycin fermentation, most of the present-day commercial production of vitamin B_{12} is by direct bacterial fermentation (Chapter 24).

References

Streptomycin

Hockenhull, D.J.D. 1960. The biochemistry of streptomycin production. Pp. 131–165 in *Progress in industrial microbiology*, vol. II (ed. by D.J.D. Hockenhull). Interscience Publishers, Inc., New York.

Hockenhull, D.J.D. 1963. Antibiotics. IV. Streptomycin. Pp. 249–267 in *Biochemistry of industrial microorganisms* (ed. by C. Rainbow and A.H. Rose). Academic Press, New York.

Rose, A.H. 1961. *Industrial microbiology*. Pp. 211–213. Butterworths, Washington.

Schatz, A., E. Bugie, and S.A. Waksman. 1944. Streptomycin, a substance exhibiting antibiotic activity against gram positive and gram negative bacteria. Proc. Soc. *Expt. Biol. Med.,* 55, 66–69.

Waksman, S.A. (ed.) 1949. *Streptomycin. Nature and practical applications.* Williams and Wilkins, Baltimore.

Woodruff, H.B., and L.E. McDaniel. 1954. Streptomycin. Pp. 264–293 in *Industrial fermentations,* vol. II (ed. by L.A. Underkofler and R.J. Hickey). Chemical Publishing Co., Inc., New York.

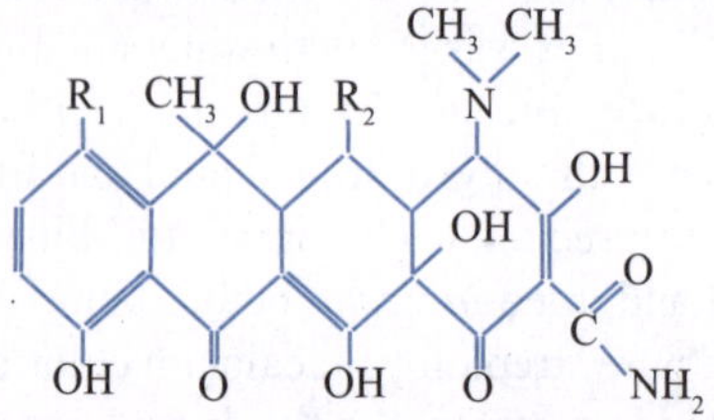

Figure 17.21 The tetracyclines. Tetracycline has hydrogens at R_1 and R_2; chloro-tetracycline (Aureomycin) has chlorine at R_1 and hydrogen at R_2; and oxytetracycline (Terramycin) has hydrogen at R_1 and a hydroxyl at R_2.

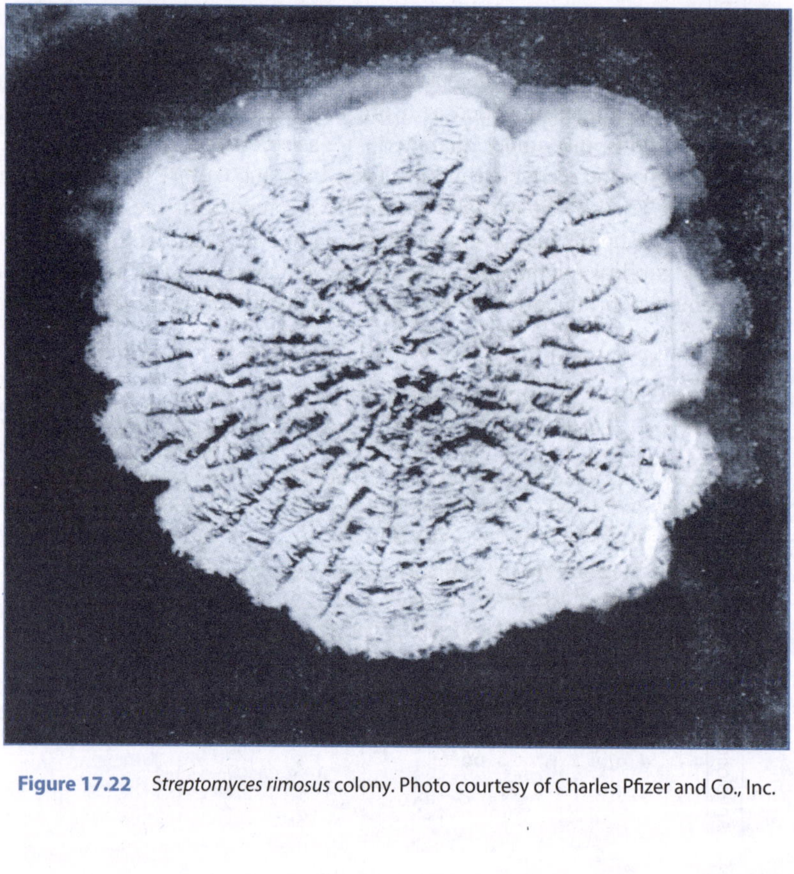

Figure 17.22 *Streptomyces rimosus* colony. Photo courtesy of Charles Pfizer and Co., Inc.

Table 17.1 Other Antibiotics

Antibiotics	Produced By	Chemical Type	Sensitive Organism
	Bacteria		
Polymyxin-B	*Bacillus polymyxa*	Polypeptide	Gram neg bacteria as Ps. aeruginosa
Bacitracin	*Bacillus licheniformis*	Polypeptide	Similar to penicillin
Griseofulvin	*Fungi*		
	Penicillium griseofulvin	Polyene	Plant pathogenic fungi
	Penicillium nigricans		
	Penicillium urticae		
Fumagillin	*Aspergillus fumigatus*	Polyene	Bacteriophage and amoebae
Cephaloridine and Cephalothin	Chemically modified Cephalosporin C	Peptide	Penicillin-resistant staphylococci
Chlorotetracycline	*Streptomycetes*		
Oxytetracycline	*Streptomyces aureofaciens*	Tetracycline[a]	Broad spetrum[c]
Tetracycline	*Streptomyces rimosus*	Tetracycline[a]	Broad spectrum[c]
	Dechlorination and hydrogenation of chlorotetracycline	Tetracycline	Broad spectrum[c]
	Direct fermentation in dechlorinated medium		
Chloramphenicol	*Streptomyces venezuelae* or total chemical synthesis	b	Broad spectrum[c] gram negative bacteria including Salmonella

Table 17.1 Other Antibiotics (continued)

Antibiotic	Produced By	Chemical Type	Sensitive Organism
Kanamycin	*Streptomyces kanamyceticus*		Gram positive bacteria, penicillin-resistant staphylococci, tubercle bacillus
Erythromycin	*Streptomyces erythreus*	Macrolide	Broad spectrum but limited gram negative activity; penicillin-resistant staphylococci
Carbomycin	*Streptomyces halstedii*	Macrolide	Gram positive bacteria, penicillin-resistant staphylococci
Oleandomycin	*Streptomyces antibioticus*	Macrolide	Antibiotic-resistant staphylococci
Nystatin	*Streptomyces noursei*	Polyene	Fungal skin infections; moniliasis
Amphotericin-B Cycloheximide	*Streptomyces nodosus* *Streptomyces griseus* (special medium)	Polyene	Antifungal Pathogenic yeasts and yeast like fungi, plant parasitic fungi
Novobiocin	*Streptomyces niveus* *Streptomyces spheroides*	Glycoside	Bacteria; antibiotic-resistant staphylococci
Neomycin-B	*Streptomyces fradiae*	Glycoside	Bacteria

a See Figures 17.21 and 17.22.

b See Figure 17.23.

c Active against bacateria, rickettsiae, and certain large viruses.

OTHER ANTIBIOTICS

Additional antibiotic fermentations are outlined in Table 17.1, and more extensive lists can be found in Peterson and Peterson (1954) and in Chain (1958). Of these antibiotics, at the present date the most important include chloramphenicol, the tetracyclines, the polymyxins, erythromycin, carbomycin, kanamycin, nystatin, amphotericin and griseofulvin.

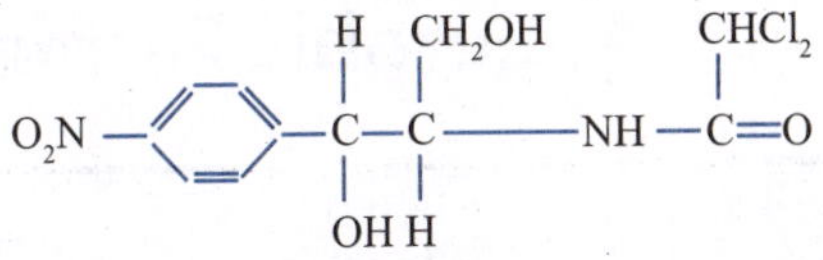

Figure 17.23 Chloramphenicol (Chloromycetin).

References

Other antibiotics

Chain, E.B. 1958. Chemistry and biochemistry of antibiotics. *Ann. Rev. Biochem.,* **27,** 167–222.

Di Marco, A. and P. Pennella. 1959. The fermentation of the tetracyclines. Pp. 45–92 in *Progress in industrial microbiology*, vol. I (ed. by D.J.D. Hockenhull). Interscience Publishers, Inc., New York.

Hickey, R.J. 1964. Bacitracin, its manufacture and uses. Pp. 93–150 in *Progress in industrial microbiology*, vol. V (ed. by D.J.D. Hockenhull). Gordon and Breach Science Publishers, Inc., New York.

Hoeksema, H., and C.G. Smith. 1961. Novobiocin. Pp. 91–139 in *Progress in industrial microbiology*, vol. III (ed. by D.J.D. Hockenhull). Interscience Publishers, Inc. New York.

Peterson, W.H., and M.S. Peterson. 1954. Pp. 344–358 in *Industrial fermentations,* vol. II (ed. By L.A. Underkofler and R.J. Hickey). Chemical Publishing Co., Inc., New York.

Rhodes, A. 1964. Griseofulvin: production and biosynthesis. Pp. 165–187 in *Progress in industrial microbiology,* vol. IV (ed. by D.J.D. Hockenhull). Gordon and Breach Science Publishers, Inc., New York.

Smith, C.G., and J.W. Hinman. 1964. Chloramphenicol. Pp. 137–163 in *Progress in industrial microbiology*, vol. IV (ed. by D.J.D. Hockenhull). Gordon and Breach Science Publishers, Inc., New York.

Stark, W.M., and R.L. Smith. 1961. The erythromycin fermentation. Pp. 211–230 in *Progress in industrial microbiology*, vol. III (ed. by D.J.D. Hockenhull). Interscience Publishers Inc., New York.

CHAPTER 18
Anaerobic Fermentations

Anaerobic fermentations are those fermentations that are carried out in the absence of oxygen by strictly anaerobic or facultatively anaerobic bacteria or yeast. In this regard, anaerobic fermentations, to date, have not been demonstrated for members of the order Actinomycetales, which includes the anaerobic Actinomyces genus, or for the fungi, although representatives of both of these large groups of organisms carry out aerobic fermentations. Thus, the property of anaerobic growth is associated with strict anaerobes, such as members of the genus Clostridium, and with facultative anaerobes, such as the lactic acid bacteria and yeasts. The strict anaerobes usually lack catalase activity, and the little peroxidase activity that they may possess cannot remove the highly toxic hydrogen peroxide as fast as it is produced during aerobic growth. In contrast to these organisms, certain organisms normally considered as being aerobic are capable of anaerobic growth, if they can reduce nitrate or sulfate in the medium to obtain oxygen atoms. These organisms, however, usually are not considered in discussions of anaerobic fermentations, because they employ similar mechanisms of terminal respiration for both aerobic and anaerobic growth, but grow better in air. In certain instances, fermentations utilizing facultative anaerobes, such as the yeasts, employ aeration during inoculum build-up to increase cell numbers before anaerobic fermentation conditions are imposed. Thus, the rate and amount of cell growth is usually greater for aerobic conditions of growth than for anaerobic.

Microorganisms growing anaerobically recover less energy per unit of carbon substrate utilized than do aerobes. Also, there is a tendency in these fermentations for carbon substrates to undergo only partial decomposition so that various organic acids, organic amines, and so forth accumulate in the growth medium; obviously, these products can present problems in pH maintenance of the fermentation. Thus, the incomplete untilization of substrate and low cellular-energy yields for these fermentations often require that much carbon substrate be decomposed for the growth and maintenence of the microbial cells. This phenomenon, however, can be beneficial to fermentation yields, if the relatively greater passage of substrate carbon through the metabolic sequences of the organism causes a resultant conversion of large amounts of substrate carbon to fermentation product.

There have been many fewer industrial fermentations developed for anaerobic microorganisms than for aerobic. In part, this is because there are fewer known species of anaerobic microorganisms than aerobic. However, a specific difference in the anaerobic and aerobic metabolism of microorganisms also plays a part, since the products of anaerobic fermentations usually are those of the major normal metabolic sequences of the organisms during anaerobic metabolism; that is, they are the normal decomposition products for a given carbon substrate as associated with a particular microorganism. While this may also be true for aerobic fermentations, it often is the case with aerobic fermentations that partially decomposed carbon substrate is shunted to normally minor biosynthetic sequences of the cells so that the structures of the fermentation products bear little resemblance to the normal catabolic intermediates of the carbon substrate. Thus, based on this reasoning, the possibilities for new types of fermentation products from aerobic organisms are probably greater than for anaerobic organisms.

Anaerobic fermentations are intriguing for commercial use, because they do not require the expense of large volumes of sterile air or the expense of energy input into the fermentation in the form of vigorous impeller action. However, anaerobic fermentations also are of interest from another standpoint. Various anaerobic microorganisms possess the ability to degrade cellulose, a substrate available in inexpensive forms as by-products of agriculture, wood utilization, and so forth; relatively few cellulolytic anaerobic microorganisms, other than the spore formers, have been studied in relation to their fermentation potential for these substrates. This results, in part, from the extreme oxygen sensitivity of some of these forms. Thus, one of the best natural anaerobic fermentation vats is the rumen of the cow, and anaerobic, cellulose-decomposing highly oxygen-sensitive bacteria, particularly those not forming spores, are highly active in the rumen. Similar organisms probably also are active in soil, but have received relatively less study. Although difficult to handle and control on an industrial scale, these organisms could well open the way to future industrial anaerobic fermentations utilizing inexpensive cellulosic and other by-products as carbon substrates.

The commercial production of acetone and butanol by species of the genus *Clostridium* will be described as representative of an anaerobic fermentation utilizing a strictly anaerobic bacterium. Brewing, industrial alcohol, and lactic acid fermentations are included as examples of industrial anaerobic fermentations which are more tolerant of oxygen.

ACETONE-BUTANOL FERMENTATION

Pasteur observed the presence of butanol in the culture broths of butyric acid-producing bacteria, and later, others observed that acetone also was present. Previous to World War I, there was interest in England in determining whether similar microorganisms could be employed to produce N-butanol as a fermentation product to be used in the synthesis of butadiene for synthetic rubber. Therefore, a *Clostridium* organism was studied extensively in association with a potato medium, and a successful process was developed in 1913 to 1914 Great interest was associated with this fermentation during World War I, but not for the butanol that it produced. There was great demand for acetone, which is a by-product of this fermentation, to dissolve cordite for the manufacture of explosives. However, the fermentation yielded more butanol than acetone, which was slightly discouraging, because there was only limited demand for the butanol so that much of it had to be either stored or disposed of while retaining the acetone. After the war, the demand for acetone markedly decreased, and the fermentation would have assumed little further importance had it not been found that butanol was a good solvent of the nitrocellulose lacquers used on automobiles.

At the present time, butanol finds extensive use in brake fluids, antibiotic recovery procedures, urea-formaldehyde resins, amines for gasoline additives, and as esters in the protective-coatings industry. However, the market for fermentation-produced acetone and butanol has decreased markedly in recent years so that relatively little is still manufactured by fermentation. Thus, both of these compounds are easily produced by chemical synthesis. Acetone is a by-product of the manufacture of isopropanol or of phenol (from cumene), and it also occurs as a by-product of the oxidation cracking of propane. Butanol is synthesized from ethylene. The vitamin, riboflavin (which is another by-product of the acetone-butanol fermentation) also is finding less demand from this source, because of the development of aerobic fermentations yielding high levels of this vitamin, and because it now can be prepared by chemical synthesis or extracted from natural materials. Finally, the increased costs of fermentation carbon substrates, both molasses and corn, also have adversely influenced the economic situation of the acetone-butanol fermentation.

The history of the particular *Clostridium* strains utilized in the acetone-butanol fermentation is of interest. Thus, the initial English process employed a potato medium, but only relatively low solvent yields were realized.

This picture was changed, however, when Weizmann in 1919 isolated a *Clostridium*, later classified as *Clostridium acetobutylicum*, which fermented various starchy substrates, including ground corn, with good yields of solvents. The patent on this process was very profitable for Weizmann, because this process was successfully used during World War I to produce acetone. In the United States, Weizmann's process was employed at Terre Haute, Indiana, and, after the war, additional large production facilities were built at Peoria, Illinois. Later, other *Clostridium* species were isolated which provided high solvent yields on molasses media; Weizmann's *Clostridium acetobutylicum* performed less well on molasses. Actually, various strains of *Clostridium* were isolated for the molasses fermentations and, although various species names were appended to these organisms in the patent literature, they all in reality closely resembled Weizmann's *Clostridium acetobutylicum*. A typical molasses organism is *Clostridium saccharoacetobutylicum.*

Microorganism

Clostridium acetobutylicum and related acetone-butanol-producing bacteria are anaerobic, motile, spore-forming rods whose spores are quite heat resistant (Figure 18.1). The spore measures approximately 1 by 1.5 microns and the vegetative cell approximately 1 by 4 microns. The spore is located at or near one end of the vegetative cell and, in the proper medium, it is formed about the time the nutrients of the medium become exhausted.

Many bacteria produce small amounts of N-butanol, but only certain *Clostridium* species produce this compound at commercially acceptable levels. These *Clostridium* species bacteria first synthesize butyric and acetic acids, then they convert these products to butanol and acetone, respectively. There are two groups of butyric acid-producing *Clostridium* species, both of which are nonpathogenic. One group, typified by *Clostridium butyricum*, produces acetic and butyric acids and gas (carbon dioxide and hydrogen) without reducing the acids to the corresponding solvents. In contrast, the other group, typified by *Clostridium acetobutylicum*, is able to carry out the further reduction of the solvents to acids. In regard to the latter type of organism, there is considerable variation from one strain to another in relation to the substrates utilized and the ratios of the various solvents produced. Some strains are strongly proteolytic and amylotic and, therefore, they can ferment corn without further additions of nutrients. Other strains, however, lack these abilities, and these strains must be provided with various of the more simple substrate molecules. For instance, various molasses cultures, which only poorly ferment starchy nutrients, in addition, require that some ammonium nitrogen be added to the medium.

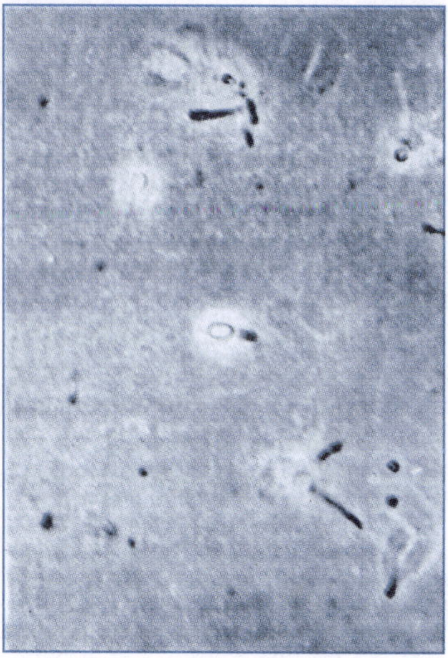

Figure 18.1 Spores and sporangia of *Clostridium acetobutylicum* as the organism is grown in corn-mash medium and observed by oil-immersion phase microscopy.

The acetone-butanol fermentation yields several products in addition to the acetone and butanol. These extra products include isopropanol, ethanol, formic acid, acetic acid, butyric acid, acetylmethylcarbinol, carbon dioxide, hydrogen, and a yellow oil, which is a complex mixture of higher alcohols, higher acids, and esters. However, butanol, acetone and ethanol are normally considered to be the principal products of the fermentation, although certain strains of butanol-producing *Clostridium* produce isopropyl alcohol instead of part or all of the acetone. Nevertheless, for a particular organism and medium, the major solvents occur in well-defined ratios and, as a result, strains of the organism are usually selected that have the ability to produce the highest possible ratio of butanol over acetone and ethanol.

Fermentation Mechanism

Although the acetone-butanol fermentation has received extensive study, the actual sequence of chemical events leading from substrate carbohydrate to the various fermentation products is still not completely clear. While it is known that acetic and butyric acids are produced first and then converted to acetone and butanol, respectively, it also is known that some of the enzymatic steps involved are reversible. This became apparent when the use of isotopically labeled acetic and butyric acids revealed that some of the carbon of each acid ended up in the alternate solvent; some of the acetic acid carbon was present in the butanol and some of the butyric acid carbon in the acetone. However, aside from this uncertainty in the reaction mechanism, a general picture of the biosynthetic sequence has evolved. Thus, glucose is degraded via the EMP scheme to pyruvate, and the excess reducing power liberated is evolved as gaseous hydrogen. The pyruvate is converted to acetyl-CoA (acetyl-coenzyme A) plus carbon dioxide and hydrogen. Part of the acetyl-CoA is converted directly to acetic acid, and additional acetyl-CoA is condensed to yield acetoacetyl-CoA which is then converted sequentially to *β*-hydroxybutyric acid, crotonic acid, and butyric acid (Figure 18.2). CoA probably is involved at each of these steps. The butyric acid then is reduced to N-butanol. The acetoacetic acid combined with acetyl CoA is also decarboxylated to yield acetone; thus, this solvent does not arise directly from acetic acid even though the level of acetic acid in the fermentation decreases as acetone accumulates. There is some question as to the origin of isopropyl alcohol; it has been proposed that acetone is reduced directly to this alcohol or that the β-hydroxybutyric acid is decarboxylated to yield the alcohol.

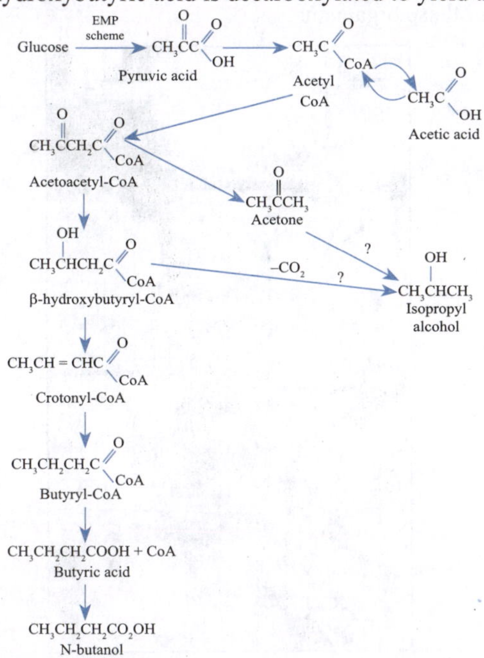

Figure 18.2 Sequence of known and postulated chemical reactions in the acetone-butanol fermentation.

Culture Maintenance

The clostridia, being spore formers, are easily maintained as soil stocks since, in contrast to the vegetative cells, the spores are not sensitive to oxygen. The spores keep indefinitely in soil, although some questions has been raised as to whether the solvent-producing power (the ability to convert the acids to solvents) of the organisms might decrease on prolonged storage. Should this "degeneration" occur, it would be necessary to rejuvenate the culture as described later.

The acetone-butanol clostridia also undergo degeneration as a result of continuous transfers of the cultures. Thus, continuous successive transfers at 24-hour incubation intervals, after several transfers, may bring on a complete loss of solvent-forming ability, and before this point, may increase the relative proportion of the acetone component of the neutral solvents. A degenerate culture demonstrates sluggish growth during the fermentation, as well as poor conversion of the acids to the corresponding solvents, although acid production in itself is not necessarily affected. Obviously, this phenomenon of culture degeneration precludes, to a large extent, the use of continuous fermentations for these organisms.

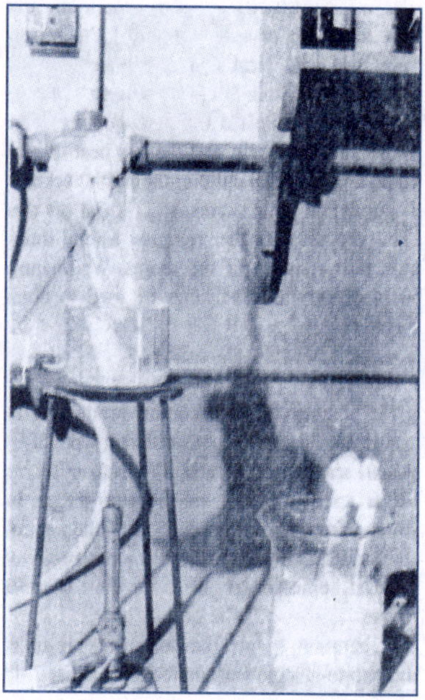

Figure 18.3 Heat shocking of *Clostridium acetobutylicum* spores in corn mash. The tubes are held in boiling water for 90 seconds then immediately transferred to an ice bath for cooling.

Degenerate cultures can be rejuvenated by heat shocking, a procedure that makes use of the fact that there seems to be a direct correlation between the heat resistance of the spores and the solvent-forming ability of the vegetative cells. Heat shocking is accomplished by subjecting spores suspended in a tube of medium to boiling water for approximately 90 seconds, followed by rapid cooling (Figure 18.3). This procedure kills vegetative cells and the less heat-resistant spores. Thus, to rejuvenate a *Clostridium culture*, the heat-shocked spores are incubated until sporulation again occurs, and the culture then is again heat shocked. This process is further repeated several times so as to select for the most heat resistant of the spores. Weizmann suggested that 100 to 150 successive heat shockings be used to obtain a high solvent-yielding culture.

The Fermentation

In discussing the commercial fermentation production of acetone and butanol, we must consider two slightly different types of *Clostridium* species, *Closridium acetobutylicum* and *Clostridium saccharo-acetobutylicum*, and their respective corn and molasses media. In general, inoculum growth and fermentative production of the neutral solvents are carried out at 31 to 32ºC for the *Clostridium saccharo-acetobutylicum* molasses types and at approximately 37ºC for the *Clostridium acetobutylicum* corn types.

For inoculum preparation, spores from soil stocks are added to deep tubes of semisolid potato-glucose medium for the molasses cultures and to deep tubes of potato or corn medium (about 5 percent corn meal in water) for the corn types. The spores are added to the bottoms of these tubes (or the soil with its spores sinks to the bottom) so that the submerged location of the spores and the high reducing power of these media can protect the vegetative cells from oxygen after germination has occurred. The inoculated tubes are heat shocked and rapidly cooled to incubation temperature. The tubes then are incubated approximately 20 hours and used as inoculum for a larger batch of medium: corn or molasses media for the respective types of culture. The molasses medium contains molasses, calcium carbonate, ammonium sulfate, phosphate, and sometimes cornsteep liquor. Further increased volumes of inoculum are produced by successive transfers of approximately 2 to 4 percent inoculum by volume to larger and larger volumes of media, again with approximately 20 to 24 hour incubation periods at each transfer. During these transfers, the concentration of corn in the corn mash is increased to approximately 6 1/2 percent. At each of these stages of inoculum transfer, the reducing conditions of the medium, the immediate use of freshly sterilized and cooled media before air becomes reincorporated, and the active evolution of fermentation gases provides the anaerobic conditions required for growth of the organism. In addition, the larger inoculum and production tanks often are provided with a blanket of inert gas, or fermentation gas derived from concurrent fermentations, added at slightly positive pressure to the head space of the fermentor so as to help in maintaining anaerobic conditions. This gas also aids in foam control and in preventing contamination. The larger inoculum tanks as well as the production tanks in addition are fitted with an agitator to aid in mixing the inoculum through the medium.

The various inoculum stages for molasses cultures, and particularly the last stage before being transferred to the production fermentor, are checked for pH values, Brix values (density), rate of gas evolution, presence of facultative anaerobes by aerobic plating on an agar medium, and microscopic appearance of the culture and presence of contaminants by hanging-drop preparation. Tests for corn-culture inoculum include rate of gas formation, pH, microscopic observation, aerobic plating, and titratable acidity. The final inoculum stage for molasses medium is incubated 26 to 28 hours before addition to the production fermentor, while the final inoculum stage for corn cultures is incubated until the titratable acidity determination demonstrates a distinct acid break (to be discussed later), indicating a lack of gross contamination. Approximately 2 to 4 percent inoculum is added to production fermentors containing freshly steamed molasses medium and, on an average, slightly less inoculum to fermentors containing freshly steamed corn medium. In certain instances, however, much higher inoculum levels are employed with molasses medium so that the high numbers of cells and their vigorous activity can allow the use of only partially sterilized medium. The inoculum is added first to the production fermentor followed by the medium, since this sequence provides mixing of the inoculum through the medium. However, in an alternate inoculation procedure only part of the medium is added to the inoculum, and the inoculum is allowed to initiate growth before the rest of the medium is added.

Corn meal for the corn fermentation is prepared by passing corn through a magnetic field to remove dust and metallic debris, followed by degerming of the corn. Corn oil is recovered from the separated germ. The degermed corn then is ground to a relatively fine state in a roller or hammer mill. To prepare the corn-mash production medium, 8 to 10 percent corn meal is added to water with or without "stillage" followed by heating approximately 20 minutes at 65°C to gelatinize the starch before sterilization of the medium. The molasses production medium contains 6 percent sugar calculated as sucrose, either black-strap or high-test molasses, and to this is added ammonia and ammonium sulfate, calcium carbonate, super phosphate (a phosphate source) and, sometimes, cornsteep liquor. The calcium carbonate is added to prevent development of gross acidity, although excess calcium carbonate can hinder solvent formation, and most of the ammonia actually is added within the first 18 to 24 hours of the fermentation. Overcooking of this molasses medium during sterilization must be avoided to prevent a slow and incomplete fermentation.

"Slopping back" is a procedure in which "stillage" (also known as "slop") from preceding butyl fermentations is used to provide 30 to 40 percent of the total aqueous volume for the preparation of fresh medium. In reality, this stillage is the aqueous residue remaining after the neutral fermentation solvents have been stripped (distilled) from completed fermentations for recovery. The slopping-back procedure adds certain nutrients to the medium, including protein and some residual carbohydrate, and lowers the requirements for supplementary nutrients. Slopping back also reduces the amount of stillage that must be evaporated for preparing feed supplements and, to some extent, it aids in foam control. However, care must be taken in this practice, because toxic fermentation by-products and unfermentable residues can accumulate to unacceptable levels in the fermentation medium with continued employment of this practice. Thus, the procedure is discontinued if slow fermentations are encountered.

The acetone-butanol fermentations are conducted in production tanks having a capacity of between 50,000 and 500,000 gallons total volume, and the duration of the fermentation is approximately 2 to 2 1/2 days. Some foaming occurs, but only small amounts of antifoam oil are used, because of the cost involved and because of the problems created by the oil in the solvent-recovery stills and in the preparation of animal feed.

The fermentation (Figure 18.4) passes through three phases. In the first phase, there is rapid growth and production of acetic and butyric acids, and carbon dioxide and hydrogen are evolved in large amounts with hydrogen initially being the major gaseous product. The pH value of the fermentation, initially at 6 to 6.5 for corn medium and 5.5 to 6.5 for molasses medium, decreases and then remains fairly constant for the rest of the fermentation; buffers from the hydrolyzed corn or other proteins and other buffers of the medium tend to prevent changes in pH value. Towards the end of this phase, after approximately 13 to 17 hours of incubation, "titratable acidity" increases to a maximum, and adaptive enzymes are produced for converting acidic products to neutral solvents. This titratable acidity is determined as the milliliters of 0.1N alkali (sodium or potassium hydroxide) required to neutralize the acids in a 10 ml sample of fermentation broth, and it is reported as milliliters 0.1N acid per 10 ml sample.

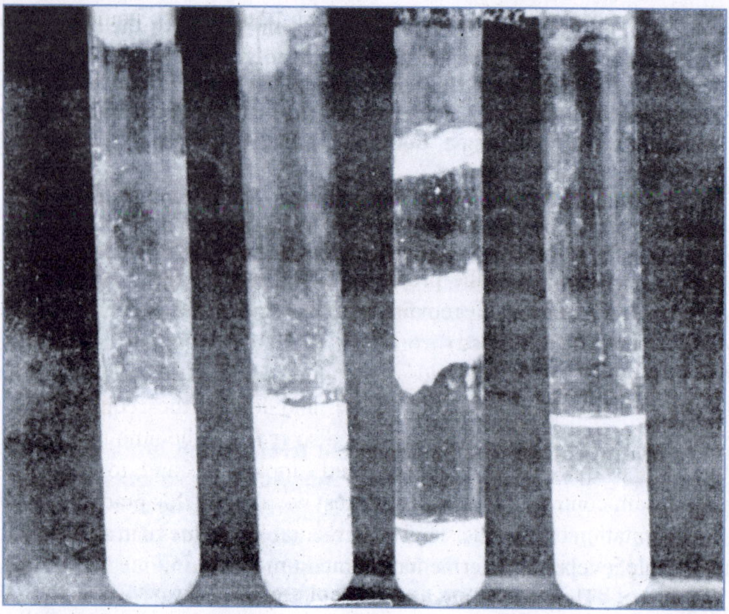

Figure 18.4 Progress of the acetone-butanol fermentation by *Clostridium aceto-butylicum* in corn mash. The tube at the left is freshly inoculated. The next two tubes show increasing rates of gas formation, with the medium in the third tube separated into segments by the evolved fermentation gases. The tube at the right contains a completed fermentation, and it will be noted that much of the starch and protein of the medium has been hydrolyzed.

In the second phase of the fermentation, there is a sharp decrease in titratable acidity, the "acid break", which coincides with the initiation of a rapid conversion of the acids to neutral solvents. This acid break is not observed, however, if the fermentation has become contaminated by acid-producing bacteria. Shortly after the acid break, the rate of gas evolution becomes maximum, but then gradually slows as the fermentation progresses.

During the third phase of the fermentation, the rate of gas evolution decreases markedly, accompanied by a decreased rate of solvent production. Also, the titratable acidity slowly increases so that the final pH of the corn fermentation is approximately 4.2 to 4.4, and of the molasses fermentation, approximately 5.2 to 6.2. Many of the cells autolyze at this point and, as a result, riboflavin is released from the cells into the medium.

Yields

The neutral solvents in the completed fermentation broth comprise about 2 percent by weight of the broth (measured by volume), and this yield corresponds to approximately a 30 percent conversion of carbohydrate to neutral solvents. However, the actual ratios of the solvents differ slightly depending on the fermentation medium. In a corn medium, the ratios of butanol, acetone, and ethanol are 6, 3, 1 trespectively, but in molasses medium these ratios are 6.5, 3 and 5 respectively. Although these neutral solvents represent the fermentation products of interest, it may come as a surprise to learn that the fermentation gases, 3 parts carbon dioxide and 2 parts hydrogen by volume, actually are the major products of this fermentation, since they account for approximately half of the sugar of the medium. Thus, the total weight of these gases exceeds that of the solvents by more than one and one-half times.

The total obtainable yields of butanol, the desired product, are influenced strongly by the toxicity of butanol for the fermentation organism. Thus, the highest concentration of butanol possible with commercially used strains is 13.5 g per liter and, in fact, extensive studies by Ryden (1958) did not demonstrate commercial feasibility for producing greater than this amount of butanol. This butanol toxicity is manifested by a retardation or slowing of the fermentation and, as a result, this toxicity fixes the usable carbohydrate concentration initially present in the medium at approximately 6 percent calculated as sucrose.

Product Recovery

The harvested fermentation broth, containing approximately 2 percent total solvents, is passed through a "beer still," which is a continuous still comprising approximately 30 perforated plates in order to strip off the solvents. The fermentation broth enters the still from the top and descends across and through the plates in opposition to upflowing steam which vaporizes the solvents. The steam and solvents then are collected and condensed by cooling in order to provide a solution containing approximately 40 percent by weight total mixed solvents (some authors state 20 to 30 percent mixed solvents). The individual solvents in this solution are further separated by fractional distillation, with the acetone and butanol occurring in separate fractions. However, the ethanol and isopropanol are still present as a single fraction, which is sold as a general solvent. It should be noted that this isopropanol is not necessarily a direct product of the fermentation, since some conversion of acetone to isopropanol occurs during storage of the harvested fermentation broth before solvent stripping. In addition to the various fractions listed above, there is a high-boiling fraction composed of higher alcohols and esters. Also, the residual stillage contains riboflavin and other B vitamins produced during the fermentation, as well as considerable quantities of bacterial cells, and it can be concentrated and dried to serve as a vitamin feed supplement.

The recovered fermentation gases, at one time or another, have been used in various ways. The carbon dioxide has been converted to dry ice, and methanol and ammonia have been prepared from these gases. At present, however, the chief commercial use for the these gases seems to be the employment of the hydrogen for chemical reductions.

Contamination

Microbial contamination has proven to be more troublesome with corn medium than with molasses medium. Nevertheless, with either medium, every attempt is made to detect contamination during inoculum production so that clean inoculum can be employed for the production fermentors. Thus,

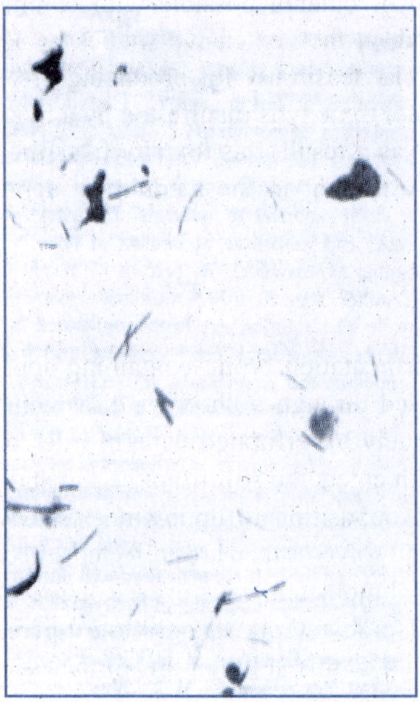

Figure 18.5 A 24-hour corn-mash culture of *Clostridium acetobutylicum* heavily contaminated with *Lactobacillus leichmannii*. The latter organism appears as long slender rods.

microscopic observations, aerobic platings, and determinations of titratable acidity and gas evolution are followed closely. The principal bacterial contaminants of the fermentation are the lactic acid-producing bacteria, and particularly the *Lactobacillus leichmannii* type (Figure 18.5) which produces large amounts of this acid, but also produces a slime that causes foam. These contaminants degrade substrate carbon, and the resulting high concentration of lactic and other acids prevents formation of the clostridium adaptive enzymes required for converting the acetic and butyric fermentation products to neutral solvents. Thus, the lack of an acid break in the corn fermentation and a slowing or cessation of gas formation in both media are good evidence for contamination by these organisms.

Phages also constitute a serious threat to acetone-butanol fermentations regardless of whether molasses or corn media are employed. The first indication of a phage attack for corn medium is a slow or sluggish fermentation with decreased fermentation gas evolution, and for a molasses medium, a slowing or even cessation of gas evolution, darker colored medium, and only a few cells observable by microscopic examination. In regard to the latter determination, the surviving bacteria also demonstrate loss of motility. After onset of the phage attack, most of the bacteria may be killed and lysed within a few hours, although the fermentation may start up again after 24 to 48 hours further incubation because of the presence of a few phage-resistant cells among the normal population of the organism. However, neutral solvents will not be produced in the latter fermentation unless the phage attack has occurred during phases 2 or 3 of the fermentation, that is, after the adaptive enzymes have been produced for converting fermentation acids to neutral solvents.

Cleanliness of operation of a fermentation production plant is an asset to preventing phage attacks of this type. Nevertheless, phage infections still occur, with the phage being brought in by the dust of the air and by Clostridium spores lysogenic for phage. To combat a phage attack, phage-resistant clostridia can be recovered from a fermentation that has survived a phage attack, or the *Clostridium* culture can be exposed in successive transfer to a bacteria-free culture filtrate containing phage. In the latter instance, however, culture degeneration must be kept in mind. Also, since the various *Clostridium* phage are highly strain specific, it is advantageous to have on hand several different phage-resistant strains of the solvent-producing *Clostridium*.

Clostridium strains surviving a phage attack may be lysogenic. In this instance, the spores as well as the vegetative cells are lysogenic and, in fact, this phage-producing ability even survives heat shocking of the spores. These lysogenic strains can be a nuisance in the production plant since their free spores are a good source for recontamination by the particular phage, if the solvent-producing bacterial strain being employed at the time is not resistant to this phage. Nevertheless, a good procedure for maintaining a particular phage is to prepare spore soil stocks of a *Clostridium* strain lysogenic for this phage.

References

Acetone-Butanol

Beesch, S.C. 1952. Acetone-butanol fermentation of sugars. *Ind. Eng. Chem.*, **44,** 1677–1682

Beesch, S.C. 1953. Acetone-butanol fermentation of starches. *Appl. Microbiol.*, **1**, 85–95.

McCutchan, W.N., and R.J. Hickey. 1954. The butanol-acetone fermentations. Pp. 345–388 in *Industrial fermentations*, vol. I (ed. by L.A. Underkofler and R.J. Hickey). Chemical Publishing Co., Inc., New York.

Prescott, S.C., and C.G. Dunn. 1959. *Industrial microbiology*, 3rd ed. Pp. 250–284. McGraw-Hill Book Co., Inc., New York.

Rose, A.H. 1961. *Industrial microbiology*. Pp. 160–166. Butterworths, Washington.

Ross, D. 1961. The acetone-butanol fermentation. Pp. 71–90 in *Progress in industrial microbiology,* vol. III (ed. by D.J.D. Hockenhull). Interscience Publishers, Inc., New York.

Ryden, R. 1959. Development of anaerobic fermentation processes: acetone-butanol. Pp. 123–148 in *Biochemical engineering* (ed. by R. Steel). Heywood & Co., Ltd., London.

Weizmann, C. 1919. U.S. Patent 1, 315, 585.

Wilkinson, J.F., and A.H. Rose. 1963. Biochemistry of industrial microorganisms. Pp. 407–410 (ed. by C. Rainbow and A.H. Rose). Academic Press, New York.

BREWING

Brewing, the production of malt beverages, is one of the oldest of fermentations, dating back thousands of years and probably originating in the Nile Valley. In early times, the type of local agriculture most likely influenced the particular fermented beverage produced in any particular locality, with cereal grains being employed for beer, fruits for wine, and honey for mead. These early fermentations were spontaneous, since no inoculum was employed, and the resulting uncertainty of these fermentations placed them in the class of an art. Thus, much folklore became associated with the art of brewing and, even today, with our advanced knowledge of fermentation microbiology, there still is much art associated with brewing because of the complexity of the fermentation and associated processing. In early times, variations in flavor that could not be controlled because of lack of knowledge of the fermentation were covered up by the addition of spices, herbs, and so forth. These amendments, however, usually are not required today.

Brewing is a complex fermentation process, because a multitude of products of the process must be considered, because several of these products do not result from microbial activity, and because the exact nature of certain of the latter products still is not known. The fermentative products of the yeast, however, are known, and these include ethanol, carbon dioxide, glycerol, acetic acid, and higher alcohols and acids. Obviously, the ethanol and carbon dioxide are of prime importance. Nevertheless, the finished product contains 8 to 15 percent solids of which a major portion is directly derived from various residual components of the medium and from interactions of these components during the various steps of the processing. It is apparent, then, that the exact composition and preparation of the medium as well as all controls over processing are of extreme importance.

Brewing also differs from most other industrial fermentations, because flavor, aroma, clarity, color, foam production, foam stability, percentage of alcohol, and satiety all are factors associated with the finished product. Thus, since people differ in their likes as to the relative balance of these factors in the finished product the resulting variations in the brewing process all are commercially profitable. Regardless of these variations, however, a typical present-day American beer may be described as having a bland flavor and a pH of 4.3, and it contains, on an average, 3.58 percent alcohol by weight, 1.12 percent sugar as maltose, 0.33 percent protein, and 2.27 volumes of carbon dioxide in the packaged product.

Various malt beverages, including beer, ale, porter, stout, and malt tonics, are available, although the process of manufacture is basically similar for these beverages, and the products themselves bear some similarity. Lager beer, the type most commonly produced, refers to a fermented beer that has been allowed to age in the cold and, for this beer, bottom-fermenting yeasts are utilized in contrast to the top-fermenting yeasts employed in the manufacture of ales. Pilsner refers to a beer light in body and color and containing approximately 3.4 to 3.8 percent alcohol. Most American beers are included in this category. The seasonal Book beer is brewed in the winter for sale at Easter time, and the carmalized or roasted malt used in its production provides its dark color, sweet taste, and heavy body. Ale, stout, and porter employ top-fermenting yeasts. High levels of hops are utilized in ale manufacture, and the alcohol content of the finished product can be as high as 8 percent by weight. Stout and porter employ heavy worts without malt adjuncts, resulting in a dark-colored, heavybodied, high alcohol-content beverage.

As a result of the foregoing considerations, the various characteristics of a finished malt or other alcoholic beverage are difficult if not impossible to duplicate by chemical synthesis or by mixing chemically synthesized products with natural materials, even though the ethanol itself can be easily synthesized chemically. In addition, there is a consistently high demand by the public for this type of fermentation product. Thus, these considerations place alcoholic-beverage fermentations in a unique situation in regard to fermentation industries, in general in that they are among the most stable of the various fermentation processes practiced today.

Medium Components

The compounding of the medium for the brewing of beer presents special problems, since the medium must supply not only the carbon and nitrogen substrates, vitamins, growth factors, and so forth for the yeast but, in addition, must contribute to the aroma, flavor, foam characteristics, color, clarity, stability, and so forth of the finished product. This picture is further complicated by the fact that the yeast is not able to directly utilize certain of the nutrients of the medium. For instance, starch is the primary carbon source of the medium, but its carbon becomes available to the yeast only after it has been totally degraded to maltose and glucose through the action of malt amylase. However, the latter enzymic reaction, in addition to the maltose and glucose, also yields dextrins, which are partial degradation products of the starch. These dextrins are not available to the yeast, but they are important, nevertheless, because of their association with the flavor of the product. The nitrogen source of the medium can also be classed in the yeast nonavailability category, since it is supplied mainly as protein, and the yeast does not possess proteolytic activity. Thus, the protein, through malt proteolytic activity, first must be degraded totally to amino acids and short-chained peptides for utilization by the yeast but, as with the carbon source of the medium, a portion of the protein must remain only partially degraded to peptones and larger peptides so as to contribute flavor, foam characteristics, and so forth to the final product. Thus, these partial and total degradations of both the carbon and nitrogen substrates of the medium are accomplished by employing the amylase and protease enzymes, respectively, of malt as prepared from barley. However, the malt, in addition to these enzymes, also provides the protein nitrogen compounds and, in most instances, part to all of the starch of the medium, although some of the starch may be supplied as "malt adjuncts." "Hops" also are added to the medium to provide various of the characteristics of the finished product, although the extractives from the hops, for the most part, are not in themselves substrates for yeast activity.

Malt. Malt is prepared from carefully selected barley. This barley is first cleaned and then steeped in water for periods of up to two days. The excess water then is drained from the soaked barley, and the barley is further incubated for periods of approximately four to six days to allow formation of a short rootlet and acrospire. This germination step allows the formation of highly active α-amylase, β-amylase, and proteolytic enzymes, as well as various flavor and color components. At the end of the incubation period, the temperature is raised just high enugh to stop germination but without harming the desired enzymes, although higher temperatures may be employed at this point to obtain darker-colored carmalized malts (with reduced enzyme activity) for stout and bock beer fermentations. This "green malt" is then carefully dried and stored. The preparation of a good malt is an exacting task requiring careful selection of barley and close supervision of the malting process. Therefore, many brewing companies do not produce their own malt but rely on separate companies that specialize in this art.

The malt contributes amylases, proteases, starch, protein, additional yeast nutrients and growth factors, and flavor characteristics to the medium. Thus, during preparation of the medium, approximately 65 percent of the weight of the added malt is extracted to become medium components. After extraction, the residual debris of the malt is separated so that it does not become a component of the medium.

Malt adjuncts. American-grown barleys contain considerable protein. If these barleys are employed in the medium as the only source of carbon and nitrogen, the resulting beer is dark colored, somewhat unstable, and too filling for the average taste. This situation is corrected by diluting the malt protein with additional starch added as starch-containing malt adjuncts. This additional starch does not present a problem, as might be expected, because the malt produced from American-grown barleys contains enough amylase activity for hydrolysis of this extra starch.

The additional carbon substrate provided by the malt adjuncts may be either as starch or as sugar. The various sources of these malt adjuncts are grits or meal prepared from rice and degermed corn, prepared starches such as flaked corn, dextrose sugar and syrups. The starch of grits or meal must first be gelatinized by boiling before it can be saccharified by the amylases of the malt, although flaked corn, a prepared starch additive, is available alrerady gelatinized. It is prepared by passing corn hominy grits through heated pressure rollers to provide a thin sheet of gelatinized starch. Approximately 80 to 90 percent of the weight of these starchy adjuncts is extracted into the wort (the fermentation medium). Dextrose sugar (prepared from starch) and syrups (from the corn wet-milling industry and available in various ratios of sugar to dextrin to suit the particular needs of the brewer) contain little or no starch and, therefore, they usually are added to the wort after the amylolytic and proteolytic activities of the malt have been inactivated.

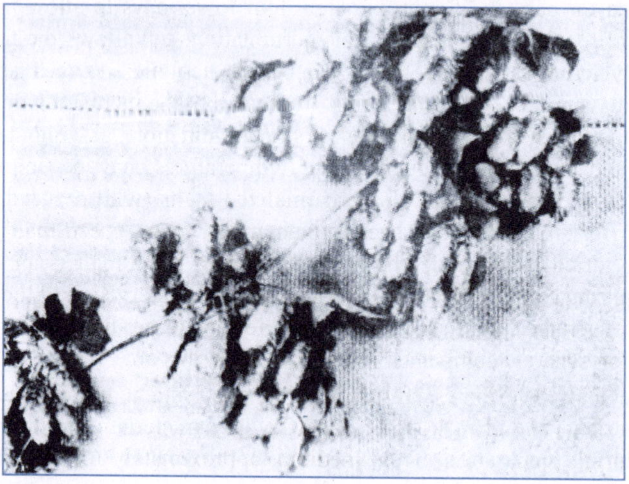

Figure 18.6 Hop cones as they appear on the female hop plant. Photo courtesy of S.S. Steiner, Inc.

Hops. Hops are the dried female flowers of the hop plant (Figure 18.6), which is grown extensively in Oregon, Washington, California and Idaho. Approximately one-quarter pound of hops is used per barrel of beer and upto two pounds per barrel of ale.

The hops provide the beer with its aromatic and pungent character, as well as having a stabilizing effect. The hops also provide tannin substances, to help coagulate protein degradation products in the wort, and alpha resins and, to a lesser extent, beta resins, which provide a bitter flavor as well as preservative action against many Gram-positive bacteria. Gamma resins also are extracted from the hops, but apparently these resins produce little effect since they are precipitated early in the processing. Some pectin is also extracted, and it is thought that this extractive may be involved in the foam characteristics of the finished product.

Water. Large amounts of water are employed in the production of beer and, in fact, each barrel of beer requires, on an average, 10 to 12 barrels of water. Obviously, only a small portion of this water ends up in the finished product; the rest is utilized in various fermentation and processing steps. The composition of the water is of extreme importance as regards its effects on flavor and other properties of the finished product. In fact, the geological location of a brewery often depends on the quality of the available water. For instance, water containing higher than normal levels of carbonates produces a heavy-flavored, dark-colored product. In contrast, the absence of carbonates but the presence of calcium sulfate allows the production of light beers and pale ales with a light flavor and absence of harshness. The characteristics of a good water for brewing are a pH of 6.5 to 7, less than 100 ppm calcium and magnesium carbonates, trace amounts of magnesium (preferably as the sulfate), 250 to 500 ppm calcium sulfate, 200 to 300 ppm sodium chloride, and 1 ppm or less of iron.

Preparation of Medium

The fermentation medium, or wort, is prepared in four successive operations. The adjuncts are first cooked to gelatinize their starch, then they are added to water along with malt in an approximate ratio of 2/3 malt to 1/3 adjuncts. This mixture is subjected to mashing (Figure 18.7), a procedure by which the various enzymes of the malt are allowed to act over a range of temperatures. On completion of mashing, the wort is separated from the undissolved husks andinsoluble protein matter and then boiled with hops at 1/4 lb per barrel of wort.

Mashing. The particular mashing procedure employed has a profound influence on the finished beer and, therefore, careful control of the mashing process is essential. Mashing extracts those materials from the malt and malt adjuncts which can be solubilized under the particular mashing conditions being employed, and also allows the malt amylases and proteases to degrade starch and protein, respectively. A portion of the starch must be partially degraded to dextrins and the rest totally degraded to maltose and glucose. In like manner, the protein must be partially degraded to peptones and peptides as well as totally degraded to amino acids. The degree of enzymatic hydrolysis of these compounds is influenced strongly by temperature and, to some extent, by pH. Thus, an elevated temperature during mashing tends to provide less degradation of these compounds as compared to a lower mashing temperature. The mashing temperature program, therefore, is adjusted to yield defined mixtures of partially and totally degraded enzymatic products.

The temperature optima for the alpha and beta amylases of malt occur within the range of approximately 57 to 77°C. However, the starch substrate for these enzymes is, in reality, a mixture of two polysaccharides, amylose and amylopectin. The amylose is a straight-chain glucose polymer, while the amylopectin is a glucose polymer with many branched chains. The beta amylase, with a temperature optimum at 57 to 65°C, cleaves maltose units from the ends of linear glucose polymers (as in amylose) but can degrade

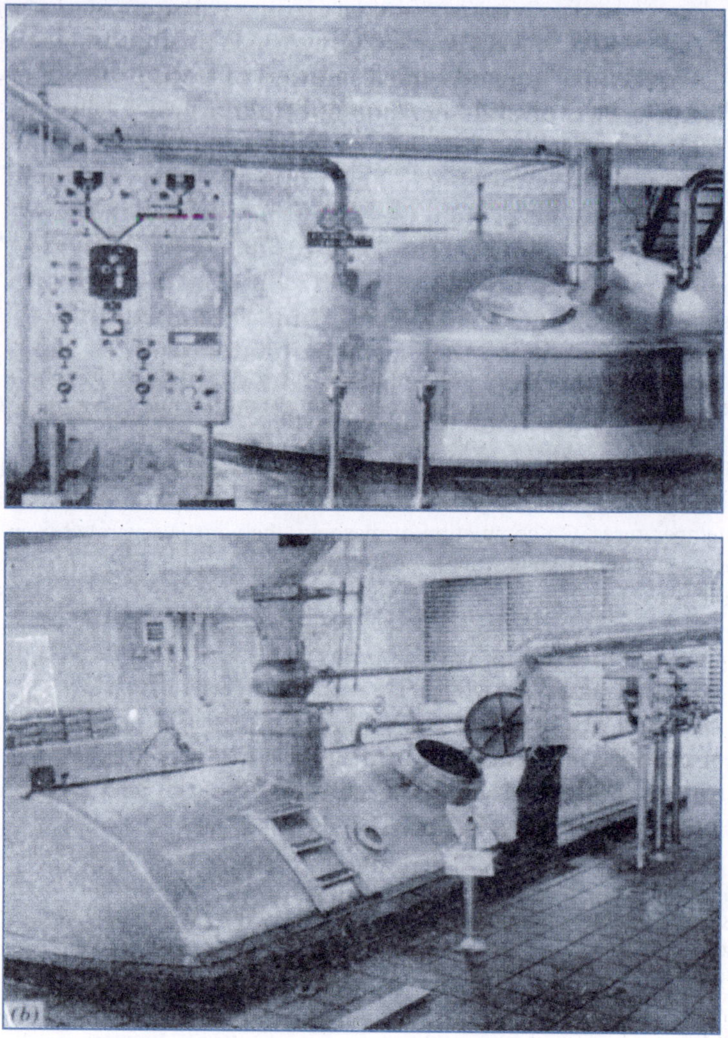

Figure 18.7 Two types of mash tubs. Photos courtesy of C. Schmidt and Sons, Inc.

only the short side chains, not including branches, of amylopectin; enzymatic activity stops at the branching points. Alpha amylase, with a temperature optimum in the range of 70 to 75°C, cleaves starch at random, in the process yielding large-fragment dextrins with or without branching units so as to make straight chains available for beta amylase activity. The alpha amylase also, but more slowly, attacks the dextrins to yield smaller fragments. However, some of the straight- and branched-chain fragments of the amylopectin are apparently resistant to degradation by both enzymes, and these fragments end up as nonfermentable dextrins.

Proteolytic activity of the malt follows a somewhat similar temperature picture. Temperatures of approximately 60°C allow formation of the higher molecular-weight peptones and peptides but, at approximately 50°C, the enzymatic activity yields a higher proportion of amino acids and low molecular-weight peptides. The lower temperature protein-degradation products are essential for yeast growth since yeasts in themselves do not possess proteolytic enzymes.

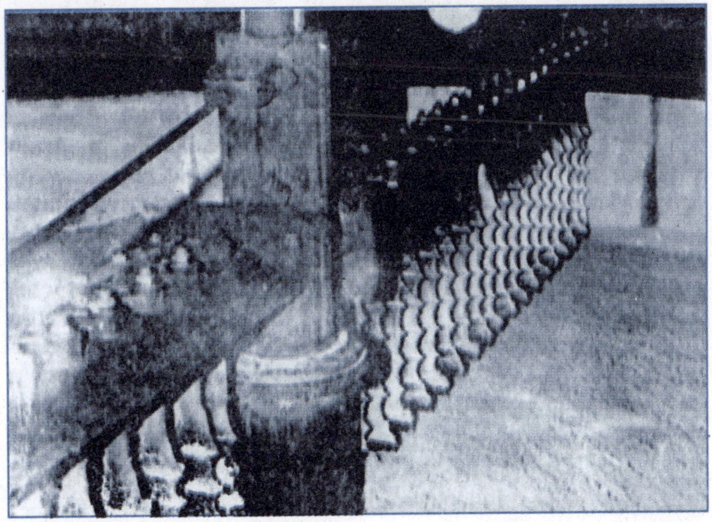

Figure 18.8 Inside of lauter tub partially filled with mash. The blades on the rotating arm move the mash across the slotted bottom of the tub (see Figure 18.9). Photo courtesy of the Pittsburgh Brewing Co.

The peptones and peptides resulting from the proteolytic activity of the malt provide flavor, foam, and foam stabilization. The dextrins, being nonfermentable, provide low-alcohol beer and certain flavor characteristics but, at the same time, their colloidal nature can impede aeration and cause slow filtration of the wort.

Careful control of pH during mashing is essential. Thus, peak enzymatic activity occurs at the pH optimum for the individual enzymes, and these optima are often different for different enzymes. As a result, the mashing pH picture can affect the relative activities of the various enzymes. The pH picture also controls, in part, the amounts of extractives obtained from the malt and malt adjuncts, as well as the extraction of tannins and bitter resins from the barley husks. In addition, the pH picture affects colored extractives and plays a role in the later ease of clarification and filtration. Where required, the pH values are adjusted by the addition of lactic, sulfuric or phosphoric acids.

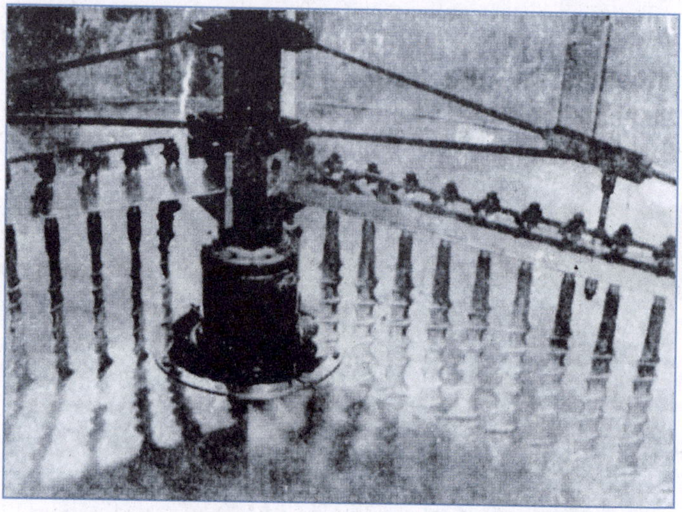

Figure 18.9 Empty lauter tub with many sort partain slots in its bottom. Photo courtesy of C. Schmidt and Sons, Inc.

A mashing procedure typical of those employed in the United States is as follows. A mixture in water of adjuncts and some of the malt is heated over a 40-minute time interval progressively from 45 to 100°C. A separate malt mash (malt plus water) is held at approximately 40°C for one hour, then its temperature is raised over a 20-minute period to 70°C by adding, at intervals, portions of the heated adjunct mash. This combined mash is held 20 minutes at 70°C, then quickly raised to 75°C and held an additional 30 minutes in order to provide a wort with a sugar degree of approximately 70 percent. This value is defined as the ratio of the fermentable to nonfermentable reducing substances present in the wort calculated as maltose and expressed as percent.

Separation of wort. The husks and other grain residues in the wort, as well as precipitated proteins and other solids, are removed from the wort by passing it through a lauter tub. This tub is a straining tank (Figures 18.8 and 18.9) with a false bottom slotted or perforated to allow passage of the wort. In certain instances, however, a filter press is employed in order to allow the use of more finely ground malt during mashing, a procedure that increases the yields of extractives.

Wort boiling. The filtered wort is boiled with stirring or agitation for approximately 1.5 to 2.5 hours, and portions of the hops are added at various times during the boiling, including near the end of the boiling period (Figure (18.10). There are various reasons for the boiling of the wort, in addition to that of extracting materials from the hops. The boiling coagulates that residual and partially hydrolyzed protein still present after the mashing process which, if not removed, could cause turbidity in the finished product. In addition, boiling inactivates the enzymes that were active during mashing, causes carmalization of some of the sugar, and concentrates and sterilizes the wort.

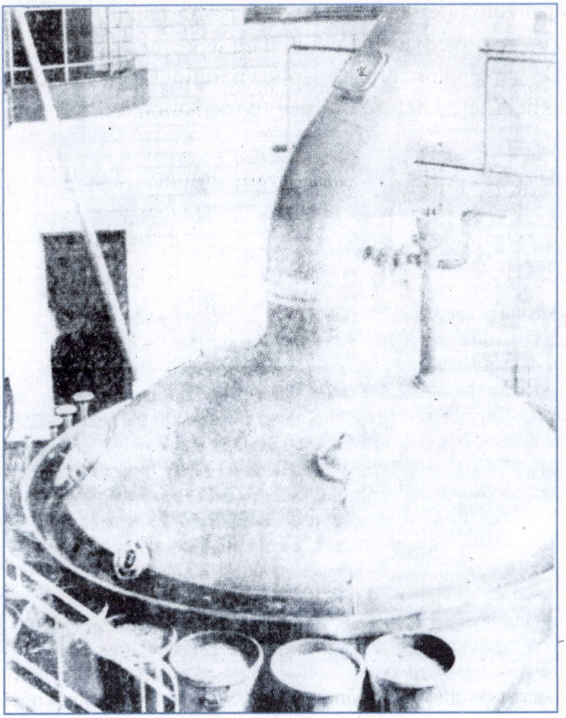

Figure 18.10 Boiling brew kettle with baskets of hops ready for addition. Photo courtesy the Pittsburgh Brewing Co.

The boiling of the wort extracts tannins, essential oil, bitter acids and resins from the hops. The essential oil, which provides aroma, is volatile and, actually, much of it is lost during boiling. However, some essential oil is retained in the wort because of the hop additions made near the end of the boiling process. This method of hop addition also is useful in another way, since it controls the amount of resins which are extracted from the hops. While the different hop extractives each have individual influences on the finished product, in general, the hop extractives (particularly the tannins) help in coagulating unwanted protein, in protecting the wort during fermentation against contamination by Gram positive bacteria, in foam formation, and in the establishment of the characteristic bitter flavor and aroma of beer. However, in regard to the latter point, overextraction of the hops can provide further unwanted bitter flavors.

At termination of boiling, the hops and coagulated materials are strained from the wort and, as a result, it is assumed that any unstable compounds which might precipitate later during processing or in the finished product, will have been removed at this point. The wort then is aerated and cooled (Figure 18.11) while maintaining aseptic conditions. The cooled wort may or may not then be filtered before use as a fermentation medium.

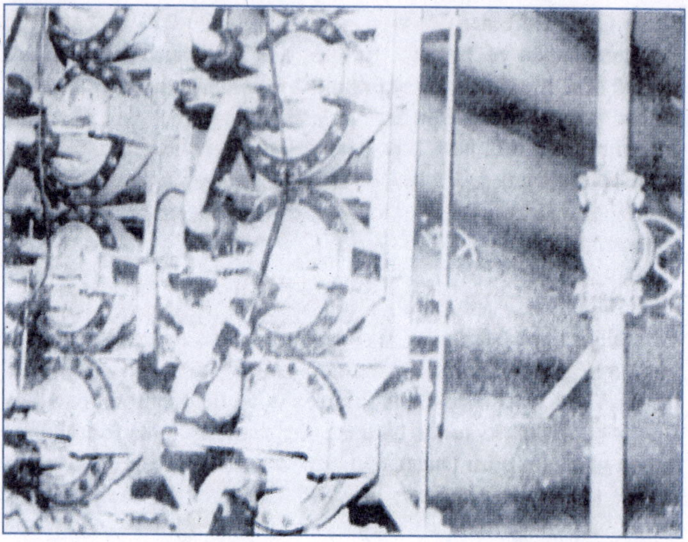

Figure 18.11 Jacketed tubes for cooling of the wort to fermentation temperature. Photo courtesy of the Pittsburgh Brewing Co.

Microorganism

Brewing utilizes strains of *Saccharomyces carlsbergensis*, a bottom yeast, and *Saccharomyces cerevisiae*, both bottom and top-yeast strains. A top yeast rises to the surface during the fermentation while a bottom yeast settles to the bottom. Top yeasts are used for the production of ale (in open tanks), and distillers', bakers' and wine yeasts also are top yeasts. However, beer and sometimes ale fermentations employ bottom yeasts.

Yeast strains are specially selected for their fermenting ability and for their ability to flocculate at the proper time near the end of the fermentation. As a result, a separate industry may select and propagate these strains as well as produce the inoculum, although these functions also can be carried out by the brewery itself. Brewing is different from many other industrial fermentations in that the cells for pitching (inoculating) are often those recovered from a previous fermentation (Figure 18.12). In other words, fresh inoculum is not necessarily prepared for each fermentation run and, in fact, fresh-yeast inoculum usually is required only when contamination presents a real problem or when the vigor of the yeast has begun to decline. Before being employed as inoculum, the yeast cells from a previous fermentation are washed (with phosphoric acid, tartaric acid, or ammonium persulfate) by settling, a procedure that reduces the pH value to approximately 2.5, and removes considerable bacterial contamination, if present. Thus, each pound of yeast added to the fermentation at inoculation yields approximately 3 to 4 pounds liquid yeast at harvest, and the excess yeast not required for further use as inoculum becomes a by-product of the fermentation.

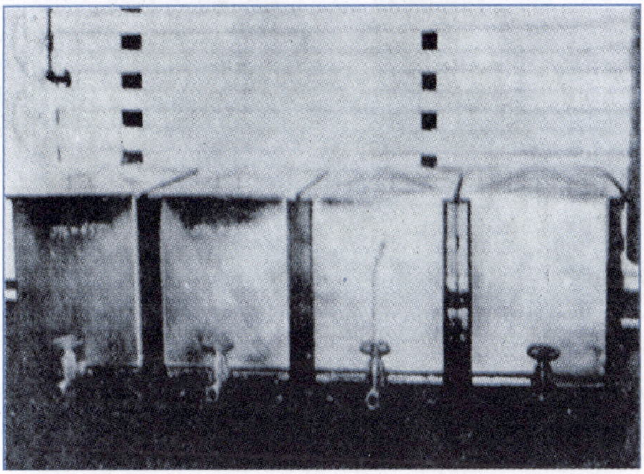

Figure 18.12 Brinks for storage of yeast inoculum between fermentations. Photo courtesy of the Pittsburgh Brewing Co.

Fermentation

The aerated wort is cooled to approximately 10 to 11°C and then placed in a closed fermentation tank containing cooling coils (Figure 18.13). Although an open tank can be used, the closed tank is preferred so that evolved carbon dioxide can be collected for later carbonation of the product. Approximately three-quarters to one pound of yeast are added for each 31 gallons (a barrel) of wort, and within 24 hours after pitching, foam begins to appear on the surface of the medium, first along the wall of the tank and then gradually across the surface. The carbon dioxide evolution then increases so that the yeast cells become suspended in the medium. At this point, the wort is often transferred to a second fermentation tank so that dead and weak yeast cells, precipitated proteins, and insoluble hop resins can be left behind as a deposit on the bottom of the original settling or starting tank or trapped in the foam. This procedure also provides some additional aeration to the medium. However, if the boiled and cooled wort has been filtered before initiation of fermentation, the transfer of the fermentation to a second tank may not be required.

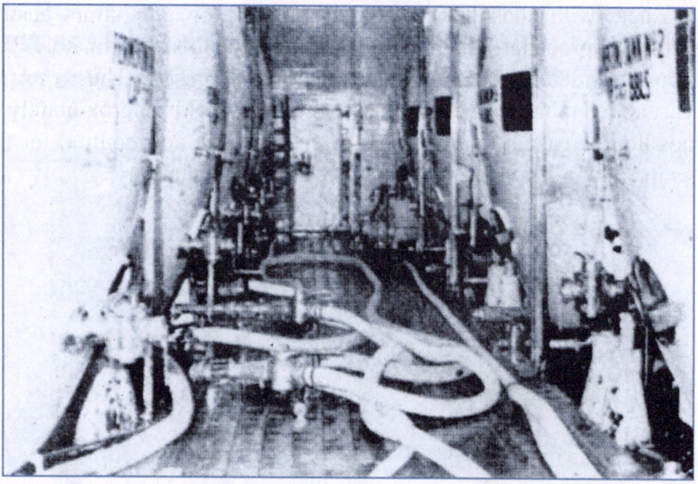

Figure 18.13 Beer fermentation tanks. Photo courtesy of the Pittsburgh Brewing Co.

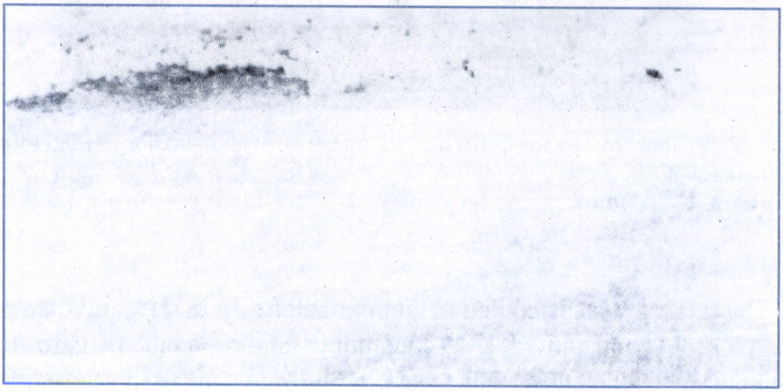

Figure 18.14 Surface foam within a beer fermentation tank. Photo courtesy of C. Schmidt and Sons. Inc.

By approximately 40 to 60 hours after pitching, the surface foam layer becomes very thick (Figure 18.14) and can measure up to almost 12 inches in depth. It is during this time that the most rapid yeast-cell multiplication occurs, and considerable heat, which is associated with this high metabolic activity, is evolved. This heat evolution causes a temperature rise to approximately 12 to 13°C, the peak temperature for this fermentation. Thus, it should be noted that the brewing fermentation is again unusual as regards the use of these very low incubation temperatures. Ale fermentations also employ low temperatures but start at a slightly higher temperature of approximately 13 to 16°C.

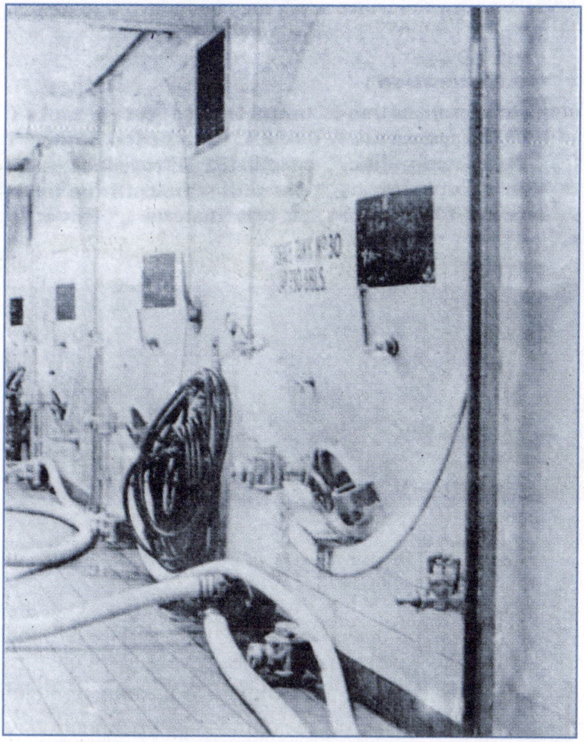

Figure 18.15 Beer cold-storage maturation tanks. Photo courtesy of the Pittsburgh Brewing Co.

By approximately the fifth day of fermentation, there is no longer enough carbon dioxide evolution to support the heavy foam and, therefore, the foam begins to collapse. Also, the decreased evolution of heat by the cells allows the medium to be cooled by the cooling coils. From seven to nine days, the last phase of the fermentation, the yeasts become inactive and flocculate, the "yeast break". An ale fermentation, however, is usually completed by approximately five to seven days. The yeasts settle to the bottom, and the medium is further cooled to hasten settling. At this time, some of the surface scum may be removed to help improve flavor.

Cold-Storage Maturation

The completed fermentation is transferred to storage tanks (Figure 18.15) and held at approximately 0 to 3°C for a period of time. During this "cold-storage maturation," coagulated nitrogenous substances, resins, insoluble phosphates, and yeast cells sediment from the beer. In addition, esters are formed, and the beer matures so that it loses its harshness.

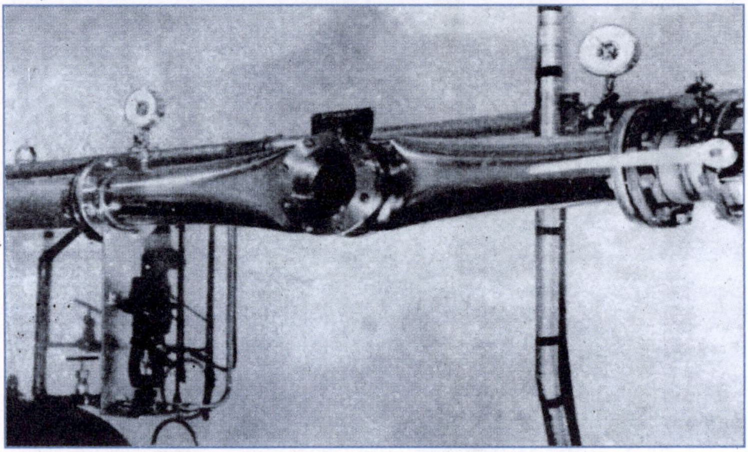

Figure 18.16 Pin-point carbonator for incorporation of carbon dioxide into beer. Photo courtesy of C. Schmidt and Sons, Inc.

During this maturation process, "chillproofing" is commonly practiced to help prevent turbidity development on later exposure of the finished beer to cold. Much of this turbidity can be attributed to unstable protein in the beer, and chillproofing can mean merely the removal by precipitation or adsorption of these unstable residual proteins or partial protein hydrolysate products. More often, however, chill proofing is practiced by employing proteolytic enzymes to reduce the molecular size of the residual proteins and protein hydrolysate products so as to insure their solubility even at cold temperatures.

Antioxidants also usually are added during cold-storage maturation to prevent later oxidative changes in the beer which affect flavor. Sulfur dioxide (sulfites) and ascorbic acid are commonly used to accomplish this end.

Carbonation

Carbonation of the beer is accomplished either by injection of cleaned carbon dioxide recovered from the evolved fermentation gas, or by the "Krausen" process in which actively fermenting yeast is added to provide the so-called "natural carbonation." Addition of carbon dioxide (Figures 18.16 and 18.17), which is the most common practice, provides a final dissolved carbon dioxide content of approximately 0.5 percent in the beer. This carbon dioxide displaces dissolved oxygen, which is detrimental to the stability of the beer, and helps in the production and retention of foam and in the preservation of the beer.

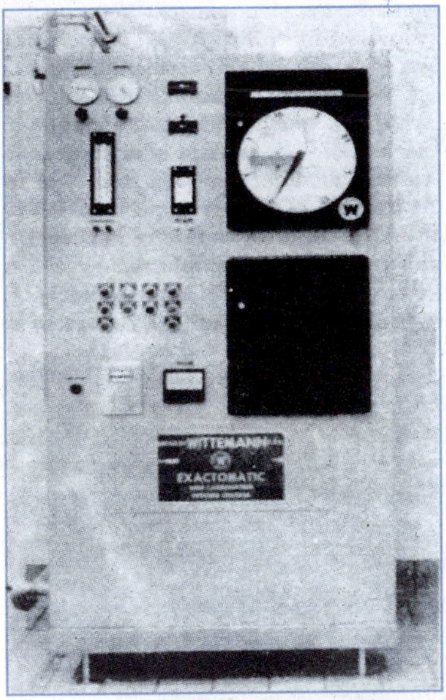

Figure 18.17 Automatic carbonating controls for beer carbonation. Photo courtesy of C. Schmidt and Sons, Inc.

The Krausening process is accomplished by the addition to beer undergoing cold-storage maturation of approximately 15 percent of active fermentation broth and cells from an early stage in the fermentation. These yeast cells are allowed to slowly ferment and remove residual sugar, a process that requires approximately three to four weeks of cold-storage maturation time. The excess carbon dioxide evolved during this period is vented so that the final level will be similar to that for carbon dioxide injection. After the sugar is gone, the beer undergoes several weeks further cold-storage maturation so as to complete the clarification of the beer.

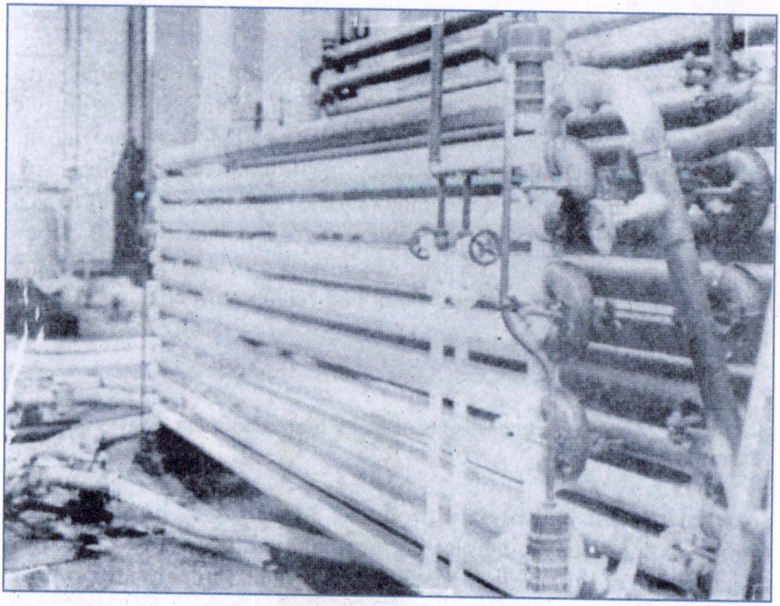

Figure 18.18 Jacketed tubes for cooling beer after completion of cold-storage maturation. Photo courtesy of the Pittsburgh Brewing Co.

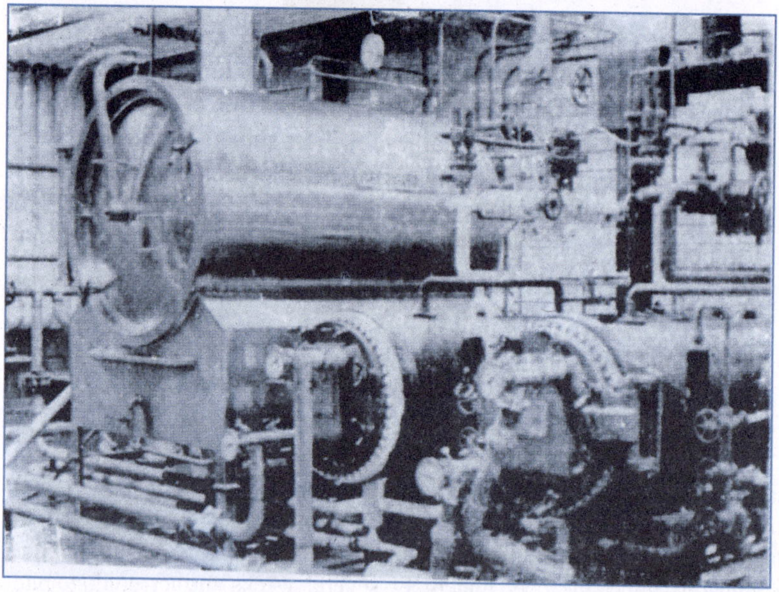

Figure 18.19 Diatomaceous earth filter. Photo courtesy of the Pittsburgh Brewing Co.

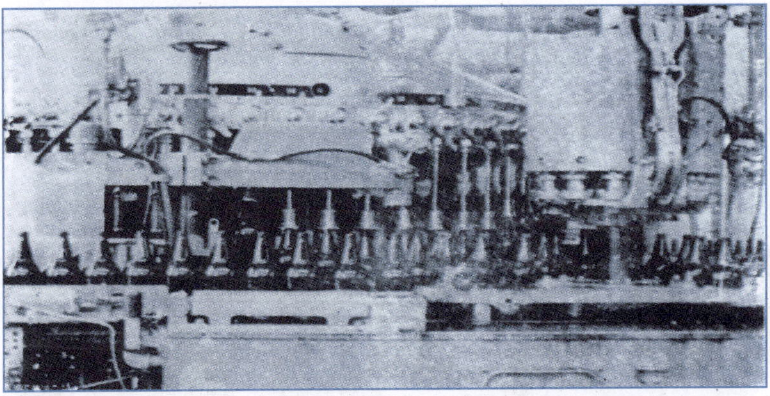

Figure 18.20 Bottles being filled with beer. Photo courtesy of the Pittsburgh Brewing Co.

Packaging

After cold-storage maturation, the beer again is passed through cooling pipes (Figure 18.18) and through a diatomaceous earth filter (Figure 18.19) before being packaged in bottles, cans and barrels or kegs (Figures 18.20 to 18.23). Air is rigorously excluded during this packaging to prevent oxidative changes in the product and, in addition, bottled beer is subjected to electronic inspection to make sure that solid impurities, turbidity, or haze are not present.

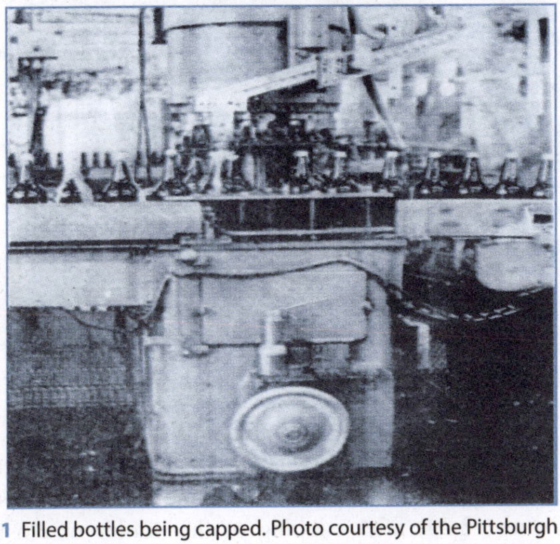

Figure 18.21 Filled bottles being capped. Photo courtesy of the Pittsburgh Brewing Co.

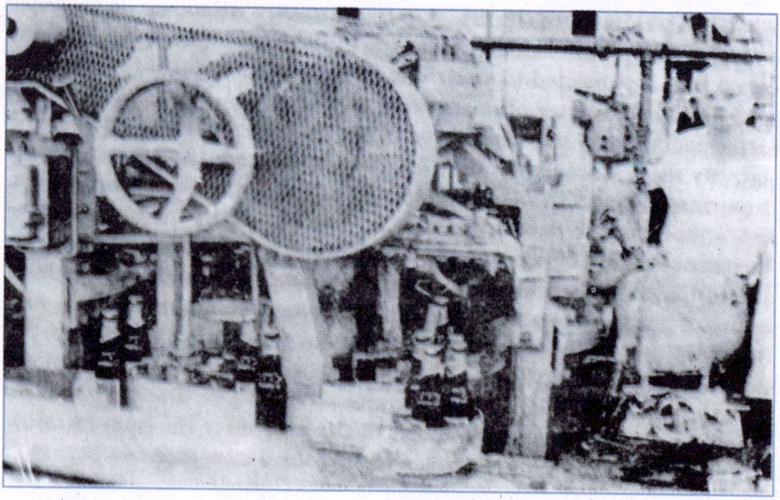

Figure 18.22 Application of labels to capped bottles. Photo courtesy of the Pittsburgh Brewing Co.

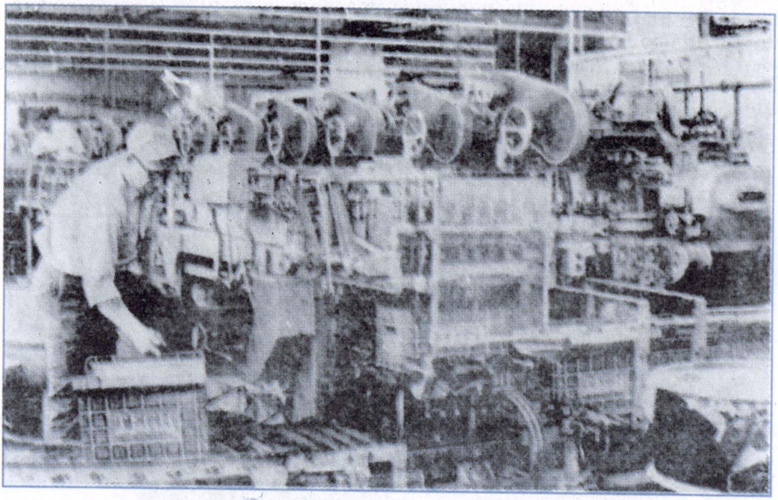

Figure 18.23 Packing of finished product into boxes. Photo courtesy of the Pittsburgh Brewing Co.

Beer packaged in barrels or kegs is not pasteurized and, hence, has a relatively short storage life. Beer for bottles and cans, however, often is pasteurized (Figure 18.24) after capping of the bottles or closing of the cans, although bulk pasteurizers are now employed by many breweries. The pasteurization of beer, however, affects its flavor and, to correct this situation, recent innovations now allow the sterilization of beer without the use of pasteurization so that the keg flavor is maintained along with good keeping quality. Thus, the beer can be passed through membrane bacteriological filters (Figure 18.25), or it can be chemically sterilized prior to packaging. For this procedure, *n*-heptyl-*p*-hydroxybenzoate at up to 12 ppm is immediately added to the beer after the final filtration step, and this compound then is effective for a considerable period.

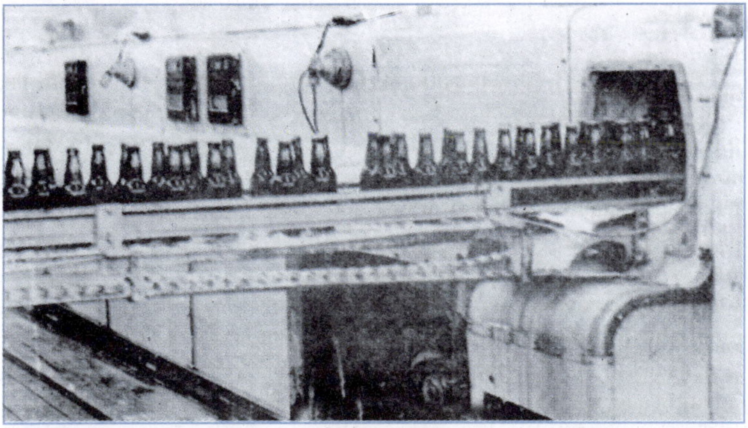

Figure 18.24 Pasteurization of beer in bottles. Photo courtesy of the Pittsburgh Brewing Co.

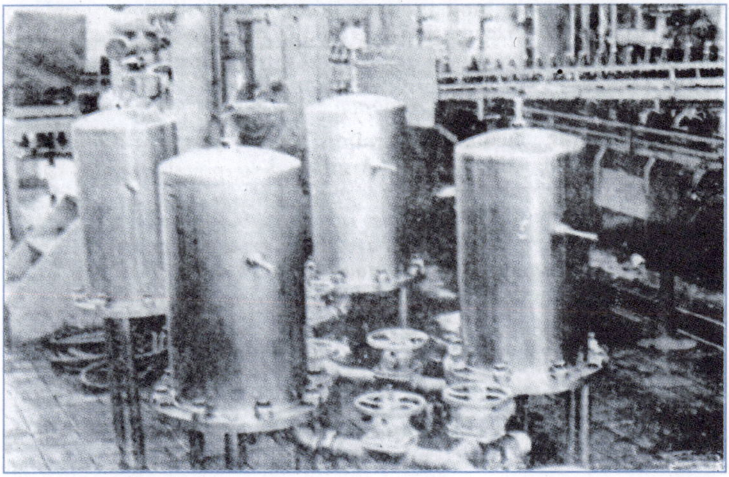

Figure 18.25 Bell Housings containing stacked membrane filters. Photo courtesy of the Pittsburgh Brewing Co.

Keeping Quality

Beer deteriorates with age, particularly as regards changes in flavor and appearance. This deterioration is caused by sunlight, storage at warm temperatures, shaking or agitation of the containers, and internal oxidation caused by residual oxygen. Turbidity is the most apparent and quickly spotted form of deterioration, and this is caused by unstable protein, protein-tannin complexes, starch, and resins becoming insoluble. Microorganisms, including yeasts and bacteria, also can produce turbidity.

Contamination

For the most part, contamination is not a problem in carefully controlled brewing operations under clean plant conditions. There are various reasons for this. The low pH of the wort, pH 5 to 5.4 (decreasing to 4.2 to 4.8 during the fermentation), is too acid for the growth of most bacteria. Also, the hop resins are particularly effective in preventing the growth of Gram-positive bacteria. The sterile wort at the beginning of the fermentation and the production of carbon dioxide and ethyl alcohol during the fermentation also tend to inhibit contaminants, as do the low incubation temperature and the anaerobic incubation conditions of the fermentation. Obviously, various of these considerations also apply to the beer during cold-storage maturation, carbonation and packaging, and the membrane filtration, chemical treatment or pasteurization of the final product further insure lack of contamination.

Regardless of these factors, however, contamination can and does occur, and gross contamination can impart turbidity, off-flavor, acidity, and ropiness to the product. Only certain groups of microorganisms are able to cause contamination. Thus, *Acetobacter* species can utilize ethanol and cause contamination, but exclusion of oxygen for these aerobes usually holds their activities in check. The facultatively anaerobic lactic acid bacteria are more serious, however, because of their ability to grow at a low pH in the absence of oxygen and to produce acidity and off flavor. Included in this group are species of *Lactobacillus*, *Streptococcus* and *Pediococcus*. Careful microscopic examination of the pitching yeast usually detects gross contamination by these bacteria, and the yeast, to a certain extent can be freed of bacterial contamination by washing with dilute tartaric or phosphoric acids or with ammonium persulfate.

Saccharomyces and other species of yeasts can also cause contamination and, when present, they utilize sugar, or even the ethanol and dextrins and, as a results, can produce additional alcohol over that usually desired in the finished product. Contamination of the pitching yeast by these "wild" yeasts may be difficult to recognize on microscopic examination of the pitching yeast, and this must be considered in decisions as to when to employ freshly propagated yeast inoculum.

Phages or viruses are not normally considered to be able to infect yeasts. However, a yeast phage (a zymophage) has been reported by Lindegren (1958). This phage caused decreased fermentative ability of the yeast.

By-Products

The spent grains separated without drying from the wort find commercial use as animal feed. However, they also are dried to about 10 percent moisture to provide an animal-feed product known as dried brewers' grains which contains protein, fat, carbohydrate, crude fiber and vitamins of the B complex.

Surplus yeast from the fermentation is sold as brewers' yeast. This product is rich in B vitamins and ergosterol, and it is utilized for human food and animal feed, as a source of concentrated vitamins, and as a starting material for the recovery of various chemicals.

Continuous Fermentation

Continuous fermentation would not appear to be applicable to brewing because of the delicately balanced properties of flavor, aroma, and so forth which must be present in the product. However, it has been reported that several breweries are successfully employing this fermentation technique, probably with specially designed fermentation tanks (Royston, 1966).

References

Brewing

Haas, G.J., 1960. Microbial control methods in the brewery, *Adv. Appl. Microbiol.*, **2,** 113–162.

Lindergren, C.C., 1958. Proc. A.M. Amer. Soc. Brew. Chem., p. 86.

Prescott, S.C. and C.G. Dunn, 1959. *Industrial microbiology*, 3rd Ed, pp. 148–173, McGraw-Hill Book Co., Inc., New York.

Rose, A.H., 1961., *Industrial microbiology*. pp. 118–131, Butterworths, Washington.

Royston, M.G., 1966. Tower fermentation of beer, *Process Biochem*., **1,** 215–221.

Tenney, R.I., 1954. The brewing industry, pp. 172–195 in *Industrial fermentations,* vol. I (ed. by L.A. Underkofler and R.J. Hickey). Chemical Publishing Co., New York.

INDUSTRIAL ALCOHOL

The production of industrial alcohol, ethanol, became commercially feasible on a large scale shortly after 1906 when the Industrial Alcohol Act was passed. This Act allowed the sale of tax-exempt alcohol, if it was first denatured to prevent its use in alcoholic beverages. Since this time, the production of alcohol has been rigorously supervised by the Internal Revenue Service, even to the point of recording the amounts of all raw materials used in its production by fermentation.

Industrial alcohol is employed extensively as a solvent, and to a lesser extent as a raw material for chemical syntheses. Also, small amounts of industrial alcohol are mixed with motor fuels such as gasoline. For many years, most of the industrial alcohol produced in the United States was by fermentation. However, in recent years, the synthesis of industrial alcohol from ethylene, as results from petroleum refinery waste gases, has made strong inroads on the market to the point that only small amounts are presently produced by fermentation. In fact, the picture may deteriorate yet further for microbially produced industrial alcohol as the costs of carbon substrates increase and the economics of chemical synthesis improve. In many parts of the world, however, a ready access to cheap carbon substrates and a relative lack of chemical synthesis technology have allowed fermentation industrial alcohol to maintain its place in the market.

Microorganism

The choice of fermentation organism for industrial alcohol production depends, to some extent, on the type of carbohydrate present in the medium. Alcohol production from starch and sugar raw materials utilizes specially selected strains of *Saccharomyces cerevisiae* and, to a lesser extent, of *Saccharomyces ellipsoideus*. Production from the lactose of whey, after protein removal, is accomplished with *Candida pseudotropicalis*. The sulfite-waste liquor fermentation employs *Candida utilis*, because of the ability of this organism to ferment pentoses, although *Saccharomyces cerevisiae* also can be utilized with this substrate. In this instance, however, the pentoses of the sulfite-waste liquor are left behind. The particular strains of these various organisms actually employed for the fermentation are selected for several properties. Thus, they must grow rapidly and be tolerant to high concentrations of sugar but, at the same time, they must be able to produce large amounts of alcohol and be relatively resistant to this alcohol.

Media

The principal media for the commercial production of fermentation industrial alcohol contain blackstrap molasses or corn but, of these, blackstrap molasses has found greater world-wide use. Industrial alcohol, in addition, is produced by the fermentation of other grains, sulfite waste liquor, whey, potatoes, and wood wastes. However, when sulfite-waste liquor is employed, the sulfur dioxide first must be removed by steam stripping followed by neutralization. Nevertheless, the continuous fermentation technique (Chapter 13) has been profitable with the latter substrate, because of the nature of the microorganism employed, and because of the presence of substances inhibitory to contaminants.

For the molasses fermentation, the molasses is diluted with water or water plus stillage to a sugar concentration of somewhere between 10 and 18 percent, as determined with a Balling hydrometer. Sugar concentrations greater than this are not employed, because the sugar becomes deterimental to the yeast, as does the resulting high alcohol concentration in the fermentation. This molasses wort is directly utilized as a fermentation medium without further nutrient additions or, if required, ammonium sulfate and ammonium phosphate can be added. The pH value of the medium is adjusted to 4 to 5, but more usually to 4.8 to 5, by adding sulfuric or lactic acids, or by allowing lactic acid bacteria to bring about an initial lactic acid fermentation. Of these reagents, the lactic acid is particularly beneficial to the fermentation, since it is inhibitory to the growth of butyric acid bacterial contaminants, and a pH value of less than 5 also inhibits the lactic acid bacteria. Other possible microbial contaminants for the fermentation are inhibited by the low pH, high sugar concentration, and anaerobic conditions of the fermentation, and by the high alcohol production by the yeast. Thus, as a result of these considerations, the molasses medium is not sterilized or, at most, it is only pasteurized.

Starchy media, such as those provided by corn, rye, and barley, must undergo initial starch hydrolysis. This is accomplished by mashing with barley malt, as for the brewing fermentation, by application of dilute acid, or by utilization of fungal amylolytic enzymes such as those associated with species of *Aspergillus* and *Rhizopus*. In most instances, however, the starch hydrolysis is accomplished with malt. Somewhere in the range of 30 percent barley malt and 70 percent corn are mixed with water or water plus stillage, and mashing procedures similar to those for brewing are carried out, but with the temperature program adjusted to yield the maximum amount of the fermentable sugar, maltose. The mashing process converts approximately 80 percent of the corn starchto maltose, although the residual dextrins are slowly converted to maltose during the actual fermentation by malt amylases still present in the wort. Again, the wort is not sterilized but may be pasteurized.

Fermentation

Industrial alcohol production is carried out in very large fermentors (up to 125,000 gallons), and the inoculum for these fermentors is added in the range of 3 to 10 percent with an average of about 4 percent. The temperature of the fermentation is set initially at somewhere between 21 and 27°C, but heat evolution during the fermentation raises the temperature to 28 to 30°C, with the temperature being held in this range through the use of cooling coils. Some fermentations, however, are conducted at temperatures as high as 33°C, although ethanol evaporation from the fermentation can become serious at temperatures much over approximately 27°C. The fermentation lasts approximately 2 to 3 days, with the actual time period being dependent on the substrate utilized and on the temperature of incubation.

During inoculum build-up, the yeast cells are highly aerated to provide rapid cell multiplication, and various semicontinuous methods of inoculum build-up have been devised. Aeration, however, is not applied to the fermentation itself, and the fermentation medium quickly becomes anaerobic, because of the withdrawal by the yeast of oxygen from the medium, and because of the rapid evolution of carbon dioxide starting shortly after pitching (inoculation).

The fermentation broth at completion of the fermentation contains in the range of 6 to 9 percent alcohol by volume and, based on various reports, this alcohol yield reflects a 90 to 98 percent theoretical conversion of substrate sugar to alcohol. Remember that, via the EMP scheme, 1 mole of a 6-carbon sugar theoretically yields 2 moles of ethanol and 2 moles of carbon dioxide. Also, when stating alcohol yields, one must be careful not to become confused by the statement of alcohol concentration as percent as contrasted to "proof." The latter is a common method of designating alcohol concentration, and it is twice the percentage in volume of ethanol as dissolved in water; for example, 95 percent ethanol is 190 proof.

As stated previously, continuous fermentation with sulfite-waste liquor is presently employed on a commercial scale. Although continuous fermentation with molasses or grain substrates would appear to have commercial feasibility, this technique, as yet, has not found extensive application with those substrates. There also is some possibility for the use of a type of replacement culture which is, in effect, merely the reuse in further fermentations of the yeast recovered from previous fermentations.

Product Recovery

Ethanol is separated from the fermentation broth in continuous stills resembling those utilized for the recovery of acetone and butanol, and ethanol of 95 percent concentration is obtained by successive distillations in these stills. To obtain alcohol concentrations greater than 95 percent, however, requires special distillation techniques, because of the ability of alcohol to form an azeotropic mixture containing 5 percent water. Thus, to prepare absolute ethanol, the 5 percent water is removed by forming an azeotropic mixture of benzene, water, and ethanol, which then is distilled with increasing temperature increments. This procedure removes first the azeotropic benzene-water-ethanol mixture, and then an ethanol-benzene azeotropic mixture so that absolute ethanol remains. The absolute ethanol, as well as 95 percent ethanol, is marketed with and without denaturation.

A high-boiling fusel oil fraction also is recovered during distillation of the fermentation broth, and this fraction accounts for approximately 0.5 percent of the crude distillates, the actual yield fluctuating somewhat with the fermentation medium employed. This fusel oil is made up of several components, but mainly it is a mixture of *n*-amyl and isoamyl alcohols. It finds commercial use as a lacquer solvent.

Other products of the fermentation, except for the carbon dioxide which is often collected for commercial reuse, are present in only small amounts. Thus, trace amounts of succinic acid and slightly larger amounts of glycerol occur. Some acrolein also may be present in the distillate, having been formed by microbiological contaminants attacking the glycerol.

References

INDUSTRIAL ALCOHOL

Hodge, H. M. and F. M. Hilderbrandt, 1954. Alcoholic fermentation of molasses, pp. 73–94 in *Industrial fermentations*, vol. I (ed. by L. A. underkofler and R. J. Hickey) Chemical Publishing Co., Inc., New York.

McCarthy, J. L., 1954. Alcoholic fermentations of sulfite waste liquor, pp. 95–135 in *Industrial fermentations*, vol I (ed. by L. A. Underkofler and R. J. Hickey), Chemical Publishing Co., Inc., New York.

Prescott, S. C. and C. G. Dunn, 1959. *Industrial microbiology*, 3rd Ed., pp. 102–147, McGraw-Hill Book Co., Inc., New York.

Rose, A. H., 1961. *Industrial microbiology*. pp. 147–151, Butterworths, Washington.

Saeman, J. F. and A. A. Andraesen, 1954. The production of alcohol from wood waste, pp. 136–171 in *Industrial fermentations*, vol. I (ed. by L. A. Underkofler and R. J. Hickey). Chemical Publishing Co., Inc., New York.

Stark, W. H., 1954. Alcoholic fermentation of grain, pp. 17–72 in *Industrial fermentations*, vol. I (ed. by L. A. Underkofler and R. J. Hickey). Chemical Publishing Co., Inc., New York.

LACTIC ACID

Man has long observed the souring of milk, but it was only in 1780 that Scheele discovered lactic acid, the chemical that causes this phenomenon. Although others had demonstrated the microbiological nature of souring, it remained for Pasteur, 77 years after Scheele's initial work, to investigate the fermentation and describe a causative organism. Today we know, moreover, that many microorganisms are able to produce at least small amounts of lactic acid, and that this acid is present in many fermented foods and beverages.

The first commercial production of lactic acid in the United States by a microbiological process was in 1881 as a means for obtaining its calcium salt, calcium lactate. Today, most of the commercial lactic acid still results from microbiological processes, since the chemical synthesis of lactic acid has not been able as yet to make appreciable inroads on the market. However, because of the relatively high (and still increasing) costs of the fermentation, commercial lactic acid is finding competition from organic acids other than lactic in instances in which these other acids can be used equally well. The costs of lactic acid production are attributable not so much to the fermentation itself as to the processes required for its recovery and purification, since this acid is difficult to separate from the impurities of the fermentation medium, and since very high purity lactic acid is required for certain applications such as the production of plastics. In addition to these costs, the expense of the equipment employed for the recovery and purification of lactic acid must be considered, since this equipment must be fabricated to resist the corrosive nature of this acid.

Lactic acid has a pleasant, sour taste, but no odor. It is completely miscible with water, alcohol, and ether, although it is insoluble in chloroform; thus, it does not crystallize from solution as do other acids. Also, its low melting point means that it is a liquid at most commonly encountered temperatures. It is a weak acid with good solvent properties, and it polymerizes readily for the production of polymers. In addition many of its salts are quite soluble in water. Thus, these various properties have allowed lactic acid to find wide commercial usage. It provides acidity in food and beverage applications and serves as a preservative in foodstuffs. Crude grades are used for the deliming of hides in the leather industry, and it is utilized for fabric treatment in the textile and laundry industries. Its ability to form polymeric polylactic acids finds application in production of various resins. Calcium lactate is employed in baking powders, as an animal- and poultry-feed supplement, and as a means for providing a calcium source in pharmaceutical preparations. Copper lactate is used in electroplating. Finally, various chemical derivatives of lactic acid are used in the production of plastics.

Isomers

The lactic acid molecule (Figure 18.26) contains one asymmetric carbon atom, and this carbon atom allows the occurrence of two optically active isomers plus an optically inactive mixture of the two isomers, a racemic mixture. D(–)-lactic acid has the D-configuration about the asymmetric carbon atom, and it is levorotary. This means that, when placed in a plane of polarized light, it rotates the light to the left. L(+)-lactic acid has the L-configuration at the asymmetric carbon and is dextrorotary. A racemic mixture of the D-and L-forms, however, is optically inactive, because the rotations of light neutralize each other. It is interesting to note, moreover, that the various lactic acid salts possess reversed optical rotations : the salt of D(–)-lactic acid is dextrorotary while that of L(+)-lactic acid is levorotary. It should also be pointed out that the L-configuration of the acid is metabolized by the animal or human body while the D-configuration is not metabolized and is largely excreted.

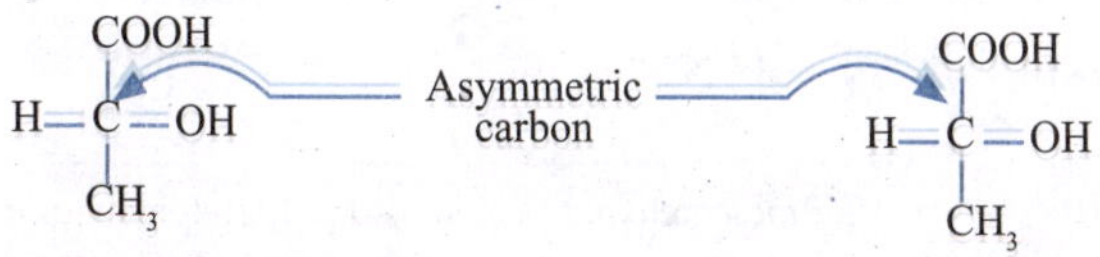

D(–)Lactic acid L(–)Lactic acid

Figure 18.26 Optically active isomers of lactic acid.

Microorganisms differ in their ability to produce either D(–)-lactic acid, L(+)-lactic acid, or the racemic mixture, and the particular acid formed seems to be a characteristic of the individual microorganism. However, from an industrial fermentation standpoint, the lactic acid recovered from the fermentation broth usually is the racemic mixture. Thus, this occurrence is attributed in large part to the fact that the fermentation microorganism or contaminants of the fermentation produce an enzyme known as "racemase" which converts either of the optically active isomers to the optically inactive racemic mixture, although trace impurities in the medium also have been reported to bring about racemization. In contrast to most other microorganisms, the fungus *Rhizopus oryzae* produces only L(+)-lactic acid, apparently without further racemization. However, this fungus has not found particular industrial application because of the slowness of its fermentation and its relatively low yields as compared to fermentations by the lactic acid bacteria.

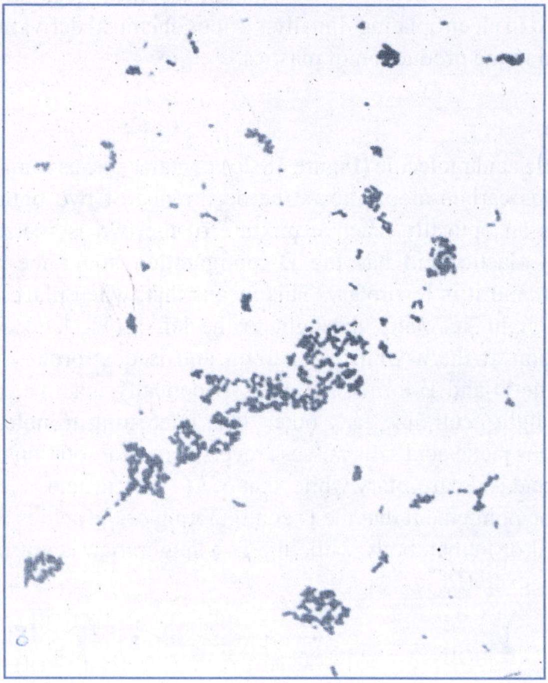

Figure 18.27 *Leuconostoc mesenteroides* as observed at 1250-fold magnification.

Microorganisms

Most microorganisms producing lactic acid are classed as being "heterofermentative." Thus, they produce some lactic acid, but at the same time, and probably by way of the pentose phosphate metabolic pathway, they also produce carbon dioxide, ethyl alcohol, acetic acid, and trace amounts of a few other products. These organisms are of little use for industrial lactic acid fermentations, because too much of the substrate carbon is directed toward products other than lactic acid. *Leuconostoc mesenteroids* (Figure 18.27) is a good example of a heterofermentative lactic acid bacterium.

Commercial lactic acid production utilizes "homofermentative" strains of lactic acid bacteria which produce only trace amounts of end products other than lactic acid. Thus, these bacteria utilize the EMP scheme to produce pyruvic acid which is then reduced by their lactic dehydrogenase enzyme to lactic acid. As a result of the use of this pathway the percent conversion of sugar to lactic acid is virtually equivalent to the theoretical yield of two moles of lactic acid for every mole of hexose sugar utilized by the organism.

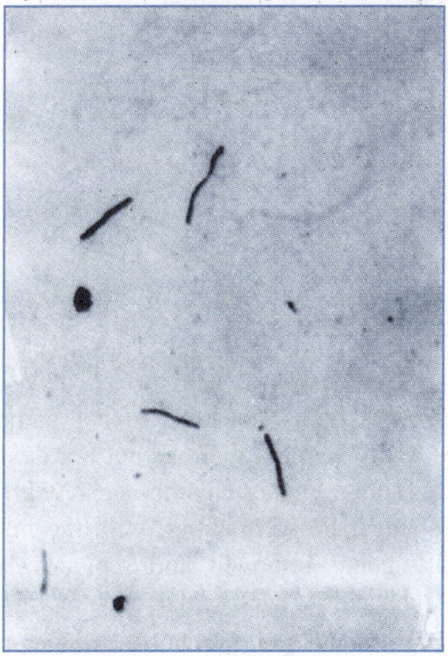

Figure 18.28 *Lactobacillus* delbrueckii as observed at 1250-fold magnification.

The most common bacterium for the industrial production of lactic acid is *Lactobacillus delbrueckii* (Figure 18.28); it is employed in fermentations utilizing corn dextrose media. Other bacteria of industrial importance include *Lactobacillus bulgaricus*, which utilize lactose as a carbon source and finds use in lactic acid production from whey media, and *Lactobacillus pentosus*, which is able to utilize the pentoses of sulfite-waste liquor for lactic acid production. Other homofermentative species of poential industrial importance are *Lactobacillus casei, Lactobacillus leichmannii* (Figure 18.29), and *Streptococcus lactic* (Figure 18.30). All of these bacteria are considered to be anaerobes, although they can withstand some oxygen.

However, *Streptococcus lactis* is less sensitive to oxygen and, therefore, can also be considered as a facultative aerobe.

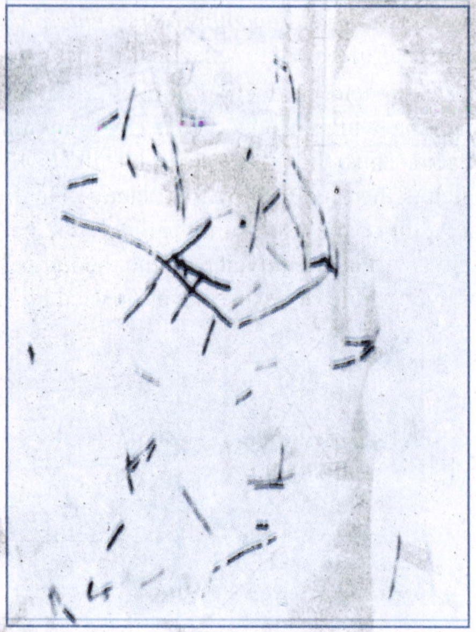

Figure 18.29 *Lactobacillus leichmannii* as observed at 1250-fold magnification.

Lactobacillus delbrueckii is unusual in that strains freshly isolated from natural sources easily ferment maltose but not dextrose; they must be adapted to ferment this sugar. This is accomplished by growing the organism in successive transfer on maltose medium, with the maltose in the media formulation gradually being removed and replaced by dextrose. Some isolates, however, are difficult to acclimatize even by this procedure.

The lactic acid bacteria are well known for the fact that they synthesize very few of the vitamins and other growth factors required for their growth, and this consideration has allowed extensive use of these organisms as specific biological assay agents for various growth factors. By the same token, however, media for the growth of these organisms or for the fermentative production of lactic acid therefore must provide a wide range of growth factors to supplement their inefficient biosynthetic capabilities.

Stock-culture maintenance for lactic acid bacteria requires greater care than for some other types of microorganisms. Thus, these bacteria die out quickly in soil stocks, and this procedure, therefore, cannot be utilized. Agar slants containing excess calcium carbonate are a possibility, but with this procedure frequent transfers are required to maintain viability of the culture.

Sterile 5 percent corn mash with excess calcium carbonate also is a possibility, and in this medium these bacteria remain viable for longer periods of time. Lyophilization, which is a good procedure for the maintenance of most other types of bacteria, also can be employed for the lactic acid bacteria, but a fairly high death rate is encountered. Probably the best way to maintain stock cultures of these organisms is to grow them in litmus milk containing $CaCO_3$, and to freeze the litmus milk before enough acid formation has occurred to affect the color of the litmus.

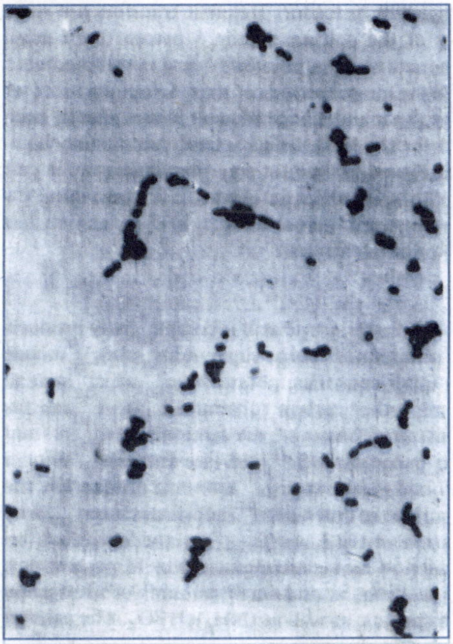

Figure 18.30 *Streptococcus lactis* as observed at 1250-fold magnification.

Medium

In the United States, lactic acid is commercially produced from media containing semirefined corn sugar (dextrose), molasses, or whey, although in other countries, potato starch, which requires preliminary hydrolysis, and other carbon substrates have at times been employed. Of these substrates, however, the semirefined sugars, maltose, lactose, sucrose, and particularly dextrose (see Inskeep, Taylor and Breitzke, 1952) have found greatest use for lactic acid production, the reason being that the impurities in crude carbon substrates interfere with the recovery and purification of the lactic acid from the completed fermentation. A typical production medium contains 10 to

15 percent dextrose, 10 percent calcium carbonate, and small amounts of nitrogenous substances, such as malt sprouts, as well as $(NH_4)_2\ HPO_4$. The calcium carbonate is employed to neutralize the lactic acid as it is produced, because the lactic acid bacteria do not tolerate high concentrations of acid. Growth factors are supplied by the malt sprouts or other organic nitrogenous substrates, but the concentration employed in the medium is maintained at the lowest possible level to prevent an accumulation of impurities that might interfere with the lactic acid recovery from the fermentation broth. Heat-labile growth factors have been reported as being present in malt sprouts, and the addition of nonheat-sterilized malt sprouts in small amounts does increase yields. High sugar concentrations are not employed in the fermentation medium, because the calcium lactate produced at these sugar concentrations tends to crystallize from the medium late in the fermentation, in the process slowing the fermentation. Also, the microorganisms must remove almost all of the sugar from the medium by the end of the fermentation so that residual sugar does not interfere with the lactic acid recovery.

Production

Lactic acid fermentations are carried out in tanks made of wood or lined with stainless steel, because most other fabrication materials cannot withstand the corrosive nature of lactic acid. Five percent *Lactobacillus delbrueckii* inoculum is added to the fermentor, and the fermentation temperature is adjusted to 45 to 50°C. This initial temperature is lower (approximately 30°C), however, if the fermentation organism is *Lactobacillus pentosus, Lactobacillus casei*, or *Streptococcus lactis*. The pH value during the fermentation is maintained between 5.5 and 6.5 by the calcium carbonate in the medium or at 6.3 to 6.5 by automatic pH control involving the addition of calcium hydroxide as required. Fermentations utilizing grain mash, however, can accommodate slightly greater acidity build-up because of the buffering action of the grain mash. The medium is not aerated, but agitation is employed to keep the calcium carbonate in suspension so that it will react with the lactic acid as it is produced during the fermentation. The fermentation is usually completed in six days or less depending on the amount of time required for the organism to deplete the sugar of the medium. The resulting lactic acid yields commonly are in the 80 to 90 percent range based on sugar, although good fermentations yield 93 to 94 percent conversion of sugar to lactic acid.

Contamination is not a particular problem with *Lactobacillus delbrueckii* lactic acid fermentations because of the high incubation temperature. Thus, most of the potential contaminants for the fermentation do not grow at temperatures of 45°C or greater. However, near the end of the fermentation, after the activity of the lactic acid bacteria has decreased, butyric-acid-producing organisms can cause contamination.

Continuous lactic acid fermentations have been practiced to a limited extent on a commercial scale, but these fermentations encounter difficulty because the residual sugar in the partially fermented medium, as withdrawn during continuous fermentation, hinders recovery of the lactic acid.

Extraction and Recovery

At harvest, additional calcium carbonate is added to the medium, the pH is adjusted to approximately 10, and the fermentation broth is heated and then filtered. This procedure converts all of the lactic acid to calcium lactate, kills bacteria, coagulates proteins of the medium, removes excess calcium carbonate, and helps to decompose any residual sugar in the medium. Various procedures then are employed for the recovery and purification of the lactic acid. In one procedure, the heated and filtered fermentation broth is concentrated to allow crystallization of calcium lactate, follwed by addition of sulfuric acid to remove the calcium as calcium sulfate. The lactic acid then is recrystallized as calcium lactate, and activated carbon is used to remove colored impurities. As an alternative to the latter step, the zinc salts of lactic acid are sometimes prepared because of the relatively lower solubility of zinc lactate. In another procedure, the free lactic acid is solvent extracted with isopropyl ether directly from the heated and filtered fermentation broth. This is a counter-current continuous extraction, and the lactic acid is recovered from the isopropyl ether by further counter-current washing of the solvent with water. In a third procedure, the methyl ester of the free lactic acid is prepared, and this is separated from the fermentation broth by distillation followed by hydrolysis of the ester by boiling in dilute water solution (the methyl ester decomposes in water). The lactic acid then is obtained from the aqueous solution by evaporation of the water, and the methanol is recovered by distillation. In a fourth procedure, secondary or tertiary alkylamine salts of lactic acid are formed and then extracted from aqueous solution with organic solvents; the solvent is removed by evaporation, and the salt then is decomposed to yield the free acid. An older procedure, not utilized commercially to any extent today, involves direct high-vacuum steam distillation of the lactic acid from the fermentation broth, but decomposition of some of the lactic acid occurs.

It is of particular importance that the recovery processing equipment be resistant to the corrosive action of the high concentrations of lactic acid which accumulate. Therefore, special stainless steel equipment is most often employed for this purpose.

Lactic acid is sold in various commercial grades, and the better grades require that well-purified substrates be utilized in the fermentation medium in order to reduce the levels of impurities present during recovery which, without great difficulty, cannot be separated from the lactic acid. Also, in this regard, the sugar should be depleted from the medium by harvest of the fermentation. One of the commercial grades of lactic acid, "crude" or "technical" grade, is a colored product prepared for commercial usage at concentrations in water of 22, 44, 50, 66 and 80 percent. It is prepared by employing sulfuric acid to remove the calcium from the calcium lactate derived from the heated and filtered fermentation broth, followed by filtration, concentration, and refiltration to remove additional calcium sulfate. Thus, this grade of lactic acid contains many of the impurities from the fermentation medium, and it finds many industrial uses where purity of the product is not essential as, for example, in the deliming of hides in the leather industry. The "edible" grade of lactic acid is straw-colored and is marketed 50 to 80 percent strengths. Thus, it receives additional refining over that of technical lactic acid. Colorless, high-purity lactic acids are the "plastic" grade, marketed at 50 to 80 percent strengths, and "U.S.P." lactic acid, marketed at 85 percent strength. Other commercial preparations of lactic acid are calcium lactate, sodium lactate, and copper lactate (a salt that is used in electroplating).

The final recovered yields of technical-and edible-grade lactic acids, based on the original carbohydrate of the medium, are approximately 85 to 90 percent and 80 percent respectively. Plastic and U.S.P. grades are prepared by further refining of technical-grade lactic acid and, therefore, slight to moderate further yield losses are incurred during this refining.

References

Lactic Acid

Inskeep, G. C., G. G. Taylor, and W. C. Breitzke, 1952. Lactic acid from corn sugar. *Ind. Eng. Chem.,* **44,** 1955–1966.

Prescott, S. C. and C. G. Dunn., 1959. *Industrial microbiology*, 3rd Ed., pp. 304–331. McGraw-Hill Book Co., Inc., New York.

Rose, A. H., 1961. *Industrial microbiology,* pp. 172–177, Butterworths, Washington.

Schopmeyer, H. H., 1954. Lactic acid, Pp. 389–419 in *Industrial fermentations*, vol. I (ed. by L. A. Underkofler and R. J. Hickey), Chemical Publishing Co., New York.

Wilkinson, J. F, and A. H. Rose, 1963. Fermentation processes, pp. 395–397 in *Biochemistry of industrial microorganisms* (ed. by C. Rainbow and A. H. Rose), Academic Press, New York.

CHAPTER 19

Environmental Control of Metabolic Pathways

The ratios of the various products that accumulate during a fermentation, or even the presence *per se* of special fermentation products, in certain instances can be altered by manipulation of the normal cultural conditions of the fermentation. These manipulations can result in a shunting of intermediate carbon compounds of major metabolic pathways through little-used side metabolic sequences of the cell. Alternatively, these manipulations may provide chemically altered fermentation products without actually utilizing other than the normal metabolic pathways of the cell. These manipulations also can change the respiratory mechanism utilized by the cell, the energy recovery to the cell during metabolic reaction, and even the permeability of the cell to substrates and fermentation products. Finally, these manipulations can allow the functioning of only individual enzymes of a metabolic sequence, both in the intact cell and in the cell that has been disrupted to release its enzymes to the fermentation medium.

Several examples might be cited to demonstrate how fermentations. manipulation can be applied to microbial fermentations. Thus, the inclusion in fermentation media of penicillin precursors and of cobalt increases the formation, respectively, of specific penicillins and of vitamin B_{12}. Another example is that of a mutant of *Micrococcus glutamicus* which, under normal fermentation conditions, produces L-glutamic acid, but which produces L-glutamine in the presence of excess ammonium ion and a pH of 5.5. Under the latter conditions, the glutaminase enzyme, which normally removes amide nitrogen from glutamine to yield glutamic acid, becomes inactivated. Moreover, with this organism, the latter fermentation conditions also are optimum for the enzyme glutamine synthetase which converts the glutamic acid to glutamine, since the pH optimum of the glutamine enzyme is 5.5 to 6.5 (Oshima *et al.*, 1963). The yeast *Rhodotrula gracilis* provides an example of fermentative manipulation, since it can be made to accumulate up to 63 percent of its cellular dry weight as fat. This is accomplished by withholding nitrogen compounds from the cells so that a nitrogen deficiency induces fat formation instead of protein synthesis. Other examples are as follows. Low temperature incubation conditions sometimes allow the accumulation of fermentation products more unsaturated than occur at the normal incubation temperatures for these organisms (Jazeski and Olsen, 1961). The use of high inoculum levels to prevent the occurrence of more than minimal additional growth (as in the yeast-glycerol fermentation), or of replacement culture (as in the *Aspergillus niger* gluconic acid fermentation), allow the fermentative use of specific enzymes or enzyme systems of the intact cell divorced from the activities of the much greater numbers of enzymes associated with normal growth. A somewhat similar condition exists in spore fermentations (Gehrig and Knight, 1958 and 1961) in which, without undergoing germination, spores of *Penicillium roqueforti* produce methyl ketones from fatty acids. This also occurs for the spores of various other species of *Aspergillus* and *Penicillium*.

Acetone drying, autolysis, toluene treatment, and the sonic disruption of cells change or destroy the permeability barrier of the cell, in the process, freeing enzymes or making substrates more readily available to the enzymes. Also, certain enzymes of metabolic sequences may be destroyed or disarranged from the normal cellular spatial sequential arrangement of the enzymes. Thus, toluene lysis of *Aerobacter aerogenes* cells has been employed to make available α,ϵ-diaminopimelic acid decarboxylase enzyme for a lysine fermentation.

The diauxie phenomenon and cooxidation can allow the accumulation of fermentation products not normally expected. In the diauxie phenomenon, two carbon substrates are provided. One substrate, readily attacked by the microorganism, is utilized for rapid growth, while the second substrate, requiring enzymatic adaptation before it can be utilized, is not attacked until the first substrate has been depleted from the medium. In a sense, the production of penicillin by *Penicillium chrysogenum* fits this picture in that the glucose of the medium is first utilized for growth while the lactose, after glucose depletion, is utilized as a starvation carbon source during penicillin production.

The concept of cooxidation (Leadbetter and Foster, 1959 and 1960; and Foster, 1962) is of particular interest as regards the manipulation of fermentations. This concept is based on the premise that the microorganism uses one carbon substrate for growth but, at the same time, and because of its having access to this carbon source, it is able to only partially oxidize a second carbon substrate which, normally, it would not attack. The first demonstration of this concept was with *Pseudomonas methanica*, which was shown to grow at the expense of methane, but which was unable to grow on ethane, propane, or butane. However, if any of the latter gases was present with methane, the organism utilized the methane for growth, but at the same time oxidized the larger molecular-weight gas. Davis and Raymond (1961) further demonstrated cooxidation by showing that a *Nocardia* species growing at the expense of *N*-alkanes gained the ability to oxidize alkylbenzenes. The fermentation possibilities for cooxidation in hydrocarbon fermentations as well as in fermentations employing sugar and other substrates are only now beginning to be realized.

Other examples of fermentation manipulation to obtain desired products are the use of metabolic poisons (particularly heavy metals to reduce or destroy the activities of specific enzymes), media adjusted to pH values remote from those normally employed for the growth of the organism, product inhibition (negative feed-back control and repression), and tie-up or removal of a fermentation product. While metabolic poisons, or enzyme poisons, may be added to the medium to affect the activities of specific enzymes, they also may already be present in the medium and require removal to allow the activity of specific enzymes. Thus, iron is usually removed or tied up in blackstrap molasses used for citric acid production by *Aspergillus niger* (Chapter 26). One or another form of product inhibition (the use of the fermentation product to inhibit the activities of enzymes in order to shut off alternate pathways leading to product formation) is not often employed as such in fermentations, but is involved for auxotrophic mutants such as those of *Microccocus glutamicus* which synthesize large amounts of specific amino acids (Chapter 20).

The tie-up or removal of a fermentation product finds specific uses in fermentations, and would be used more widely if the mechanics of specific applications could be worked out. Sometimes, the fermentation product is quite toxic to the fermentation organism and should be tied-up or removed to circumvent its toxicity. A specific example is *n*-butanol toxicity to *Clostridium acetobutylicum* in the acetone-butanol fermentation (Chapter 18), although no means has yet been found to reduce this toxicity. However, in the *Aspergillus niger* gluconic acid fermentation (Chapter 21) various means are known for circumventing the toxicity of the acid. Sometimes, the enzymatic equilibria for the final enzymes in the sequence for product formation do not favor accumulation of the product and, thus, tie-up or removal of the product can allow increased product accumulation. In other instances, the normal fermentation product is not desired, and removal or tie-up of this product forces the microorganism to utilize an alternate relatively minor metabolic sequence. An example of this situation is the yeast glycerol fermentation in which various procedures are used to tie up or destroy acetaldehyde so that the electrons normally involved in its reduction to ethanol are shunted to reductive enzymatic sequences leading to glycerol formation.

GLYCEROL FROM YEAST

Glycerol finds many applications in industry and commerce. At the present time, it is produced commercially by the saponification of fats and by chemical synthesis from propylene or propane, but not by fermentation. However, during World War I large amounts of glycerol were produced by fermentation in Germany to provide glycerol for explosives. The German fermentation process was based on earlier studies of the yeast-ethanol fermentation by Neuberg, who observed that the addition of sodium sulfite decreased ethanol yields but increased yields of glycerol. The overall reaction is shown in Figure 19.1. Further studies allowed the development of the "soluble sulfite process" for the fermentation synthesis of glycerol, and this was the process employed in Germany.

Neuberg Theoretical Reaction

$$C_6H_{12}O_6 + Na_2SO_3 + H_2O \longrightarrow \underbrace{CH_3C(=O)H - NaHSO_3}_{\text{(Fixed acetaldehyde)}} + NaHCO_3 + \underbrace{C_3H_8O_3}_{\text{(Glycerol)}}$$

Alkaline Fermentation (Cannizzaro Reaction)

$$2C_6H_{12}O_6 + H_2O \longrightarrow 2CO_2 + CH_3C(=O)OH + C_2H_5OH + \underbrace{2C_3H_8O_3}_{\text{(Glycerol)}}$$

Figure 19.1 Two yeast fermentation reactions yielding glycerol.

In the soluble sulfite process, strains of *Saccharomyces cerevisiae* or related species are added at relatively high inoculum levels to a black-strap molasses medium (the German process used highly refined beet sugar), and the cells are allowed to start a vigorous ethanol fermentation. Sodium sulfite then is added at near-toxic levels, and further additions of sodium sulfite are made during the fermentation. The sodium sulfite reacts with carbon dioxide in the medium to produce sodium bisulfite, which then fixes acetaldehyde

(Figure 19.1) so that it cannot be reduced to ethanol by electrons accumulating during sugar metabolism via the EMP scheme (Figure 19.2). Since these electrons cannot be used to reduce acetaldehyde to ethanol, they are shunted to reduction of the dihydroxyacetone phosphate of the EMP scheme to glycerol phosphate, which is then acted upon by a phosphatase to yield glycerol plus phosphoric acid (Figure 19.2). Actually , the normal alcohol fermentation without added sulfite produces some glycerol during the "initial phase" of the fermentation before enough acetaldehyde has accumulated to serve as an electron acceptor.

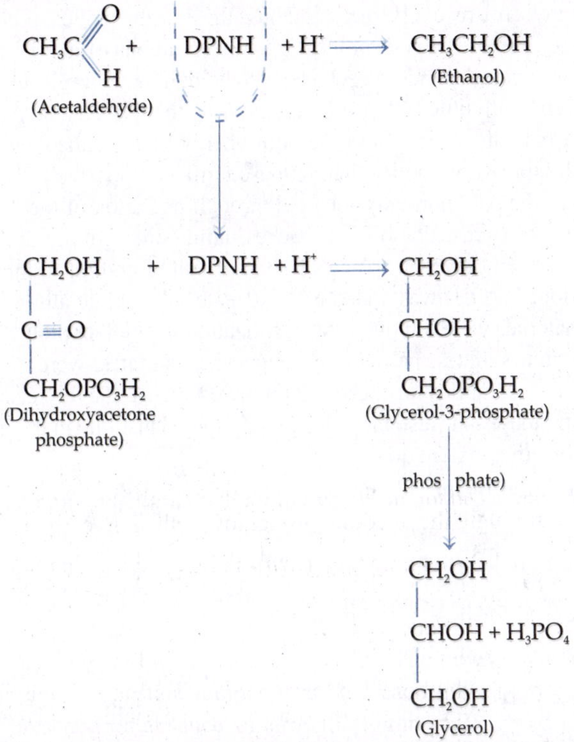

Figure 19.2. Reductions caused by DPNH during the normal working of the EMP scheme in yeast.

Glycerol has not been produced commercially by fermentation since **World War I**. However, further studies in the intervening time have yielded additional potentially good yeast glycerol fermentations. At the time of **World War I**, the American "Eoff" process was developed, which utilized an alkaline fermentation reaction, pH 7 to 8 provided by sodium carbonate, to bring about a Cannizzaro reaction for destruction of the acetaldehyde. Through a dismutation reaction caused by the alkali, two moles of acetaldehyde yielded one mole each of ethanol and acetic acid, thus preventing the acetaldehyde from serving as an electron acceptor (Figure 19.1). The Eoff process, however, was more prone to contamination than the sulfite process because of the greater toxicity of the bisulfite of the sulfite process for contaminating microorganisms.

At termination of a glycerol fermentation, the glycerol is difficult to separate from the fermentation broth and, therefore, in recent years several variations of the soluble sulfite process have been developed in an attempt to improve this poor glycerol recovery picture. Thus, these fermentation procedures were designed to decrease or control the high concentrations of inorganic salts in the fermentation medium and, in each instance, a high inoculum level, in the range of 10 percent, with little cell proliferation during the fermentation was employed to combat bisulfite toxicity and the poor energy yield to the cells caused by a lack of ATP formation (notice that, in these fermentations, the cells recover only a portion of the ATP normally released through operation of the EMP scheme). In one of these fermentation approaches, ammonium sulfite and ammonium bisulfite were employed in place of sodium sulfite and, at termination of the fermentation, $Ca(OH)_2$ was added to precipitate salts, while ammonia and other volatile materials were removed by volatilization. In another procedure, calcium or magnesium sulfates, particularly magnesium sulfates, were employed. The relatively low solubility of these salts allowed their relatively easy removal at harvest, and these salts also provided less dissolved bisulfite in the medium, thus reducing bisulfite toxicity to the yeast.

A variation of the alkaline fermentation process bubbled air, nitrogen, or oxygen through the medium to remove ethanol, carbon dioxide, and acetaldehyde. This procedure was said to allow multiplication of the yeast cells, and a better physiological state for the cells. Also, the yeast cells could then be reused for fresh fermentations.

Theoretically, in the various yeast glycerol fermentations, approximately half of the sugar should end up as glycerol and the other half as fixed or decomposed aldehyde. In practice, however, the yields of glycerol are only 20 to 25 percent or slightly less based on sugar utilized, because the inhibition of the ethanol fermentation is not complete so that some ethanol and carbon dioxide are produced, and because the poor recovery picture for glycerol has not yet been improved.

GLYCEROL FROM BACILLUS SUBTILIS

Bacillus subtilis is commonly considered to be an aerobic microorganism, although certain strains are facultatively aerobic. Aerobic growth of this organism or glucose yields glycerol, 2,3-butanediol, acetoin, ethanol, lactic acid, carbon dioxide, and a few other products. However, anaerobic growth, accomplished by bubbling nitrogen gas through the medium, provides glycerol and 2,3-butanediol as the main fermentation products without resort to acetaldehyde tie-up or destruction, and the glycerol yields for this fermentation are reported to be similar to those for the various yeast glycerol fermentations.

References

Davis, J. B., and R. L. Raymond. 1961. Oxidation of alkyl-substituted cyclic hydrocarbons by a Nocardia during growth on *n*-alkanes. *Appl. Microbiol.,* **9**, 383–388.

Foster, J. W. 1962. Bacterial oxidation of hydrocarbons. Pp. 241–271 in *The oxygenases* (ed. by O. Hayaishi). Academic Press, Inc., New York.

Gehrig, R. F., and S. G. Knight. 1958. Formation of ketones from fatty acids by spores of *Penicillium roqueforti. Nature*, **182,** 1237.

Gehrig, R. F., and S. G. Knight. 1961. Formation of 2-heptanone from caprylic acid by spores of various filamentous fungi. *Nature*, **192,** 1185.

Jazeski, J. J., and R. H. Olsen. 1961. The activity of enzymes at low temperature. Proc. Low Temp. Microbiol. Symp., pp. 139–140. Campbell Soup Co., Camden, New Jersey

Leadbetter, E. R., and J. W. Foster. 1959. Terminal oxidation of gaseous hydrocarbons by *Pseudomonas methanica* (Sohngen). *Bacterial. Proc.*, **1959,** 118.

Leadbetter, E. R., and J. W. Foster. 1960. Bacterial oxidation of gaseous alkanes. *Arch. Microbiol.*, **35,** 92–104.

Oshima, K., K. Tanaka, and S. Kinoshita. 1963. L- glutamic acid fermentation.

X. The conversion of L-glutamic acid fermentation to L-glutamine fermentation. *Hakko To Taisha*, **7**, 73–78.

Prescott, S. C., and C. G. Dunn. 1959. *Industrial Microbiology*. 3rd Ed., pp. 208–217. McGraw-Hill Book Co., Inc., New York.

Rose, A. H. 1961. *Industrial Microbiology*. Pp. 153–159. Butterworths, Washington.

Underkofler, L. A. 1954. Glycerol. Pp. 252–270 in *Industrial fermentations*.

Vol. I (ed. by L. A. Underkofler and R. J. Hickey). Chemical Publishing Co., Inc., New York.

Chapter 20

Genetic Control of Metabolic Pathways

Mutation and selection programs are commonly employed for increasing the yields of fermentation products by industrially important microorganisms. While such programs often provide strains with increased yield capacity, in most instances it is not apparent as to just which biosynthetic pathways of the organism have been altered. This picture, however, is more clear with auxotrophic mutants and, in some instances, the auxotrophic mutations allow specific control over microbial metabolic pathways such that high yields of desired fermentation products accrue. An auxotrophic mutant is a cell which, through mutation, has lost the ability to produce one or more enzymes of a biosynthetic pathway and, because of this metabolic block, it requires that a specific metabolite or metabolites just beyond the block in the metabolic pathway be supplied in its growth medium. Thus, the latter is necessary, because the organism, because of the metabolic block, is in itself not able to synthesize the specific metabolite (or metabolites) required for its growth. An auxotrophic mutant can be of considerable value as a fermentation organism, because the intermediate compound or compounds of the biosynthetic sequence just preceding the metabolic block may accumulate in quantity in the culture broth due to the lack of an enzyme for bringing about further chemical conversion.

Auxotrophs have been used for industrial fermentations, but to date their application has been limited almost exclusively to amino acid fermentations. Of the various amino acids, there is real commercial demand only for L-glutamic acid and L-lysine, and fermentation processes utilizing auxotrophs (or organisms resembling auxotrophs) are employed for the production of these two amino acids. However, similar fermentation processes also are available for other amino acids if the need should arise. L-Glutamic acid is utilized in the manufacture of monosodium L-glutamate which, because of its meatlike flavour, is used as a flavouring agent. L-Lysine is an essential amino acid, but it often is present in only small amounts in foods prepared from cereal grains. To remedy this situation, L-lysine often is used to fortify such foods in order to make them nutritionally more equivalent to meant proteins. Two fermentation processes have been or are presently employed commercially for the production of L-lysine, and both of these processes utilize auxotrophic mutants. While the commercial production of L-glutamic acid does not utilize an auxotrophic mutant, the fermentation process will be described, nevertheless, because the control mechanisms involved closely resemble those for an auxotrophic mutant, and because mutation of the microorganism so that it becomes an auxotroph allows it to be utilized in the commerical production of L-lysine.

Two general phenomena are observed for most of the microorganisms, auxotrophic or not, which are employed for the commercial fermentation production of amino acids. The major portion of the amino acid accumulation occurs after maximum growth of the microorganism has been obtained, and the level of the specific growth requirement initially present in the medium is highly critical. In regard to this point, levels above or below the optimum markedly decrease yields.

Amino acids can be synthesized quite economically by chemical means. However, the various chemical syntheses usually yield a racemic mixture of the DL-isomers, although only the L-isomer is of value for flavor applications or for food or feed supplementation. The D-isomers are biologically inactive. To date, the chemical resolution of the DL-racemic mixtures has been relatively expensive, although a Japanese process is apparently in commercial use.

INDIRECT OR DUAL FERMENTATION

L-Lysine

L-Lysine was the first amino acid to be commercially produced by fermentation (Casida, 1956). This fermentation is a dual fermentation, with the first half employing an *Escherischia coli* auxotrophic mutant which, as the prototroph, lacks lysine decarboxylase and through mutation, in addition, lacks $\alpha,\in$-diaminopimelic acid decarboxylase (Figure 20.1). Because of the latter metabolic block, this organism requires small amounts of L-lysine for growth and accumulates $\alpha,\in$-diaminopimelic acid (DAP) in considerable quantity in the culture broth. The inoculum and fermentation media contain glycerol, cornsteep liquor, and $(NH_4)_2 HPO_4$, although, in addition, calcium carbonate is employed in the production medium, and the levels of all of the individual nutrients are lower in the inoculum medium. The cornsteep liquor supplies the L-lysine required by the organism for growth, although additional L-lysine recovered as crude fermentation product can be also added to the medium, if required. The pH of the medium is neutral to slightly alkaline, and incubation is for approximately three days at 28°C with high aeration.

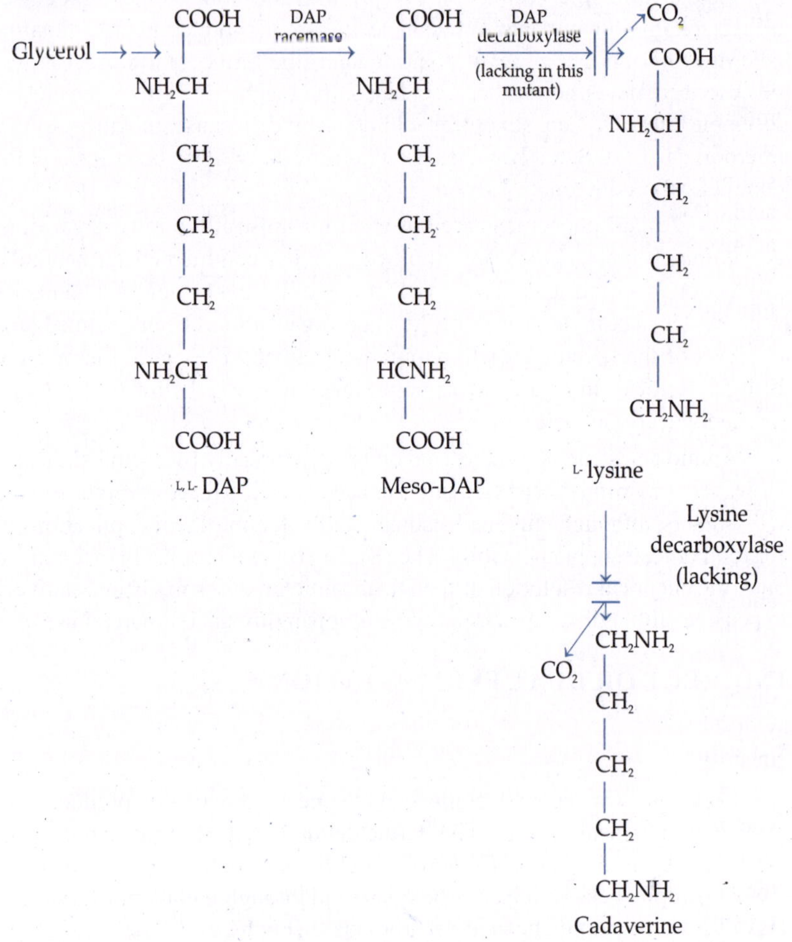

Figure 20.1 Position of metabolic block in the l-lysine metabolic pathway of an *Escherichia coli* auxotroph which accumulates α,ε-diaminopimelic acid (DAP) during growth on glycerol. The *Aerobacter aerogenes* wild-type cells, also used in this fermentation, employ a similar pathway except that the DAP decarboxylase is both present and active.

To further obtain the l-lysine, the α,∈-diaminopimelic acid must be decarboxylated by the enzyme diaminopimelic acid decarboxylase. Wild-type strains (prototrophs) of *Escherichia coli* or *Aerobacter aerogenes* (usually the latter) are employed to supply this enzyme. However, these organisms also must lack the ability to adaptively produce lysine decarboxylase so that the lysine product will not be destroyed by decarboxylation to cadaverine (Figure 20.1). These cells, as well as the *E. coli* auxotrophs, should also possess strong α-∈diaminopimelic acid racemase activity (Figure 20.1) to convert all residual, L-DAP to meso-DAP. The wild-type organisms are grown in a medium similar to that for producing the *E. coli* auxotroph inoculum, and the wild-type cells then are separated from the growth medium by centrifugation, sedimentation, and so forth and added to the complete α,∈-diaminopimelic acid fermentation broth of the E. *coli* auxotroph. In addition, toluene is aded at this point to cause cell lysis of the *E. coli* auxotroph and of the *A. aerogenes* wild-type cells in order to liberate the diaminopimelic acid decarboxylase into the medium. The α,∈-diaminopimelic acid broth, together with the lysed cells of both organisms, is then incubated without aeration for approximately 24 hours at 28°C, during which time the α,∈-diaminopimelic acid is decarboxylated to yield L-lysine.

During the production of α,∈-diaminopimelic acid by the *E. coli* auxotroph some back mutation occurs and, consequently, at termination of the fermentation, low to fairly high numbers of these backmutant cells may be present in the fermentation broth. Thus, these cells through mutation have reacquired the ability to produce the diaminopimelic decarboxylase enzyme and, hence, resemble the wild-type cells. It is possible, therefore, that enough of these cells may be present, so that if toluene is added to this half of the fermentation, enough of the enzyme will be present to convert the α,∈-diaminopimelic acid to l-lysine without further addition of the *A. aerogenes* wild-type cells (Kita and Huang, 1958). Of course, the DAP and lysine yields in such a fermentation might be expected to be low.

The *E. coli* auxotroph requires l-lysine for growth, although only very small amounts are required in relation to the high yields of α,∈-diaminopimelic acid which result. However, the level of l-lysine provided to the organism for the fermentation is critical. Thus, levels less than optimum select against the auxotroph during growth and in favor of the back mutant, since the back mutant does not require L-lysine for growth. Levels greater than optimum at the initiation of the fermentation exert feedback control over the biosynthesis of α,∈- diaminopimelic acid and, thus, also depress yields. It is not known whether this feedback control represents repression or inhibition of enzymatic activity, as described later on this chapter.

The biosynthetic sequences involved in this fermentation are outlined in Figure 20.1. Glycerol, through a series of enzymatic steps, is converted to L, L -diaminopimelic acid, which then is partially racemized by diaminopimelic acid racemase to the D, L-isomer, mesodiaminopimelic acid. Both the L, L-isomer and mesoisomer then accumulate behind the metabolic block, because diaminopimelic acid decarboxylase is not present to convert the mesoisomer to L-lysine, and because the racemase enzyme activity reaches equilibrium before all of the L, L-isomer is converted to the mesoisomer. Thus, the accumulated diaminopimelic acid consists of approximately 40 L, L-isomer and 60 percent mesoisomer. In the second half of the fermentation, as carried out by wild-type *A. aerogenes* cells, the L, L-diaminopimelic acid is completely racemized by the diaminopimelic acid racemase of both the auxotroph and wild-type cells to mesodiaminopimelic acid and then decarboxylated by the diaminopimelic acid decarboxylase to yield L-lysine. The equilibrium of the decarboxylation strongly favors the formation of L-lysine so that the L, L-isomer and mesoisomer of diaminopimelic acid are almost completely converted to L-lysine.

This fermentation, as described, requires that the prime carbon source be glycerol. However, Huang *et al* (1960) circumvented the relatively high cost of the glycerol in this fermentation by obtaining a double auxotroph of E *coli* which requires both L-lysine and L-histidine for growth. This auxotroph carries out a fermentation similar to that described above, but instead of glycerol, it utilizes lactose, sucrose, or molasses as the carbon source.

DIRECT FERMENTATION

L-Glutamic Acid

Micrococcus glutamicus, a nonmutated natural isolate, was shown by Kinoshita *et al*(1957) to produce high yields of L-glutamic acid from sugar. Although not theoretically an auxotroph, this organism requires biotin for growth, and the level provided at the initiation of the fermentation is critical. Thus, too low a level prevents growth and, hence, L-glutamic acid production, while too high a level prevents L-glutamic acid production (Figure 20.2) both by feedback control and by regulation of the cell-permeability barrier. As regards the latter case where excess biotin is provided at the initiation of the fermentation, there is heavy cell growth, but lactic acid instead of L-glutamic acid becomes the principal product of the fermentation, although other organisms related to *Micrococcus glutamicus* under similar conditions may produce both lactic and succinic acids as the major fermentation products.

Also, as regards excess biotin, *Micrococcus glutamicus* seems to have a permeability barrier at the cell membrane which prevents L-glutamic acid from leaking from the cells into the medium but at optimum biotin levels for fermentative production of L-glutamic acid, this permeability barrier does not seem to function, and L-glutamic acid accumulates in the medium.

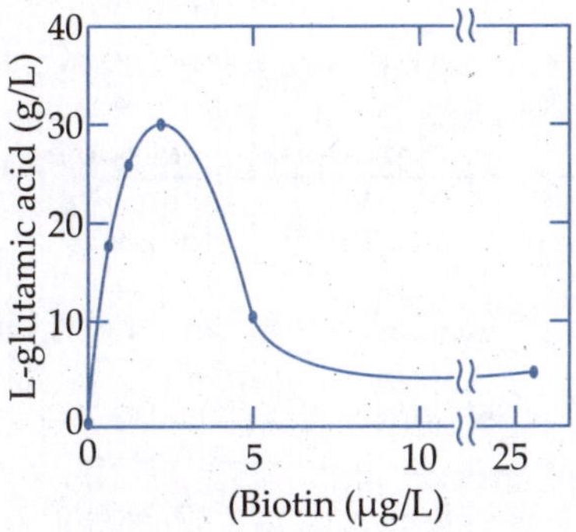

Figure 20.2 Effect of biotin level on L-glutamic acid yeild. (Anderson, Huang, Singer, and Rogoff. 1966. *Dev. Ind. Microbiol.*, **7**, 12).

The fermentation utilizes a glucose medium, high aeration, 30°C incubation temperature, a pH of 6 to 8, and intermittent additions of urea during the fermentation. It lasts two days or less with approximately 40 percent of the sugar being converted to L-glutamic acid, which represents a harvest yield of approximately 30 g per liter of L-glutamic acid.

Since the discovery and commercial utilization of this fermentation, other workers have found that several different organisms produce these high yields of L-glutamic acid and have a biotin requirement (Table 20.1). However, all of these organisms, including *Micrococcus glutamicus* but excluding a *Bacillus* species, appear to be related to each other and to be more properly classified as representatives of the genus *Arthrobacter*.

The biological control mechanisms involved in this fermentation are not really known. However, it would appear that citric acid formed from sugar is converted to α-ketoglutaric acid which is then aminated to provide L-glutamic acid. Thus, although *Micrococcus glutamicus* possesses all the enzymes of the TCA cycle, with the exception of α-ketoglutaric acid dehydrogenase, the normal TCA cycle does not seem to be functioning in this organism. Also, this organism lacks the ability to oxidize L-glutamic acid to α-ketoglutaric acid.

Table 20.1 L-Glumatic acid producing bacteria[a]

Proposed Name	Gram Stain	Morphology	Chromogenesis	Authors
Micrococcus glutamicus	+	Elliposidal sphere ; elongated form	Pale yellow to white	Kinoshita (1959)
Brevibacterium aminogenes	+	Short rod	Pale yellow to cream grey	Ota and Tanaka (1959)
Micrococcus glutamicus	+	Short rod	Pale yellow to white	Chen, Tu, and Chen (1959)
Bacillus megaterium cereus	–	Rod, single or short chains	Creamy white	Chao and Foster (1959)
Brevibacterium sp.	+	Not reported	Not reported	Kobayashi *et al* (1959)
Brevibacterium flavum	+	Short rod	Pale yellow to yellow	Okumura *et al* (1959)
Brevibacterium divaricatum	+	Straight rod	Pale yellowish grey	Su and Yamada 1960
Microbacterium salicinovorum	+	Short rod	Milky white	Doi *et al* (1960)
Unidentified	+	Rod	Not reported	Wakisaka *et al* (1961)
Arthrobacter globiformis	+	Cocci to rod		Veldkamp *et al* (1963)
Corynebacterium lilium	+	Rod	Yellow to creamy white	Lee and Good (1963)
Corynebacterium herculis	+	Rod	Pale yellow	Dunn *et al* (1964)

[a] *Source*, Anderson, Huang, Singer, and Rogoff, 1966, *Dev. Ind. Microbiol.*, 7,9.

L-Lysine

The strain of *Micrococcus glutamicus* utilized in commercial glutamic acid production was mutated to obtain as auxotroph capable of producing L-lysine by direct fermentation (Kinoshita, *et al*, 1958). This auxotroph requires L-homoserine or a mixture of L-threonine and L-methionine for growth, and produces greater than 20g per litre of L-lysine in the fermentation broth. In addition, the L-lysine is not destroyed by the organism during the fermentation, because it also lacks the ability to produce L-lysine decarboxylase. The biotin requirement of this organism was not lost as a result of the mutation and, therefore, both biotin and L-homoserine must be initially supplied in the medium. The ability to produce L-glutamic acid also was not lost through mutation. However, this fact is not as much of a problem as it would seem because, as discussed earlier, the production of this amino acid is inhibited by incorporating excess biotin in the medium.

The level of L-homoserine (or L-threonine plus L-methionine) provided initially in the medium must be optimum. Too small an amount impedes growth and, hence, L-lysine production, and an excess also prevents L-lysine production. The reasons for this are incompletely understood, and this also applies to the biosynthetic sequences leading to L-lysine formation by this organism. However, the available evidence allows a partial diagrammatic representation of the L-lysine formation as shown in Figure 20.3. As may be seen in Figure 20.3, a branching point in the biosynthetic pathway occurs at aspartic-β-semialdehyde. One branch without a mutational block leads in the direction of α, ∈-diaminopimelic acid and L-lysine. The other route, however, has a mutational block between aspartic-β-semialdehyde and L-homoserine. Since a further branching of the sequence occurs just beyond L-homoserine, it is obvious that either L-homoserine or L-threonine plus L-methionine must be supplied for growth of the organism.

Feedback control, either inhibition or repression, is probably operating on the threonine-methionine end of the sequence. However, there is as yet no good explanation as to why feedback control does not operate also on the lysine branch to inhibit production of excess lysine as occurs with the prototroph or wild type.

Negative feedback control (also known as feedback inhibition, end-product inhibition, or allosteric inhibition) is a biological control mechanism employed by microorganisms to prevent overproduction of metabolic products not needed in excess at any particular moment by the cell. In other words, it is a method for shutting down unneeded biosynthetic sequences. To explain this action, an accumulation of a slight excess of the terminal product of a biosynthetic pathway causes one of two types of control of enzymatic activity somewhere earlier in the metabolic sequence in order to slow down or stop further production of the product. A diagrammatic representation of negative feedback control is presented in Figure 20.4. Thus, in one type of negative feedback control called "repression," one to several enzymes of the biosynthetic sequence cease to be produced (enzymes 3, 4 and 5 in Figure 20.4). In contrast, "inhibition," as a negative feedback control mechanism, is a situation in which an enzyme is produced but is inactive (enzyme 2 in Figure 20.4). Thus, the product of the biosynthetic sequence causes repression of one to several of the enzymes along the biosynthetic sequence, but inhibition by the product applies only to the first enzyme of the biosynthetic sequence.

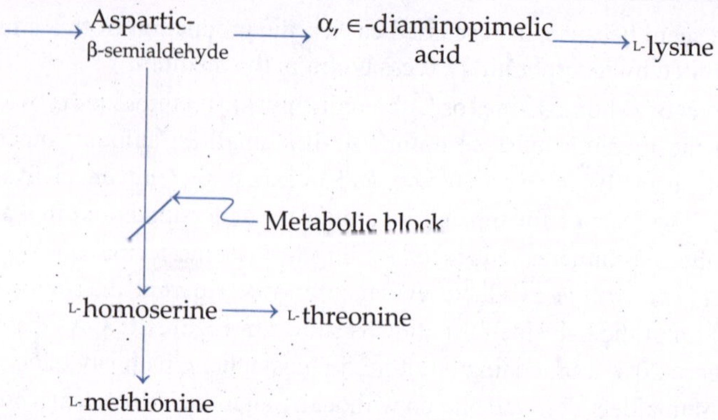

Figure 20.3 Outline of biosynthetic sequences leading to L-lysine in a *Micrococcus glutamicus* auxotroph requiring L-homoserine or a mixture of L-threonine and L-methionine for growth.

At each site along the biosynthetic sequence at which either repression or inhibition occurs, there may be more than one enzyme (multiple enzymes or isoenzymes) to carry out the particular enzymatic reaction. This presence of several enzymes to accomplish a single enzymatic reaction is explained by the fact that end products, all of which are required by the cell, often arise via branched pathways. Thus, in the absence of isoenzymes, feedback control (either repression or inhibition) of an enzymatic step occurring before the branch in a metabolic pathway could cause what might be called "regulatory suicide" (Demain, 1966.) Each isoenzyme, however, is controlled only by the product of one of the branches of the metabolic pathway so that no one product can completely stop the operation of the pathway.

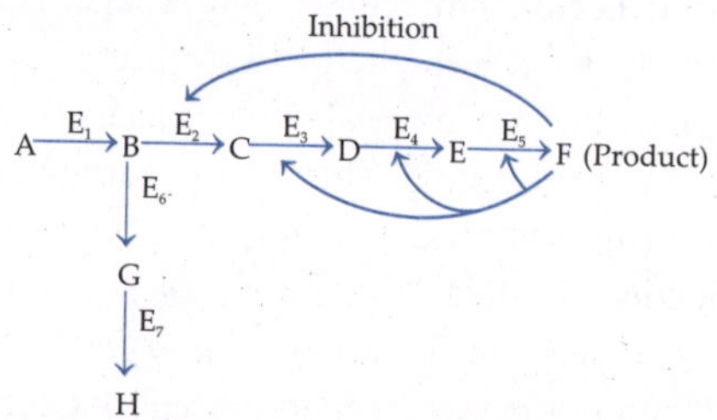

Figure 20.4 Diagrammatic representation of negative feedback control. The letters "A" through "H" represent intermediate compounds along the biosyntheti sequences, while "E_1" through "E_7" represent the respective enzymes associated with each of the steps of the sequences.

In addition to isoenzymes, there are two other means by which the cell prevents this type of regulatory suicide. In each of these instances only one enzyme, instead of several enzymes, controls the critical reaction step. In "multivalent" feedback (or "concerted" feedback), all of the end products of the branched pathway must be present in excess to allow inhibition or repression of the enzyme; an excess of only one or of a part of the end products has no effect. For "cumulative" feedback, each end product of a branched pathway is capable of limited inhibition or repression, so that the cumulative effects of all the products are required to shut down the pathway.

Other Amino Acids

Auxotrophic mutants and wild-type strains of various other microorganisms also have been studied for the production of other amino acids by direct fermentation, and the resulting respective fermentations and control mechanisms are somewhat similar to those described for *Micrococcus glutamicus* and its mutants. However, these fermentations have not as yet gained commercial usage because of a poor economic picture or lack of a market.

References

Casida, L. E., Jr. 1956. U.S. Patent 2,771,396.

Demain, A. L. 1966. Industrial fermentations and their relation to regulatory mechanisms, *Adv. Appl. Microbiol.,* **8**, 1–27.

Huang, H. T. 1964. Microbial production of amino acids. *Progress Indust. Microbiol.*, **5**, 57–92.

Huang, H. T., J. M. Griffin, and J. H. Fried. 1960. U.S. Patent 2,955,986.

Kinoshita, S., K. Nakayama, and S. Kitada. 1958. L-lysine production using microbial auxotroph. *J. Gen. Appl. Microbiol. (Tokyo)*, **4**, 128–129.

Kinoshita, S., K. Tanaka, S. Udaka, and S. Akita. 1957. Glutamic acid fermentation. *Proc. Int. Symp. Enzyme Chem.,* **2**, 464–468.

Kita, D. A., and H. T. Huang. 1958. U.S. Patent 2,841,532.

CHAPTER 21

Microbial Oxidative Transformations of Substrate

Not all fermentations involve total microbial degradation of carbon substrates to small biosynthetic building blocks, such as acetate, and resynthesis to yield the desired fermentation product. Thus, some microbial fermentations involve one-, two-, or a few-step enzymatic transformations of the substrate to provide a fermentation product closely related chemically to the substrate. Obviously, if microbial growth is associated with the transformation, a certain portion of this substrate or of an alternate substrate, if present, must also be at least partially degraded to supply carbon for the energy and growth of the cell.

The second half of the α, ∈-diaminopimelic acid-lysine dual fermentation is an example of a microbial transformation, since the α,∈-diaminopimelic acid decarboxylase from *Aerobacter aerogenes* is used to carry out a single step enzymatic decarboxylation of the α, ∈- diaminopimelic acid to L-lysine. The use of microbial transformations of this and other types is finding increased interest in the fermentation industry, because the enzymatic reactions can be employed to bring about certain chemical transformations which are expensive, or even difficult or impossible by purely chemical means. The microbial transformations involved in the fermentation production of vinegar, gluconic acid, and steroids are examples of those currently employed as industrial fermentations.

VINEGAR

The vinegar fermentation is one of the oldest fermentation known to man, occurring naturally as an unwanted spoilage of wine. Thus, literally translated, vinegar means sour wine. Technically, vinegar is a fermentation-derived food product containing not less than 4 g of acetic acid per 100 ml, and the fact that, in addition to its acid content it possesses special flavor characteristics, protects it as a fermentation product from competition by direct chemical synthesis.

The production of vinegar actually requires two fermentations, the first utilizing a yeast to produce ethanol from sugar, and the second utilizing various *Acetobacter* species in impure culture to oxidize ethanol through acetaldehyde to acetic acid. The substrate for the first fermentation can be almost any natural material that can be fermented to yield alcohol, including various fruits, berries, honey, wine, malt, and so forth. However, wine or apple cider usually are used in present-day vinegar production, with *Saccharomyces cerevisiae* or *Saccharomyces cerevisiae* var, *ellipsoideus* as the fermentation organism. Sulfur dioxide is sometimes added to the fermentation to control bacterial growth but, if utilized, it must be removed by aeration or by other means before the alcohol is further oxidized to acetic acid. At the end of the alcohol fermentation, the yeast cells and various sediments are allowed to settle, and the supernatant alcoholic broth is withdrawn. The alcohol content of this broth is adjusted, if required, to a predetermined concentration of up to 10 to 13 percent alcohol, and a small amount of vinegar may be added to increase the acidity of the broth. This addition also can add *Acetobacter* cells for those processes that require inoculation.

The microbial oxidation of ethanol to acetic acid is an aerobic fermentation process that has a high oxygen requirement. The *Acetobacter* cells themselves are highly aerobic, and their activities are harmed by the development of an oxygen deficiency in the fermentation medium. Also, the oxidation of ethanol to acetic acid per se requires considerable oxygen, as for example, the conversion of one liter of alcohol to acetic acid requires 552 g of oxygen. The oxidation of ethanol to acetic acid also evolves considerable heat, such that conversion of one gallon of ethanol to acetic acid liberates approximately 30,250 BTU's, most of which must be dissipated from the fermentation. Over the years, several fermentation processes have been developed for carrying out this oxidation, but it is only the more recent processes that have provided adequate manipulative controls for supplying sufficient oxygen to the fermentation and for the dissipation of heat.

The early vinegar fermentations, other than those in which a fortuitous souring of wine occurred, were accomplished by placing an alcoholic liquid, either wine or other fermented fruit juice, in a shallow pan or wooden vat (Figure 21.1). The alcoholic solution became inoculated by *Acetobacter* bacteria from the air, and the large surface area provided the required aeration. During an extended incubation period, a bacterial scum containing the alcohol-oxidizing bacteria developed on the liquid surface. However, vinegar eels (nematodes peculiar to vinegar) also actively multiplied in these vats.

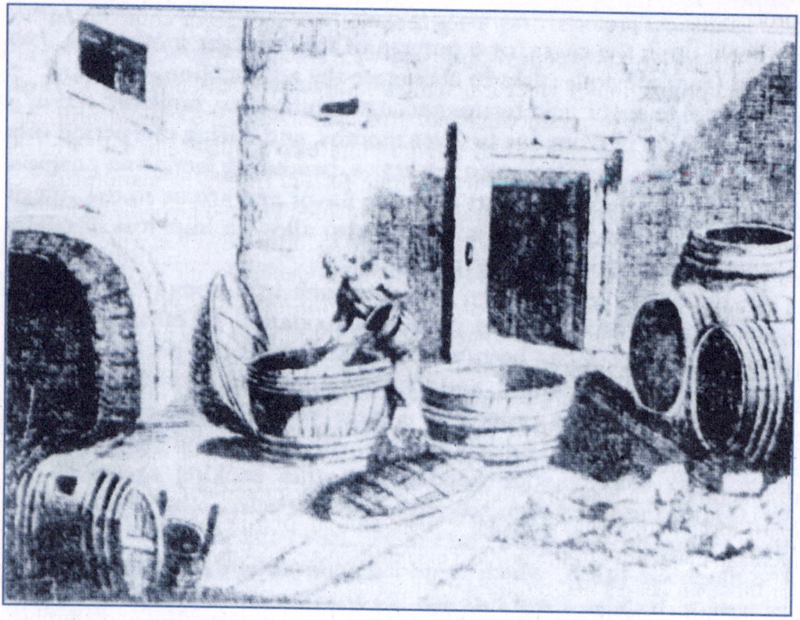

Figure. 21.1 Early vinegar manufacture in wooden vats. Photo courtesy of Yeomans Brothers Co.

In Orleans, France, vinegar production gradually evolved from the vat fermentation to the more sophisticated "Orleans process" for wine vinegars, and this process on a limited scale is still practiced to provide special fine-quality table vinegars. The fermentation vessels for the Orleans process consist of large barrels or casks placed either upright or on their sides. Holes in the walls of these vessels above the liquid level admit air. The *Acetobacter* bacteria produce considerable slime and grow as a film, or "vinegar mother," on the surface of the alcoholic broth, being supported at the surface on a floating raft composed of wooden grating. The cells in this slime layer are further held together by cellulosic strands produced by one of the *Acetobacter* species, *Acetobacter xylinum*. A natural inoculum of *Acetobacter* cells is allowed to build up in the casks, or a portion of the "vinegar mother" is transferred from previous casks to accelerate acetification. The oxidation of ethanol to acetic acid by this process is quite slow, however, requiring an incubation of from one to three months, and during this period other non-*Acetobacter* bacteria also are active, producing lactic and propionic acids which, as esters, impart a unique flavor and aroma to the vinegar. However, the long incubation period also allows a high loss of ethanol through evaporation and overoxidation.

In the early 19th century, Schutzenbach in Germany developed a more rapid process for the microbial oxidation of ethanol to acetic acid. This process has been variously known as the packed-generator process, the quick method, and the trickle method. The vinegar generator employed in this process is a large vertical tank, either open or closed at the top, and loosely packed with beechwood shavings, twigs, corn cobs, bamboo-stick bundles, or other packing agents. A bacterial film composed of mixed *Acetobacter* species, other than those for the Orleans process, grows on the surface of the supporting agent, and the alcoholic broth, which is added intermittently to the top of the generator, trickles down through the shavings so as to provide contact of the alcohol with the cells and consequent oxidation of the alcohol. The generators are provided with air inlets near the bottom to allow air to rise through the generator, with the rise of air being accelerated by the heat generated during the fermentation. This heat evolution is controlled, so as not to harm the fermentation, by the rate of addition and temperature of the added alcoholic broths or, in the more sophisticated generators, it is controlled by cooling coils or by cooling of the incoming or recycled alcoholic broth.

The alcoholic broth is recycled through the fermentor until the alcohol becomes virtually completely oxidized, or it is passed through several generators in series to successively oxidize the alcohol at each of the generators. These generators will produce a considerable concentration of acid and, in fact, they commonly produce 15 percent acid, and therefore are employed today especially for the production of white vinegar. These present-day generators are packed with beechwood shavings prepared from air-dried beechwood, 2 × 11/4 inches and loosely or tightly rolled; the recirculating generators hold approximately 2000 cu ft of these shavings. Once a satisfactory bacterial film has accumulated on the supporting agent in the generator, the generator can be operated continuously for several to many months, or until contamination by the slime-forming bacterium, *Acetobacter xylinum*, becomes a problem.

The vinegar fermentation would seem to be well suited for the application of the submerged fermentation approach. However, early attempts to accomplish a submerged fermentation were without success and, in fact, the submerged approach for this fermentation had to await the intensive aeration studies carried out on antibiotic fermentations during and after **World War II**. Submerged fermentations have now been developed, however, and are employed extensively in the commercial production of table vinegars. These submerged fermentations utilize two different fermentor designs known as the Acetator and the Cavitator (see Figures 21.2 to 21.5). Both of these fermentors provide the high aeration levels required for the vinegar fermentation and, in fact, pump and recycle their own air so that a compressor is not required. Thus, these fermentors make efficient use of their own air, stripping from

50 to 80 percent of the available oxygen from it, although a small amount of fresh air is, nevertheless, continuously bled into the fermentors. This aeration approach is particularly advantageous for the vinegar fermentation, since it lessens the loss to the atmosphere of the ethanol and of the aromatic substances present in the raw materials. Automatic temperature control is applied to dissipate the heat resulting from the ethanol oxidation and from the operation of the moving mechanical parts in the fermentors.

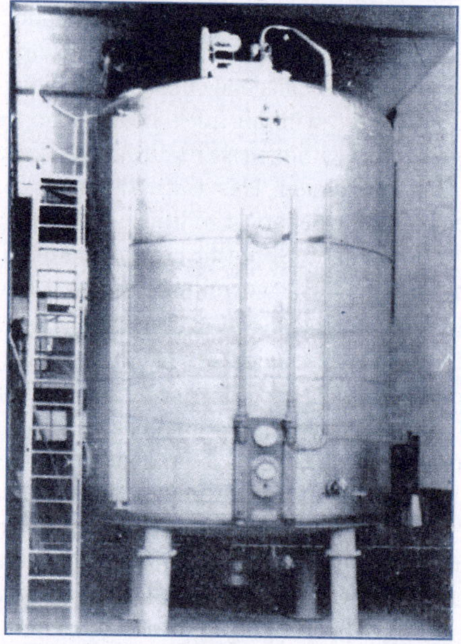

Figure 21.2. Outward appearance of the Frings Submerged Culture Acetator. Photo courtesy of Heinrich Frings and Yeomans Brothers Co.

Neither fermentor utilizes shavings or packing material of any kind, so that clogging by microbial slime (as can occur with the previously described packed vinegar generator) does not occur. Also, in this regard, conversion vinegars, or blended vinegars, are not a problem. Thus, with the packed vinegar generator, if the alcoholic substrate is changed, the resulting vinegars for a period of time will be a blend of vinegars produced from the new alcoholic substrate and from residual alcoholic materials entrained in the packing materials of the generator. Both the Acetator and the Cavitator are automated for both charging with alcoholic solution and discharging of completed fermentation broth. Also, the *Acetobacter* microflora in these units is not carried over in the fermentor from previous fermentations but is added

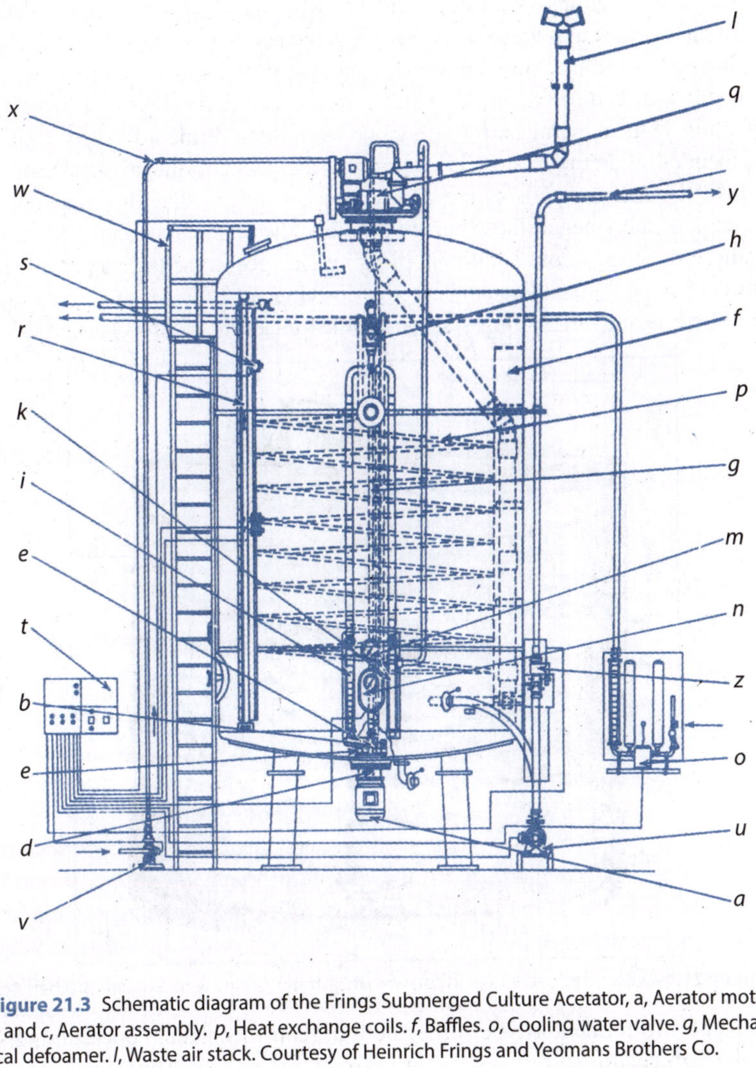

Figure 21.3 Schematic diagram of the Frings Submerged Culture Acetator, a, Aerator motor. *b* and *c*, Aerator assembly. *p*, Heat exchange coils. *f*, Baffles. *o*, Cooling water valve. *g*, Mechanical defoamer. *l*, Waste air stack. Courtesy of Heinrich Frings and Yeomans Brothers Co.

at start-up. This allows a quick start-up and even a shut-down, if this should be required. Since these fermentors are highly efficient and produce acetic acid at a rapid rate, they are considerably smaller than the packed vinegar generators, thus taking up less space in the production plant. Slime is not a problem with these fermentors, nor is the vinegar eel. Also, the rate of oxygen removal from the medium by the *Acetobacter* cells is so great that "oxidative browning" of the apple cider or wine mash does not occur. Finally, with the operation of these units there is some residual alcohol in the vinegar as it is recovered from the fermentator and, therefore, with both processes the vinegar is stored to allow aging and consequent microbial depletion of this alcohol. Thus, the vinegar as withdrawn from these fermentors also contains suspended microorganisms, in contrast to the packed vinegar generators in which the microorganisms are firmly attached to the shavings, and during storage of the vinegar, these bacteria oxidize the residual alcohol and, at the same time, bring about additional pleasing changes in the taste and aroma to produce what is considered to be a superior vinegar. After a period of storage, the bacteria and other solids settle from the vinegar to yield a clear product.

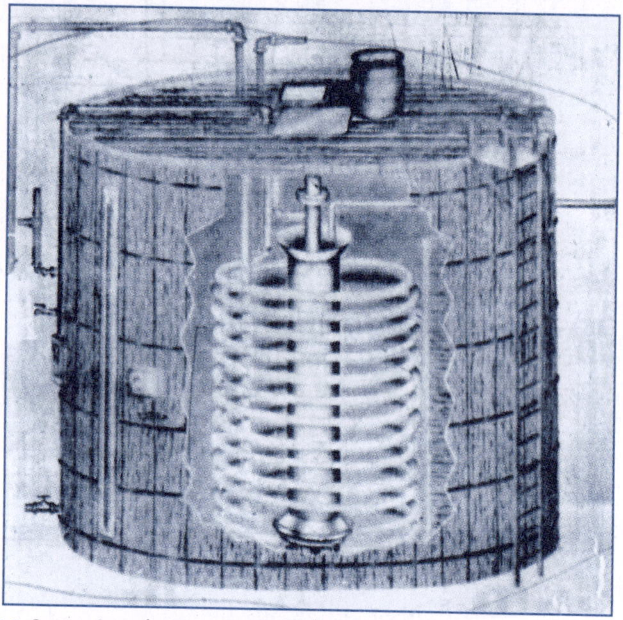

Figure 21.4 Outward appearance and cutaway of Cavitator. Courtesy of Yeomans Brothers Co.

The two fermentor types differ both in their mechanical operations and in the fermentation programs that are carried out in them. Thus, the Acetator

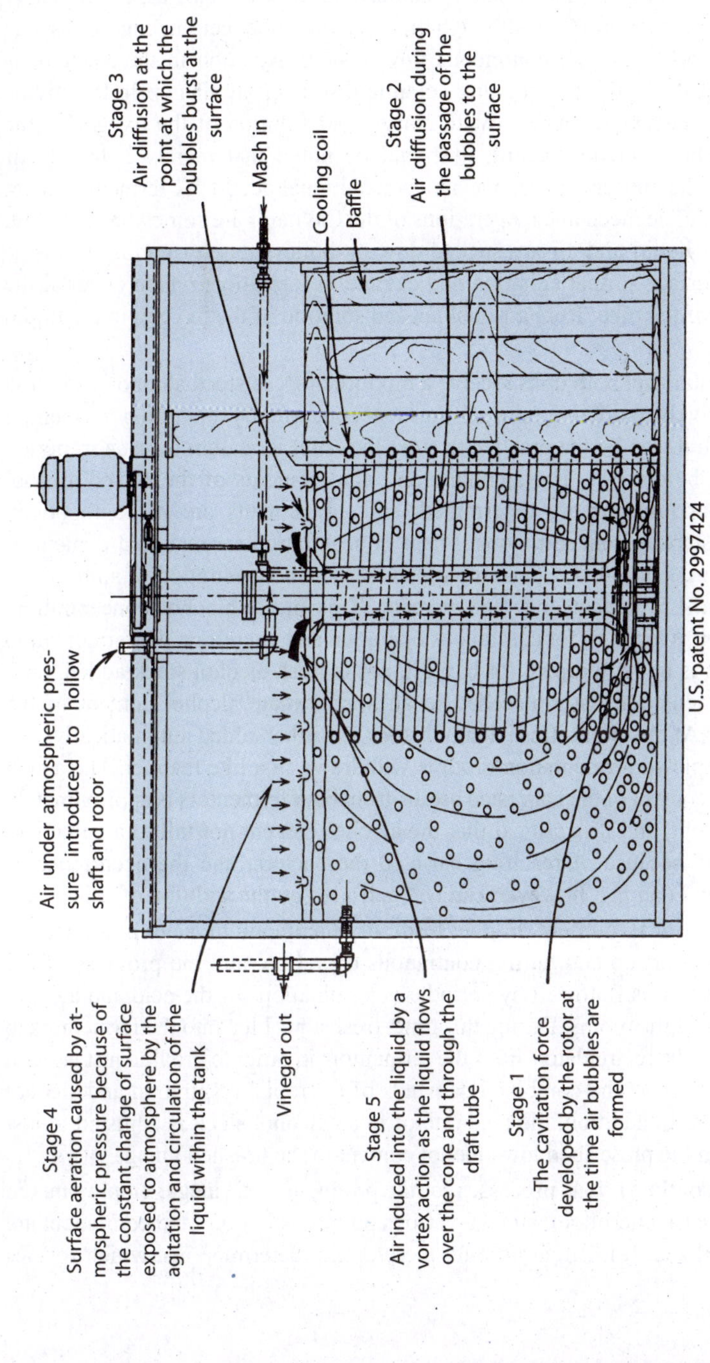

Figure 21.5 Schematic diagram of the Cavitator®, and the five steps in its operation as a gas (air) diffuser. Courtesy of Yeomans Brothers Co.

usually operates in a semibatch manner and the Cavitator as a completely continuous fermentation, although the Acetator, under certain conditions, can now be operated as a continuous flow system. Aeration in the Acetator is accomplished by a fast-rotating ceramic disc over an air nozzle to provide finely dispersed air bubbles with consequent solution of the oxygen in the liquid phase. In this regard, it should be noted that merely bubbling air through the nutrient solution as in a conventional deep-tank fermentor is not effective. The mechanical operations of the Cavitator are somewhat different. Nutrient liquid and air are sucked down a hollow tube extending from the liquid surface so that agitation and cavitation formation, which occur at the bottom of the tube, from air bubbles and solution of the oxygen in the liquid sodium.

At start-up, both units receive a mixture of fresh stock alcoholic solution and actively oxidizing vinegar from a concurrently operating fermentor, although it can be the practice to store the latter inoculum for a short period of time before use. The alcoholic and acid contents of the mixed alcohol stock and vinegar are determined, and adjustments are made to obtain proper starting concentrations. These concentrations are an acid content of approximately 1 to 1.5 percent, and an alcohol concentration of somewhere between 4.5 percent and 10.8 percent. This initial alcohol concentration, however, is too high for continuous operation and, therefore, the fermentation solution is not withdrawn for harvest, nor is fresh alcohol stock added, until the fermentation has proceeded to an approximate alcohol content of 0.5 percent. At this point, fresh alcohol stock is further added automatically, and the completed fermentation broth is withdrawn in a like manner. The actual alcohol content of the harvested broths from both fermentors is approximately 0.3 percent, and it is critical that the alcohol content not fall to a value less than this because of resulting harm to the bacteria and the occurrence of foaming. Foaming, however, can be controlled by the addition of silicones.

Additional nutrient in the form of diammonium acid phosphate is added at start-up and during continuous operation, and the progress of the fermentation is followed by periodic determinations of the acid and alcohol contents of the broths. During this time, fresh air is bled into the fermentors to mix with the recirculated air of the fermentors in order to provide just enough oxygen to meet the combined demands of microbial respiration and alcohol oxidation. In addition, the feed rate of fresh alcohol stock is adjusted to just maintain the prescribed low alcohol content in the finished vinegar.

All of the various processes for the production of vinegar employ mixed *Acetobacter* microflora, and the various nutrient solutions and equipment are not sterilized. It is often difficult, therefore, to determine just which species of *Acetobacter* actually are carrying out the ethanol oxidation and, in fact, the different processes, being naturally inoculated probably utilize different species and strains of *Acetobacter*. Nevertheless, the fermentative organisms are usually assumed to be *Acetobacter schuetzenbachii*, *Acetobacter curvum*, *Acetobacter orleanense* and related organisms. Figure 21.6 shows *Acetobacter* cells as recovered from a Cavitator ; notice the capsular material around the individual cells.

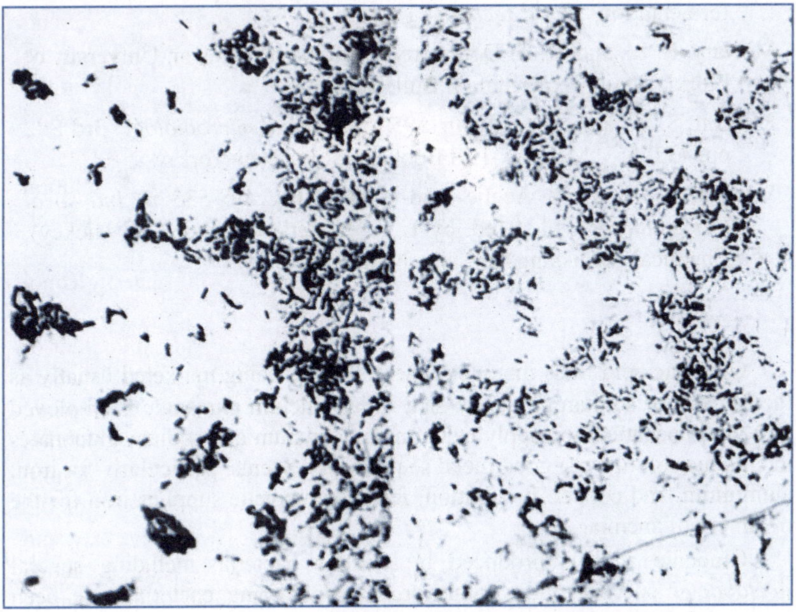

Figure 21.6 *Acetobacter* bacteria as recovered from a Cavitator and viewed at 1000-fold magnification by phase microscopy. The slime layer around each cell is evident. Culture courtesy of H. J. Heinz Co.

As is obvious, alcohol-containing solutions are required for the production of vinegar by each of these processes. It should be noted, therefore, that federal regulations must be followed in relation to these substrates.

References

Vinegar

Allgeier, R. J., and F. M. Hildebrandt. 1960. Newer development in vinegar manufacturers. *Adv. Appl. Microbiol.* **2**, 163–182.

Burgoon, D. W. Dec. 27, 1960. Mixing apparatus. U.S. 2,996,345 (Cavitator design).

Ebner, H. 1965. Vinegar-making leaps ahead. *Food Eng.*, **36**, 42–45.

Enenkel, A., and R. Maurer. Feb. 2, 1952 (application). Apparatus for the aeration of liquids. Brit. 724,791 (Acetator design).

Mayer, E. Aug. 22, 1961. Process for making vinegar. U.S. 2,997,424 (Cavitator process patent).

Mayer, E. 1963. Historic and modern aspects of vinegar making (acetic fermentation). *Food Technol.*, **17**, 74–76.

McNary, R. R., and M. H. Dougherty. 1960. Citrus vinegar. University of Florida Agric. Expt. Station Bull. 622.

Prescott, S. C., and C. G. Dunn. 1959. *Industrial microbiology*. 3rd Ed., pp. 432–453. McGraw-Hill Book Co., Inc., New York.

Vaughn, R. H. 1954. Acetic acid-vinegar. Pp. 498-535 in *Industrial fermentations*, vol. I (ed. by L. A. Underkofler and R. J. Hickey). Chemical Publishing Co., Inc., New York.

GLUCONIC ACID

Gluconic acid finds many commercial uses, being marketed usually as the calcium or sodium gluconate salt. Thus, calcium gluconate is employed as a pharmaceutical to supply calcium, and calcium and sodium gluconates in alkaline solution are good metal sequestering agents, particularly for iron, aluminium, and copper. In addition, ferrous gluconate supplies iron for the treatment of anemia.

Gluconic acid is produced by various bacteria, including several *Acetobacter* species, and various processes utilizing bacteria have been patented but not commercialized. In addition, several fungi, including *Penicillium* and *Aspergillus* species, also produce gluconic acid in good yields, and selected strains of *Aspergillus niger* presently are employed in commercial production. However, gluconic acid also is produced industrially by the direct chemical oxidation of glucose.

The fermentation production of gluconic acid by *Aspergillus niger* is a one-step enzymatic transformation of glucose to gluconic acid, with the aldehyde of glucose being oxidized to the carboxyl of gluconic acid (Figure 21.7). The enzyme mediating this oxidation is a flavorprotein that is known as glucose-oxidase, or more correctly, glucoseaerodehydrogenase. In addition to gluconic acid, hydrogen peroxide also is a product of this reaction, but the hydrogen peroxide is immediately decomposed by the catalase of *Aspergillus niger* in order to liberate an atom of oxygen. Therefore, the reaction can be considered as one mole of glucose plus an atom of oxygen yielding one mole of gluconic acid.

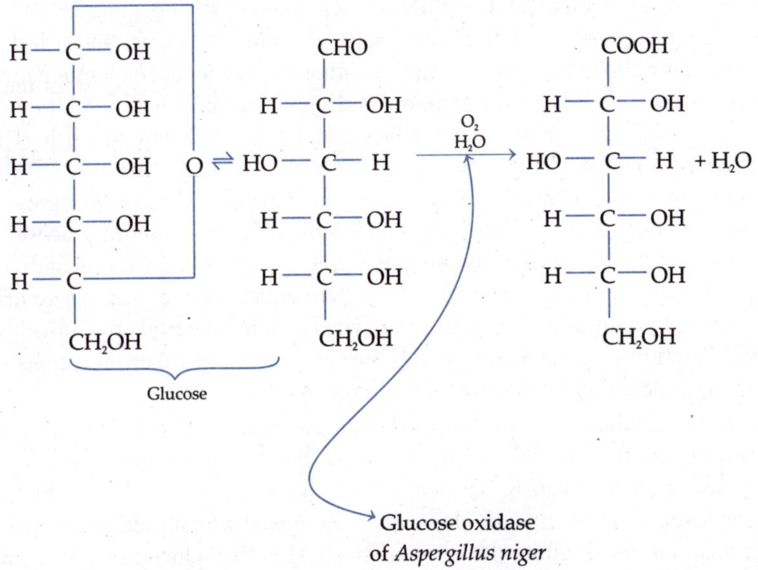

Figure 21.7 Glucose oxidation to gluconic acid by the glucose oxidase of *Aspergillus niger.*

An interesting historical note might be interjected here. Several years ago in the search for new antibiotics, it was observed that purified culture filtrates of *Penicillium notatum* contained a powerful antibiotic-like substance that was called variously Notatin, penicillin **B**, and Penatin. This antibiotic was unusual in that it was active against susceptible organisms only in the presence of glucose and oxygen. However, after much study, it was realized that the antibiotic activity was not caused by an antibiotic as such but by the hydrogen peroxide generated by the purified glucose oxidase from *Penicillium notatum* which had been separated during purification from the catalase activity that normally would have destroyed the hydrogen peroxide.

The *Aspergillus niger* gluconic acid fermentation can be accomplished by both stationary and submerged culture, but the submerged culture is presently utilized in industrial production. Once formed in an initial gluconic acid-growth fermentation, the *Aspergillus niger* myceliutm is reused in successive "replacement culture" fermentations so long as the glucose oxidase activity of the mycelium remains highly active. Thus, after the initial fermentation produces the mycelium, the successive fermentations are purely enzymatic transformations mediated by the glucose oxidase of the mycelium. This reuse of the mycelium obviously means a lessening of the requirement for inoculum build-up. Nevertheless, when inoculum is required, it is usually provided as spores, or pregerminated spores, added directly to the production fermentor.

The growth medium for gluconic acid production contains about 25 percent glucose, along with various salts, calcium carbonate, and a boron compound, although, at times, cornsteep liquor also is added. The fermentation is conducted at 30°C with aeration and agitation, and heat evolution is controlled by cooling coils, water-jacketed fermentors, and so forth. The replacement culture fermentation is conducted in a similar manner, but the medium does not contain nitrogen compounds (to prevent further growth of the mycelium) and, under these conditions, the conversion of glucose to gluconic acid is somewhere in the range of 95 percent. At the termination of either the growth or replacement culture fermentations, the gluconic acid is recovered by neutralization of the broth with calcium hydroxide so as to allow crystallization of calcium gluconate. Free gluconic acid then is recovered from the calcium gluconate by the addition of sulfuric acid.

Early studies of the *Aspergillus niger* gluconic acid fermentation demonstrated that, in the absence of boron, the maximum sugar content in the medium which can be fermented is about 16 percent. Thus, at higher sugar levels, excess calcium gluconate is produced which precipitates from the medium and inhibits the fermentation. Also free gluconic acid in the medium, not tied up as calcium gluconate, injures the mycelium particularly when the mycelium is continuously exposed to gluconic acid during reuse of the mycelium. This situation was changed, however, when it was discovered that the addition of boron compounds to the medium allows up to 35 percent glucose to be converted to gluconic acid. Thus, the boron compounds temporarily stabilize the calcium gluconate in solution and, consequently, prevent its precipitation; this allows the use of excess calcium carbonate to neutralize all or almost all of the gluconic acid that is produced. With boron additions, however, special strains of *Aspergillus niger* are required which possess high boron tolerance ; this requirement is in addition to the requirement that they produce gluconic acid without simultaneously accumulating citric, oxalic, and other acids. The boron is added to the initial and replacement culture fermentations as dry boric acid or as borax after the fermentation is well under way, but because of its toxicity, the level of incorporation is held at about 1500 ppm.

A more recent innovation to circumvent the toxicity of calcium gluconate and gluconic acid to the mycelium is a fermentation approach that, without the addition of boron compounds, yields sodium instead of calcium gluconate. Thus, by utilizing automatic pH-control equipment, the medium during fermentation is continuously neutralized by sodium hydroxide.

Another interesting recent innovation of the gluconic acid fermentation may well help in maintaining the competitive position of the fermentation.

For this approach, sucrose is employed as the carbon source, but it is first converted to glucose plus fructose. Then, by proper control of the fermentation, the glucose is oxidized to gluconic acid by *Aspergillus niger* glucose oxidase, but without destruction of the fructose so that the fructose can be recovered as a valuable by-product of the fermentation. As a matter of fact, however, the patent for this process considers the fructose and not the gluconic acid to be the main product of the fermentation (Holstein and Holsing, 1962).

References

Gluconic Acid

Holstein, A. G., and G. C. Holsing. Aug. 21, 1962. Method for the production of levulose. U.S. 3,050, 444.

Prescott, S. C., and C. G. Dunn, 1959. *Industrial microbiology*. 3rd Ed., pp. 578–597. McGraw-Hill Book Co., Inc., New York.

Underkofler, L.A. 1954. Gluconic acid. Pp. 446–469 in *Industrial fermentations,* vol. I (ed. by L. A. Underkofler and R. J. Hickey). Chemical Publishing Co., Inc., New York.

STEROID TRANSFORMATIONS

The most striking example of the use of microorganisms to carry out chemical transformations is that of the steroid transformations. Various steroids such as the steroid hormones are known to be regulators of metabolism in the animal or human body, and further valuable properties of steroids came to the fore when it was discovered that cortisone and its derivatives (for instance, prednisone and prednisolone) are effective in the treatment of rheumatoid arthritis. In addition, various other steroids have since found new pharmacological uses, including their employment as oral contraceptives.

Chemotherapeutically important steroids are prepared commercially by multistep chemical and microbiological transformations of naturally available steroids. Thus, small amounts of steroids are found in most living cells. Yeasts, and particularly strains of *Saccharomyces cerevisiae*, contain relatively high levels of the steroid ergosterol, and wool wax steroids are available in wool wax, a by-product of the wool processing industry. However, the bulk of the steroids employed as substrates for steroid transformations are extracted from several species of plants that contain considerable quantities of plant steroids (or sapogenins). These plants are indigenous to certain tropical and subtropical countries, although attempts now are being made to grow these plants in the United States.

The total chemical transformation of one steroid to another can require many steps, and the process may be costly and provide only low yields because of certain rather difficult steps in the process. Thus, the total chemical transformation of the cattle bile steroid deoxycholic acid to cortisone (Figure 21.8) requires 37 separate chemical steps.

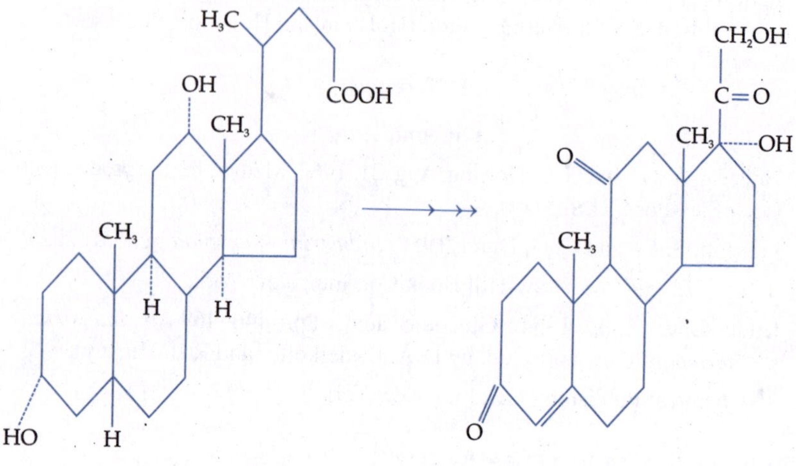

Figure 21.8 Transformation of deoxycholic acid to cortisone, a process requiring 37 separate chemical steps.

Those reactions of this and of similar transformations which are difficult to carry out chemically, however, often proceed with apparent ease when mediated by microorganisms. For instance, certain microorganisms can introduce hydroxyl groups at any of several of the carbon atoms of the steroid molecule. An example of such a transformation step is presented in Figure 21.9 in which either *Cunninghamella blakesleeana* or *Curvularia lunata* are utilized to introduce a hydroxyl group at carbon 11 on cortexolone to yield hydrocortisone. Carbon 11 of the steroid nucleus is of particular interest, since an oxygen atom at this point (Figures 21.8 and 21.9) is required for biological activity such as that required for the treatment of rheumatoid arthritis, and because introduction of an oxygen atom at this carbon is particularly difficult by purely chemical means. Other transformations of the steroid nucleus carried out by microorganisms include hydrogenations, dehydrogenations, epoxidations, and side-chain cleavage of the $-CH_2OHC=O$ function of the molecule.

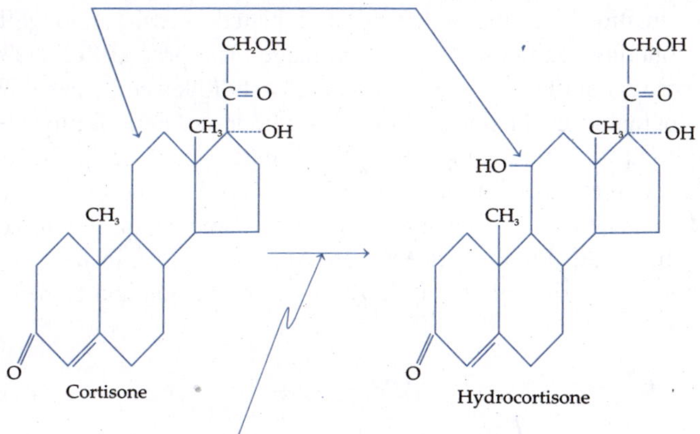

Figure 21.9 The use of micro-organisms to cause hydroxylation of cortexolone to yield hydrocortisone.

Steroid transformations are effected by fungi, bacteria, actinomycetes, yeasts, protozoa, and algae, although probably only bacteria, fungi, and actinomycetes are used commercially. Fungal and *Streptomyces* spores also carry out these transformations, and there is some indication that cell-free enzyme preparations can be used. In any event, specific organisms must be used to carry out specific transformations, and the organism should carry out the desired transformation without, at the same time, attacking other portions of the steroid molecule causing accumulation of side-reaction products. There are some indications that the enzymes responsible for the various transformations are adaptive enzymes. Thus, it has been suggested that the hydroxylating activities of fungi, and possibly other enzymatic reactions involved in these transformations, are really detoxifying mechanisms employed by the microorganisms.

The steroid transformation fermentations are carried out in stainless steel aerated fermentors, and the media employed are compounded at minimal nutritional levels to allow greater ease of extraction and purification of the transformation product. The particular medium depends on the choice of organism, although glucose or molasses are usually employed as a carbon source for growth. The steroid substrates are not water soluble and, therefore, are dissolved in a water-miscible solvent such as ethanol, acetone, or propylene glycol. Obviously, the solvent must not be toxic to the microorganism. After addition to the medium, the steroid substrate becomes colloidally dispersed throughout the medium, and it is added at low concentration to the fermentation after the organism has initiated growth, although further semicontinuous additions also may be made. The progress of the steroid transformation during the fermentation is closely followed by paper or other chromatographic evaluations of samples withdrawn periodically from the culture broth ; the chromatographically separated spots are easily observed under ultraviolet light. The fermentations usually last one to two days and yield a high percent conversion of the small amount of steroid that has actually been added to the fermentation. At harvest, the transformed steroid is separated from the culture broth by solvent extraction and is then further purified.

References

Steroid Transformations

Hanc, O. 1964. Transformation of steroids by microorganisms and biochemical reaction mechanisms. **P**p. 420–438 in *Global impacts of applied microbiology* (ed. by M. P. Starr). John Wiley and Sons, Inc., New York.

Peterson, D. H. 1955. Microorganisms and steroid transformations. in *Perspectives and horizons in microbiology* (ed. by S. A. Waksman). Rutgers University Press, New Brunswick, New Jersey.

Peterson, D. H. 1956. Microbiological conversions of steroids. *Rec. Chem. Progr.,* **17,** 211–240.

Peterson, D. H. 1964. Introduction of nuclear double bonds into steroids by microbial enzymes. **P**p. 439–448 in *Global impacts of applied microbiology* (ed. by M. P. Starr). John Wiley and Sons, Inc., New York.

Prescott, S. C., and C. G. Dunn. 1959. *Industrial microbiology*. 3rd. Ed., pp. 723–761. McGraw-Hill Book Co., Inc., New York.

Rose, A. H. 1961.; *Industrial microbiology*. **P**p. 269–278. Butterworths, Washington.

Shull. G. M. 1956. Transformations of steroids by molds. *Trans. N. Y. Acad. Sci.,* **19,** 147 – 172.

Stoudt, T. H. 1960. The microbiological transformation of steroids. *Adv. Appl. Microbiol*., **2.** 183–222.

Vischer, E., and A. Wettstein. 1958. Enzymic transformation of steroids by microorganisms. *Adv. Enzymol*., **20**, 237 – 282.

Wettstein, A., H. Hurlimann, and E. Vischer. 1964. Microbial synthesis of pharmacologically active substances. Pp. 295–326 in *Global impacts of applied microbiology* (ed. by M. P. Starr). John Wiley and Sons, Inc., New York.

Chapter 22

Hydrocarbon Fermentations

Hydrocarbons as fermentation carbon substrate sources present many possibilities for future industrial fermentations. However, they have not as yet received enough study for a critical evaluation of their real potential in the fermentation industry.

Hydrocarbons are completely reduced organic compounds containing carbon and hydrogen but not oxygen atoms in their molecules, and both coaltar and the petroleum derivatives are included in this class of substrates. Hydrocarbons may be saturated or unsaturated. Also, their molecules may be cyclic (either aromatic or paraffinic), straight or branched chains, or mixtures of the two types of structures within the same molecule.

Microbial attack on a hydrocarbon which, in the process, introduces an oxygen atom into the molecule produces a compound which, by definition, is no longer a hydrocarbon. This is an important consideration, because the unique characteristics of hydrocarbon-oxidizing microorganisms appear to be associated mainly with their ability to bring about the initial attack on the molecule. Thus, many microorganisms can attack the resulting oxygenated products of hydrocarbons and, in fact, the degradation of hydrocarbons after the initial oxidative attack seems to follow the general metabolic pathways common to many microorganisms. This point should be considered in screening programs to obtain hydrocarbon-oxidizing bacteria, since non-hydrocarbon-oxidizing microorganisms grow readily on the hydrocarbon-oxidation products and, in mixed cultures, only a few representatives of the microbial population may actually be attacking the hydrocarbon itself.

In general, the most amenable of the hydrocarbons to microbial attack are the 10 to 18 carbon, normal, straight-chain alkanes, and growth on these hydrocarbons is often rapid and voluminous. The 1 to 4 carbon gaseous hydrocarbons (methane through butane) are attacked by a lesser number of microorganisms as are the 5 to 9 carbon liquid alkanes. Branched-chain alkanes often are less easily attacked, and saturated cyclic hydrocarbons such as cyclohexane and methylcyclohexane are rarely attacked. However, in this instance, microbial oxidation has been demonstrated by application of the cooxidation fermentation technique (Ooyama and Foster, 1965). Aromatic hydrocarbons also undergo microbial degradation, but the relatively greater toxicity of many of these compounds to a certain extent limits the range of possible organisms. These various considerations, however, cannot be taken as absolute facts, because the microbial attack on hydrocarbons is known to be a relative matter. In other words, probably most any hydrocarbon can be attacked if the right organism is allowed enough incubation time. Thus, even highly toxic hydrocarbons such as toluene are known to be degraded by microorganisms.

The ability to attack and degrade hydrocarbons has been demonstrated for many different types of microorganisms. These organisms include members of the fungi, yeasts, *Streptomyces*, *Nocardia*, bacteria, and others, although this ability is particularly pronounced among various species of *Nocardia*, *Pseudomonas*, *Mycobacterium*, *Corynebacterium*, *Brevibacterium*, and the yeast *Candida*. However, among these various organisms, there is considerable specificity as to the particular range of hydrocarbons which any one microorganism can utilize although, in general, these hydrocarbon-oxidizing microorganisms would appear to utilize adaptive enzymes to bring about at least the initial attack on the hydrocarbon molecule.

Hydrocarbons as fermentation substrates present special problems because of their physical nature. They are gases, liquids, or solids all immiscible with water. Thus, for their use as a fermentation substrate, they must be passed through the medium as finely dispersed gas bubbles, emulsified in the medium as finely dispersed liquid oil droplets (Figure 22.1), or dispersed in the medium as finely divided solids. High agitation rates generally are required to disperse the liquid hydrocarbons in the fine oil-droplet state, and emulsifying agents may be added to help in achieving this end, although these agents often are similar enough in chemical structure to the hydrocarbon oxidation products that they also may be degraded by the fermentation microorganism Salts of the fatty-acid oxidation products of hydrocarbons also serve as emulsifying agents, once they have been formed during the fermentation.

The fermentation microorganism must have access to the aqueous phase of the fermentation medium, since it is in this phase that the various salts, nitrogen-containing compounds and other growth requirements are dissolved. At the same time, however, the microorganism must have access to the hydrocarbon and to oxygen. Usually, this means that the microorganism grows at the hydrocarbon-aqueous interface at the surface of the finely dispersed gas, liquid or solid hydrocarbon, although admittedly, minute amounts of various hydrocarbons do dissolve in the aqueous phase. With a relatively small ratio of liquid hydrocarbon to aqueous medium, the hydrocarbon becomes dispersed as finely divided oil droplets in the aqueous phase. At high proportions of hydrocarbon to aqueous medium, the hydrocarbon becomes dispersed as finely divided cell droplets in the aqueous Phase. At high Proportions of hydrocarbon to aqueous medium, the hydrocarbon becomes dispersed as finely divided oil droplets in the aqueous phase, however, the reverse situation is true : the phases are inverted so that finely dispersed droplets of water are suspended in the hydrocarbon. Microorganisms can grow under either situation, although to date most fermentation approaches have involved dispersions of hydrocarbons in water.

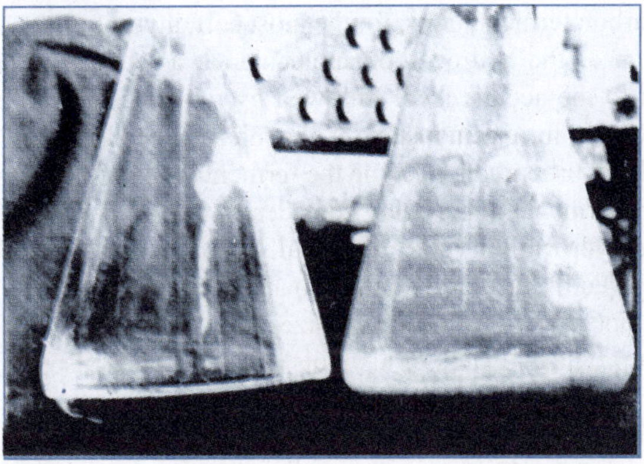

Figure 22.1 Emulsification of a liquid hydrocarbon in an aqueous medium during the growth of a hydrocarbon-oxidizing microorganism. The culture at the left with hydrocarbon floating on its surface was just inoculated, while that at the right has been incubated several days by shaking.

Another problem in hydrocarbon fermentation is that the more highly volatile hydrocarbons and the thick viscous hydrocarbons may be difficult to sterilize although, in some instances, sterilization is not required because of the toxicity of the hydrocarbon to contaminating microorganisms or the inability of these microorganisms to utilize the hydrocarbon. However, it must be remembered that contaminating microorganisms can utilize the hydrocarbon oxidation products in a fermentation and do not have to attack the hydrocarbon per se.

There are few, if any, indications that microorganisms can bring about an anaerobic attack on hydrocarbon molecules and, in fact, the oxygen requirements for a hydrocarbon fermentation are quite great. Thus, hydrocarbon fermentations usually require much greater air input and agitation than do fermentations utilizing the more conventional carbohydrate and protein substrates. In part, this may be attributed to a problem in getting oxygen to the surfaces of the microbial cells and, in part, to the fact that considerable oxygen must be incorporated into the hydrocarbon molecule during its microbial degradation. In regard to the latter point, on a theoretical basis the weight yields of products derived from hydrocarbons should be greater than the initial weight of the hydrocarbons, because of the oxygen that becomes incorporated into the product molecule. As regards the transmission of oxygen through the medium to the cells, the hydrocarbons per se usually do not constitute a barrier to air incorporation into the medium, since oxygen is quite soluble in many hydrocarbons. However, the emulsified hydrocarbon usually does provide an extra interface through which the oxygen must pass.

Hydrocarbon fermentations, for the most part, involve either an oxidative transformation of the hydrocarbon molecule, or a total degradation of the hydrocarbon to the acetate level followed by resynthesis of a fermentation product. However, in certain instances, the microbial cells, which grow at the expense of the hydrocarbon, become the fermentation product. Regardless of which type of fermentation is being considered, the initial steps of enzymatic attack on the hydrocarbon molecule usually involve first an oxidation to an alcohol, followed by further oxidation to an aldehyde and finally to an acid. Thus, fatty acids of various molecular sizes often are encountered among the fermentation products. Esters of alcohols and fatty acids also are commonly present. As stated previously, the fatty-acid salts serve as emulsifying agents for the fermentation, although they also may be further degraded by "β-oxidation." In this instance, acetic acid is split from the long-chain fatty acid leaving a residual fatty acid two carbons shorter in length, and this procedure is repeated until the entire molecule has been degraded to acetic acid. Obviously, fatty acids of varying chain lengths are intermediates in this process. There also is some evidence for ω-oxidation of straight-chain alkane hydrocarbons ; that is, oxidation occurs at both ends of a hydrocarbon molecule to yield products such as diterminal dicarboxylic acids.

The fermentative conversion of naphthalene to salicylic acid (Strawinski and Stone, 1943) by special strains of *Pseudomonas aeruginosa* for aspirin production may possibly already have found commercial usage. In this fermentation, a portion of one ring of the naphthalen molecule is removed by the organism to supply its carbon for growth and metabolism (Figure 22.2). However, naphthalene is a solid substrate and, hence, requires special handling. Also, it is added in slight excess to the fermentation medium in order to provide just enough toxicity to the P*s. aeruginosa* cells that extensive further degradation of the salicylic acid fermentation product is prevented. Claims approaching 100 percent conversion of naphthalene to salicylic acid have been made for this fermentation (Klausmeir and Strawinski, 1957).

Considerable public acclaim has been accorded a hydrocarbon fermentation process that produces the edible yeast *Candida lipolytica* (Champagant, 1963). This yeast is grown on an aqueous-salts medium with various oil fractions, including furnace oil, as the hydrocarbon substrate. Inorganic N-P-K agricultural fertilizers provide the salts and nitrogen for the aqueous medium, and the fermentation is continuous in that the hydrocarbon is recycled. During its growth, the yeast removes paraffins from the oil to bring about dewaxing, thus yielding as a by-product oil improved as to its pour-point characteristics. The yeast cells recovered from this fermentation contain a nutritionally balanced protein that should find use as a food or food supplement in the undernourished areas of the world.

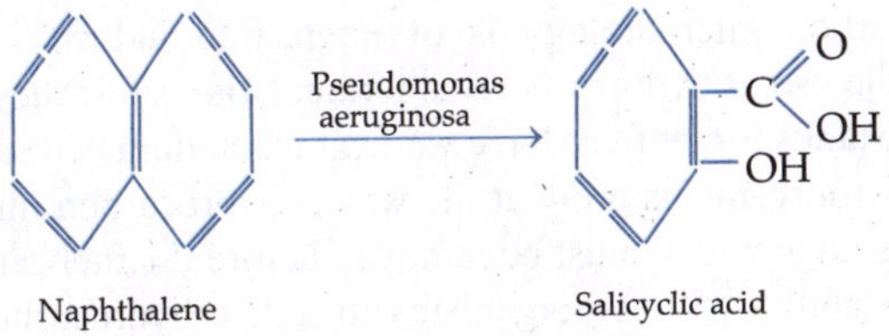

Figure 22.2 Microbial oxidation of naphthalene to salicyclic acid as mediated by special strains of *Pseudomonas aeruginosa*.

Other hydrocarbon fermentations are presently under study. *L*-Glutamic acid is a possible fermentation product (Takahashi, *et al*, 1965), as is extracellular lipase (Tagahashi, *et al*, 1963). The fermentative conversion of hydrocarbons to various aldehydes, alcohols, ketones, unsaturates, and so forth also are worthy of consideration.

The concept of cooxidation as it applies to hydrocarbon fermentations opens the way for possible new fermentation products and for the transformation of hydrocarbon substrates that normally are not easily attacked by microorganisms. The term cooxidation was applied by Foster (1962) to a phenomenon observed in earlier studies by Leadbetter and Foster (1960). Studies by these workers showed that *Pseudomonas methanica*, which grows on methane but not on ethane, propane, or butane, can oxidize these hydrocarbons while growing on methane. Thus, one hydrocarbon, methane, serves as the growth substrate while the second hydrocarbon (the ethane, propane, or butane) is merely oxidized. Davis and Raymond (1962) then showed that cooxidation also can occur with liquid hydrocarbons. Thus, a *Nocardia* species growing on the straight chain paraffin *n*-octadecane cooxidizes *n*-butylcyclohexane to cyclohexaneacetic acid. It is also possible that at least some cooxidation occurs when microorganisms grow on mixtures of hydrocarbons of the type found in petroleum distillates or crude-oil fractions, and an unexplored area for the potential use of cooxidation is in fermentations in which carbohydrate, protein, or some other oxidized substrate is employed in conjunction with a hydrocarbon.

The possibilities for hydrocarbon fermentations, therefore, present great appeal from a commercial standpoint. In addition, hydrocarbons are inexpensive and, if anything, their price should go down and not up as have the prices of more conventional fermentation substrates. Fermentations utilizing mixtures of hydrocarbons, such as kerosene, crude oils, or hydrocarbon distillation fractions, and the inexpensive hydrocarbon gases are particularly appealing. Thus, the ultimate fermentation would be that in which petroleum gas from a producing area is piped directly to a fermentation tank.

Hydrocarbon microbiology is of interest to industry for reasons in addition to the use of hydrocarbons as fermentation substrates. For example, huge storage tanks for jet fuels have water at the bottom beneath the kerosene fuel, and microorganisms grow at the water- hydrocarbon interface to form a microbial sludge which must be removed before the fuel can be used in jet aircraft. The ability of microorganisms to utilize hydrocarbons for growth is also finding some use in geologic prospecting for new oil deposits, since hydrocarbon gases emanate from these oil deposits and diffuse upward through the overlying soil. The presence of large numbers of hydrocarbon-oxidizing microorganisms in soil therefore can be taken as an indication of a possible oil reserve below. Nevertheless, a better indication is to bury culture vessels containing ethane- or propane-oxidizing microorganisms in the soil so as to detect the presence of the hydrocarbon gases by observing the resultant growth of these microorganisms. Methane-oxidizing bacteria cannot be employed for this purpose because of methane production through anaerobic processes by indigenous bacteria of the soil.

References

Beerstecher, E. 1954. *Petroleum microbiology*. Elsevier Press, Inc., New York. Champagant, A. 1963. Brit. 914,567.

Davis, J. B., and R. L. Raymond. 1962. Microbiological oxidation of hydrocarbons. U.S. 3,057,784.

Foster, J. W. 1962. Bacterial oxidation of hydrocarbons. Pp. 241-271 in *The oxygenases* (ed. by O. Hayaishi). Academic Press, Inc., New York.

Foster, J. W. 1962. tydrocarbons as substrates for microorganisms. *Antonie van Leeuwenhoek*, **28**, 241–274.

Klausmeir, R. E., and R. J. Strawinski. 1957. Microbial oxidation of naphthalene. I. Factors concerning salicylate accumulation. *J. Bacterial.*, **73,** 461–464.

Leadbetter, E. R., and J. W. Foster. 1960. Bacterial oxidation of gaseous alkanes. *Arch Microbiol.*, **35,** 92–104.

Ooyama, J., and J. W. Foster. 1965. Bacterial oxidation of cycloparaffinic hydrocarbons. *Antonie van Leeuwenhoek*, **31,** 45–65.

Rogoff, M. H. 1961. Oxidation of aromatic hydrocarbons by bacteria. *Adv. Appl. Microbiol.,* **3,** 193–221.

Strawinski, R. J., and R. W. Stone. 1943. Conditions governing the oxidation of naphthalene and the chemical analysis of its products. **J. Bacterial., 45,** 16.

Takahashi, J., Y. Imada, and K. Yamada. 1963. Lipase formation by microorganisms grown on hydrocarbons. *Nature*, **200**, 1208.

Takahashi, J., K. Kobayashi, Y. Imada, and K. Yamada. 1965. Effects of cornsteep liquor and thiamine on L-glutamic acid fermentation of hydrocarbons. IV. Utilization of hydrocarbons by microorganisms. *Appl. Microbiol.,* **13**, 1–4.

Treccani, V. 1964. Microbiol degradation of hydrocarbons. Pp. 1–33 in *Progress in industrial microbiology*, vol. IV (ed. by D. J. D. Hockenhull). Gordon and Breach Science Publishers, Inc., New York.

CHAPTER 23

Microbial Cells as Fermentation Products

In certain fermentation approaches, the microbial cells themselves are the desired fermentation product. A specific example is the production of food and feed yeast from hydrocarbons (described in Chapter 22). Other examples are bakers' yeast, *Torula* food and feed yeast, mushrooms, algae for food and feed and possibly gas-exchange reactions, *Rhizobium* bacterial legum, inoculant, and *Bacillus thuringiensis* insecticide.

BAKERS' YEAST

In historical times, the preparation of leavened bread was accomplished by inoculating fresh dough with left-over starter dough, that is, dough from a previous batch of bread. Obviously, the results did not always turn out as expected, because the sugar fermentation in the dough yielded variable amounts of carbon dioxide, or even very little carbon dioxide if the yeast was weak, was of the wrong type, or had died out. At a later date, the residual yeast from breweries and distilleries was added to dough, although this imparted a bitter taste from the hops. This situation later was rectified by growing the yeast specifically for use as a bakers' yeast, but still employing a brewing-type medium that was composed of malt, rye, and corn mash, but without hops. Present-day bakers' yeast fermentations utilize molasses media and aeration, with the aeration being employed to shunt much of the metabolic activities of the yeast to cell proliferation instead of to the fermentative production of ethyl alcohol.

Specially selected strains of *Saccharomyces cerevisiae* are employed for the production of bakers' yeast. These strains are selected for stable physiological characteristics, vigorous sugar fermentation in dough (dough-raising power), cellular dispersion in water, good keeping quality without autolysis, rapid growth and high cell yields in a fermentor, and the maintenance

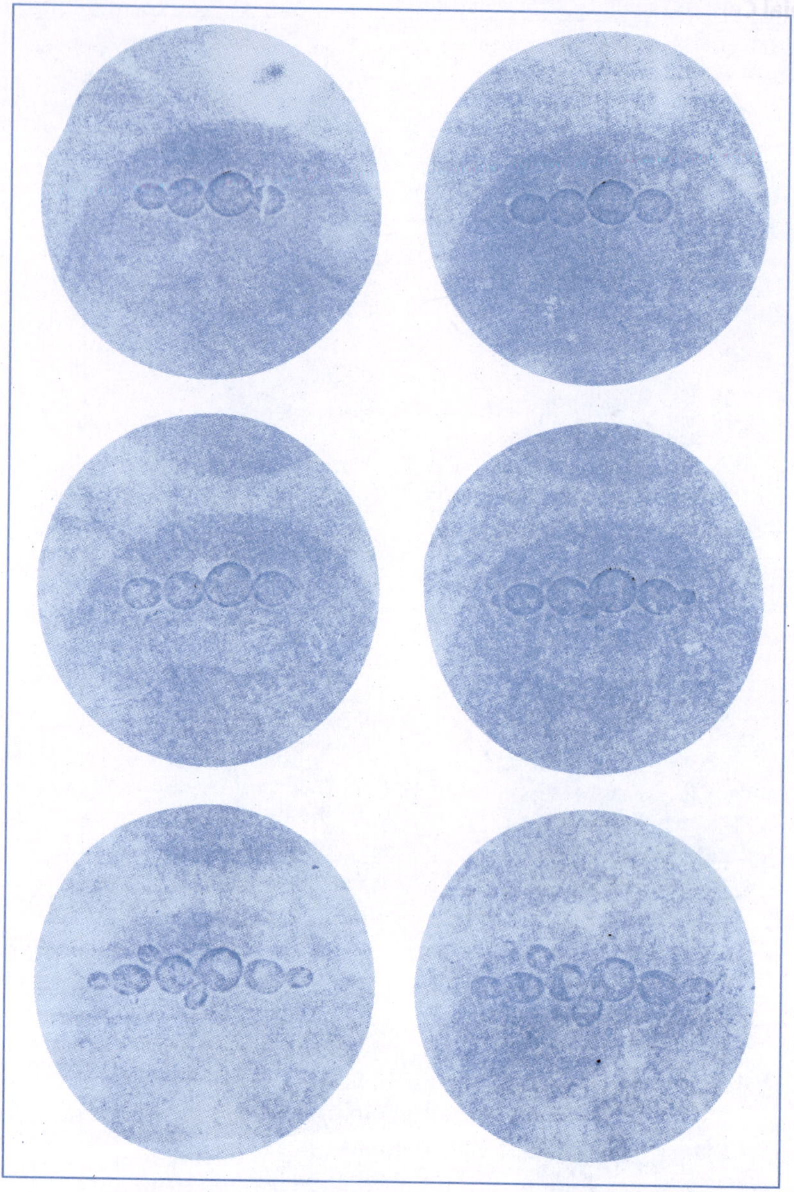

Figure 23.1 Sequential photographs at 15-minute intervals of the budding and growth of a single cell of Saccharomyces cerevisiae. Photos courtesy of the Fleishmann IV Manufacturing Division of Standard Brands, Inc.

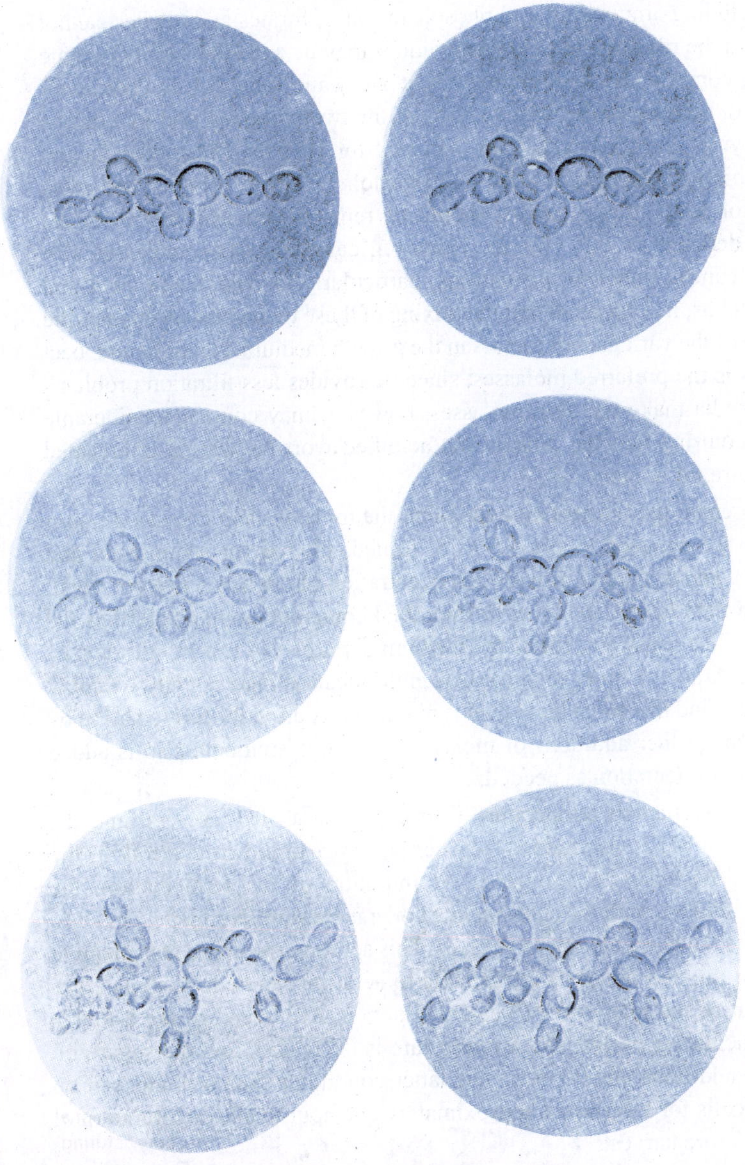

of a pleasing appearance on storage. Stock cultures of these strains are carefully maintained, and single-cell is isolations are often employed to retain the cultural constancy of these characteristics (Figure 23.1).

The production medium for bakers' yeast contains molasses and various salts, including ammonium and phosphate salts. Nitrates and nitrites cannot be used in the medium, but cornsteep liquor may be added to supply organic nitrogen compounds. A mixture of beet and cane molasses is commonly employed, because of the relative costs of the two molasses, and as a means of supplying the yeast with "bios" factors for growth. These bios factors include biotin, pantothenic acid, and inositol. Of these, biotin is the most critical for yeast growth, and it should be remembered that beet molasses often is deficient in this vitamin. However, cane blackstrap molasses also at times can be deficient in vitamins, particularly in pantothenic acid and inositol. Thus, it is apparent that the mixing of these two molasses ensures the presence of the various bios factors in the growth medium. Nevertheless, beet molasses is the preferred molasses, since it provides less filtration problems during media make-up. This molasses, however, may contain considerable sulfite, requiring that the diluted and acidified wort be aerated at elevated temperature for its removal.

To prepare the fermentation medium, the molasses and cornsteep liquor (if used) are adjusted to pH 4.5 to 5, heated, filtered (or sedimented and decanted), and diluted to provide a concentration of 0.5 to 1.5 percent sugar. This treatment lowers the level of microbial contamination and clarifies the molasses. The sugar content of the medium is purposely low at initiation of the fermentation in order to favor cell multiplication and not ethyl alcohol production, and this sugar level then is maintained during the fermentation by intermittent further additions of molasses. Aqueous ammonia also is added during the fermentation as needed.

The fermentation temperature is maintained at 30°C or less, and the culture broth pH is maintained between 4 and 5 to aid in controlling the growth of bacterial contaminants. At initiation of the fermentation, the culture is aerated, with the aeration rates then increasing during the next 8 to 12 hours as the fermentation progresses. This aeration requires a considerable volume of air, and the costs attributable to aeration can be as high as 20 to 30 percent of the total cost of yeast production. At the end of the 8-to 12-hour fermentation period, the aeration rate is decreased, and the sugar and ammonia additions are stopped. The latter conditions then are imposed on the yeast cells for a period of approximately one hour to allow maturation of the cells before harvest.

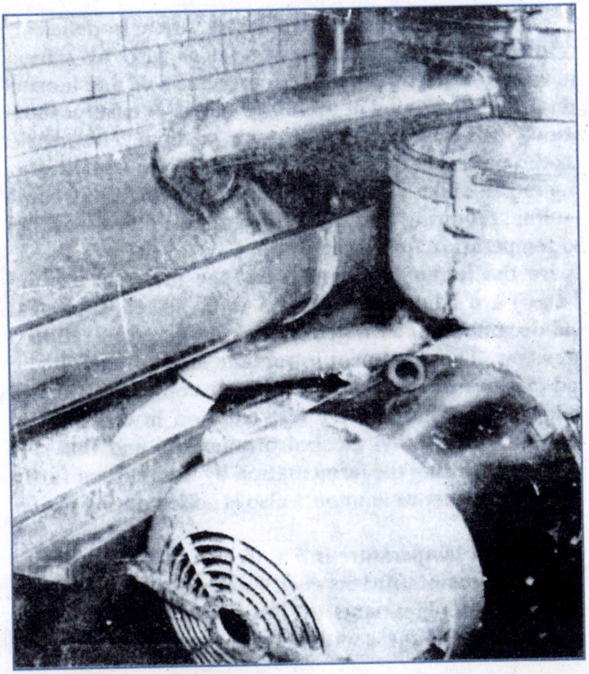

Figure 23.2 Centrifugation and washing of yeast cells. Photo courtesy of the Fleishmann Manufacturing Division of Standard Brands, Inc.

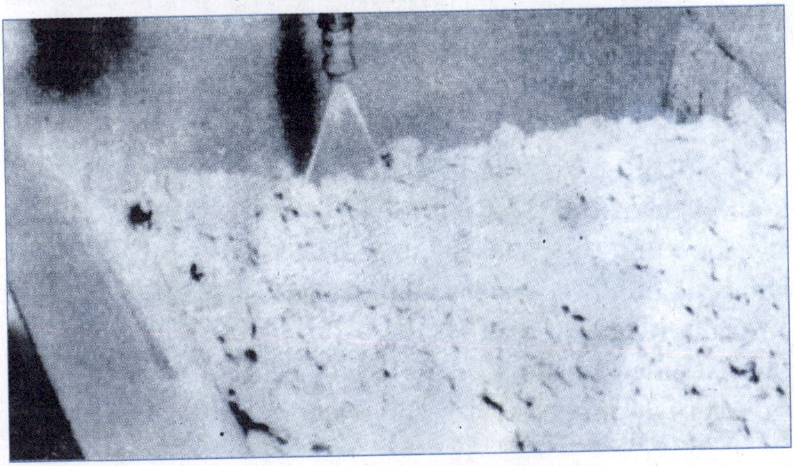

Figure 23.3 Plasticizer addition to yeast cells before mixing and extruding. Photo courtesy of the Fleishmann Manufacturing Division of Standard Brands, Inc.

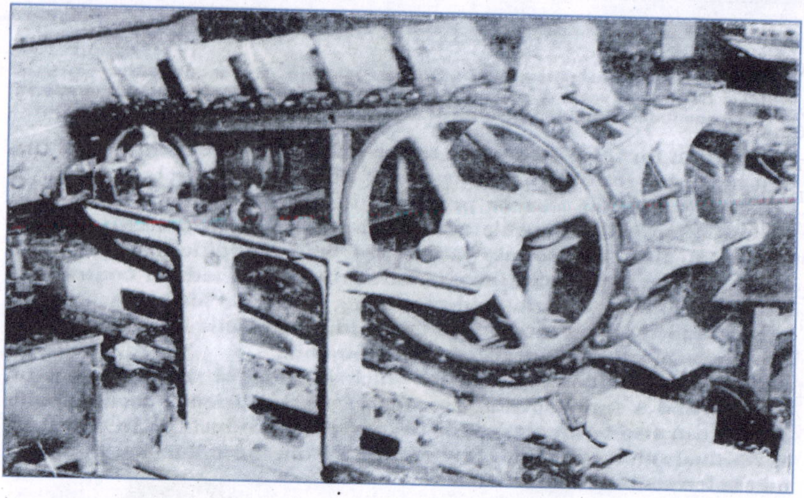

Figure 23.4 Extrusion and cutting of yeast blocks. Photo courtesy of the Fleishmann Manufacturing Division of Standard Brands, Inc.

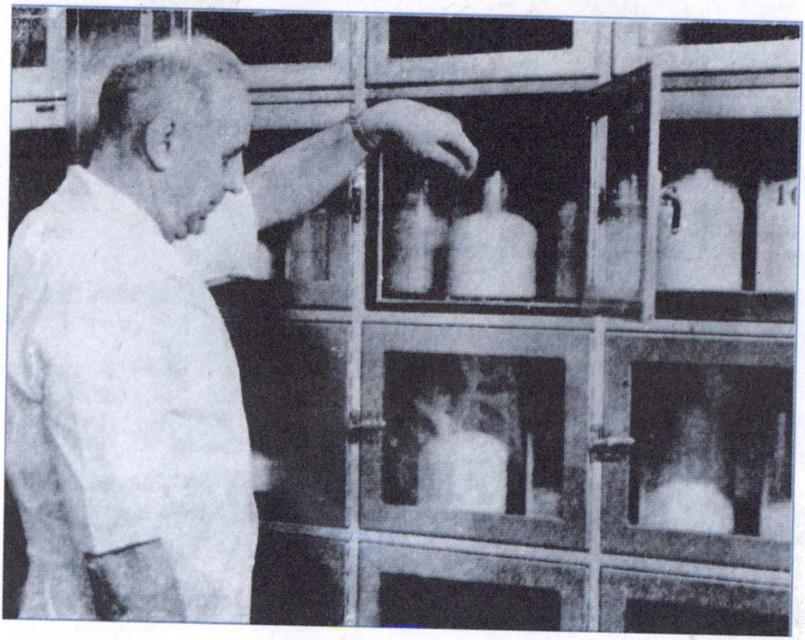

Figure 23.5 Yeast quality testing in a Dough Proof Box. The dough-raising power of individual batches of yeast is evaluated in the graduated cylinders. Photo courtesy of the Fleishmann Manufacturing Division of Standard Brands, Inc.

At harvest, the culture broth is cooled, and the cells are removed from the wort by centrifugation. The yeast cells are then washed by suspension in water and centrifugation to remove the residual impurities and color of the medium, and this washing may be repeated several times (Figure 23.2). The cells finally are separated on a filter press from the aqueous phase, mixed with plasticizer (small amounts of vegetable oils, Figure 23.2), and extruded in block from (Figure 23.4). This block then is cut into portions of commercial size and weight, wrapped, and stored under refrigeration for sale. Before sale to the public, however, samples of the yeast are tested for dough-raising power (Figure 23.5).

Bakers' yeast can also be produced in a grain-malt medium. This medium often is first inoculated with *Lactobacillus delbrueckii* and incubated at 50°C to produce lactic acid before addition of the yeast inoculum. The lactic acid favors yeast growth and aids in controlling contamination by butyric acid-producing bacteria. Molasses also, at times, is added to this medium so that additional lactic acid can be produced, which is then neutralized with ammonia.

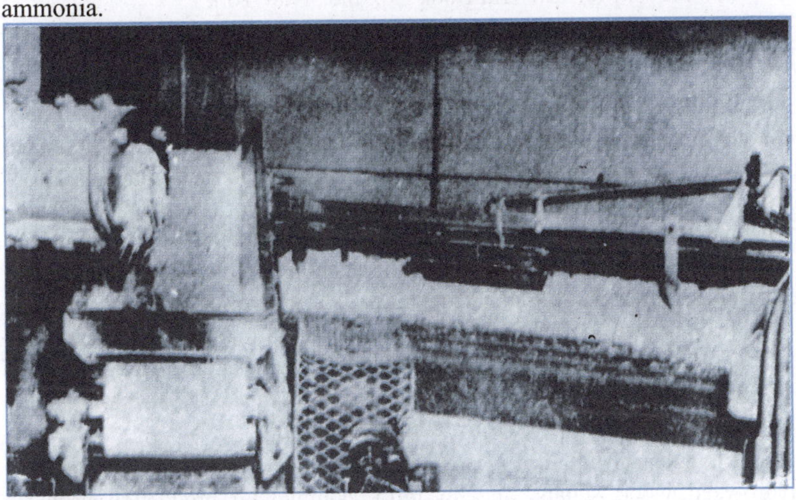

Figure 23.6 Drying of yeast for production of activated dry yeast. Photo courtesy of the Fleishmann Manufacturing Division of Standard Brands, Inc.

Sulfite-waste liquor medium to which is added a small amount of molasses and a supplementary source of yeast nutrients, such as malt sprouts, can also be employed for bakers' yeast production. In this case, the residual sulfur dioxide is first removed from the sulfite-waste liquor, and the fermentation is aerated and continuous.

"Active dry yeast" is produced by a fermentation resembling that for molasses-grown bakers' yeast, but special strains of *Saccharomyces cerevisiae* are employed. The harvested and washed yeast from the filter press is dispersed as pellets or granules and then dried (without addition of filler) to about 8 percent moisture (Figure 23.6). This yeast preparation does not require refrigeration and remains active for many months under normal atmospheric conditions. Also, it will retain its activity for considerably longer periods of time, if vacuum or inert gas packaging is employed.

References

Bakers' Yeast

Irvin, R. 1954. Commercial yeast manufacture. Pp. 273–306 in *Industrial fermentations*, vol. I (ed. by L. A. Underkofler and R. J. Hickey). Chemical Publishing Co., Inc., New York.

Prescott, S. C., and C. G. Dunn. 1959. *Industrial microbiology.* 3rd Ed., Pp. 60–70. McGraw-Hill Book Co., Inc., New York.

FOOD AND FEED YEASTS

Various yeasts are nutritionally good sources of protein and B vitamins. Therefore, yeast is commercially produced for animal feed, and it is possible that yeast may gain greater acceptance as human food (see Chapter 22 for hydrocarbon-derived yeast) since two-thirds of the world population is said to be underfed. *Saccharomyces cerevisiae* grown on a molasses medium can be used as a food or feed yeast, but the economics often are poor. Better economics, however, are associated with *Torula* yeast, also known as *Candida utilis* or *Torulopsis utilis*, because of its ability to assimilate a wide variety of carbon and nitrogen compounds, including pentoses, under relatively simple fermentation conditions. *Candida arborea* and *Oidium lactis* also have been utilized to produce feed yeast on a commercial scale.

Although *Torula* yeast grows well on media containing molasses, hydrolyzed wood sugars, and so forth, commercial production usually utilizes a sulfite-waste liquor medium in a continuous fermentation. Thus, contamination and genetic instability do not appear to be particular problems with this continuous fermentation. The sulfite-waste liquor for the medium is filtered, and the sulfur dioxide is removed by steam stripping. Diammonium acid phosphate and potassium chloride are added to the medium at make-up, and aqueous ammonia as well as fresh nutrients are continuously fed to the yeast as the fermentation progresses (Figure 23.7). The pH of the medium is approximately 5. Aeration and agitation are employed, and the temperature is maintained at approximately 37°C. Although this temperature often is higher than ambient, cooling may be required, nevertheless, since considerable heat is evolved during the fermentation. That portion of the fermentation broth continuously removed from the fermentation for cell harvest is centrifuged to separate the cells from the broth, and the cells then are washed and dried under conditions that kill the cells.

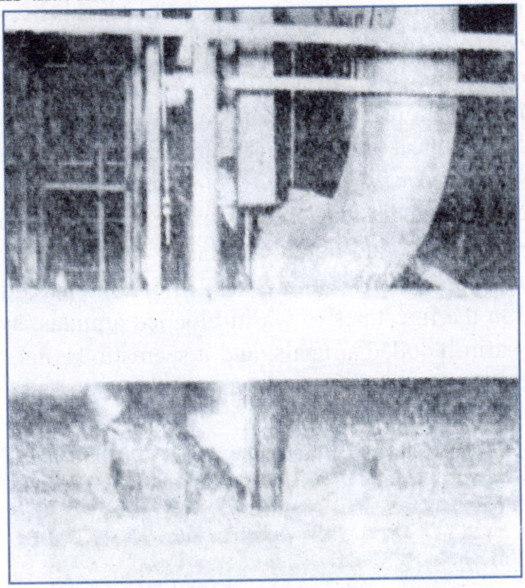

Figure 23.7 Sulfite-waste liquor being continuously added to the *Tarula* yeant continuous sulfite-waste liquor fermentation. Photo courtesy of the Rhinelander Division of St. Regis Paper Co.

Brewers' yeast also can be utilized as a feed yeast, if it is first debittered to improve its flavour. To accomplish this, the yeast is washed with water, dilute sodium hydroxide, and again with water before sodium chloride and phosphoric acid (to produce a slight acidity) are added. The yeast then is dried.

References

Food and food yeast

Prescott, S. C., and C. G. Dunn. 1959. *Industrial microbiology*. 3rd Ed., Pp. 71–87. Mc Graw-Hill Book Co., Inc., New York.

Wiley, A.J. 1954. Food and fodder yeast. Pp. 307–343 in *Industrial fermentations*, vol. I (ed. by L. A. Underkofler and R. J. Hickey). Chemical Publishing Co., Inc., New York.

BACTERIAL INSECTICIDES

Various *Bacillus* species presently are being studied for their possible use in the control of agricultural insect pests. Of these bacilli, *Bacillus thuringiensis* already is produced on a commercial scale for use as an insecticide against various *Lepidoptera* and some *Diptera*. Thus, over 100 species of *Lepidoptera* are known to be susceptible to this bacterium.

Bacillus thuringiensis is a representative of the crystalliferous bacteria, a group of bacteria in which a crystalline parasporal body accompanies sporulation. This parasporal body is a protein that can be observed in the cytoplasm of the cell near the spore (Figure 23.8). On ingestion of these cells by susceptible insects, the high pH value and reducing agents present in the gut of the insect dissolve the toxic crystalline protein. Thereafter, the gut becomes damaged and nonfunctional so that feeding ceases almost immediately, and the insect dies within 24 to 48 hours. Apparently, this protein is not dissolved in the intestines of warm-blooded animals, and it seems to be nontoxic to warm-blooded animals, and it seems to be nontoxic to worm blooded animals, plants and bees, a picture which contrasts markedly with that for various chemical insecticides.

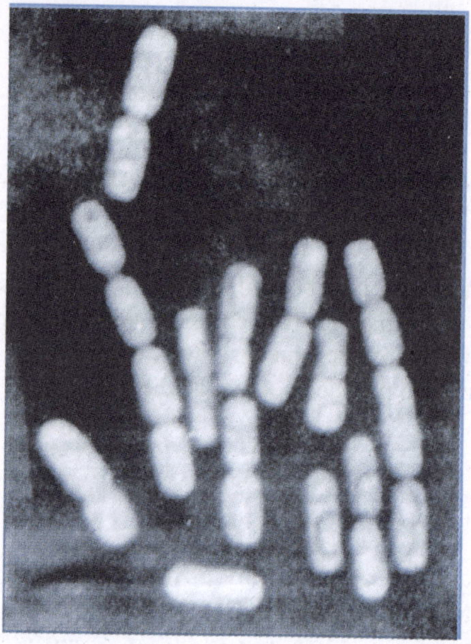

Figure 23.8 *Bacillus thuringiensis* showing the larger spore and smaller crystalline parasporal body within the sporangium. Air-dried nigrosin smear at 3880-fold magnification. (Photo courtesy of P. C. Fitz-James.)

At harvest of the fermentation, the vegetative cells and spores are mixed with bentonite or other carrier for application as a dust, or the cells and spores may be applied as a water spray. Actually, little information is generally available to the public on the proper procedures for growing *Bacillus thuringiensis* in order to obtain high yields of the crystalline toxic protein. However, the organism is reported to be easily grown and with good yields of toxin.

References

Bacterial Insecticides

Anderson, R. F., and M. H. Rogoff. 1966. Crystalliferous bacteria as insect toxicants. *Adv. Chem.* Ser., **53,** 65–79.

Angus, T. A., and A. M. Heimpel. 1960. The bacteriological control of insects. *Proc., Ent. Soc. Ont.,* **90,** 13–21.

Heimpel, A. M., and T. A. Angus. 1960. Bacterial insecticides. *Bacterial, Rev.,* **24,** 266–288.

Steinhaus, E. A. 1951. Possible use of *Bacillus thuringiensis* Berliner as an aid in the biological control of the alfalfa caterpillar. *Hilgardia,* **20,** 359–381.

LEGUME INOCULANT

The seeds of legumes, such as alfalfa, peas, clover, and so forth, are usually inoculated with proper species and strains of *Rhizobium* bacteria at the time of planting of the seed. As a result, these bacteria then become favourably located in the soil in relation to the roots of the leguminous plants for the development of legume root nodules (Figure 23.9). The bacteria within these nodules aid plant growth (Figure 23.10) by fixing gaseous nitrogen from the air into forms usable by the plant. Specific *Rhizobium* species are required for the particular leguminous plant to be grown, and to insure good nodule formation, a mixture of strains of the proper *Rhizobium* species is incorporated into the inoculant. The individual strains of *Rhizobium* are grown in aerated fermentors (Figure 23.11) and, at harvest, these strains are mixed with a slightly moist carrier such as peat and then packaged. The cells remain viable in the peat for a year or so, but the inoculant is usually used within the same growing season as prepared.

A recent innovation of legume inoculation is the preinoculation of leguminous seed before sale to the public. In this process, the *Rhizobium* bacteria are vacuum impregnated into the seed or applied to the exterior of the seed along with a protective coating to prevent death of the bacterial cells.

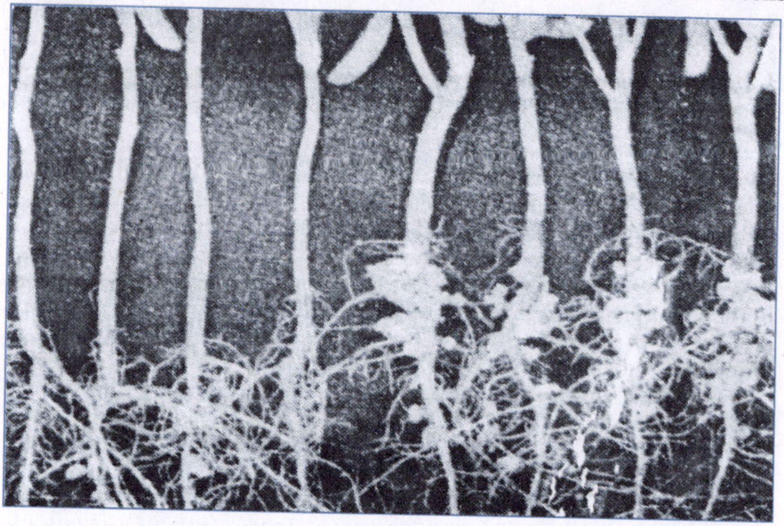

Figure 23.9. Nodulated roots of soybeans. The roots at the left were not inoculated ; those at the right were inoculated with effective strains of rhizobia and demonstrate good nodulation. Photo courtesy of the Nitragin Co.

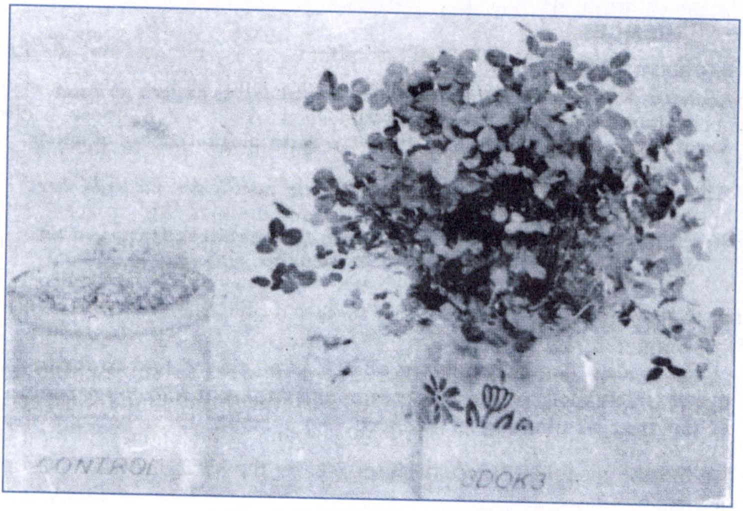

Figure 23.10. Growth of Red Clover inoculated with effective strains of rhizobia (on the right) as compared to uninoculated Red Clover (on the left). Photo courtesy of the NitragIn Co.

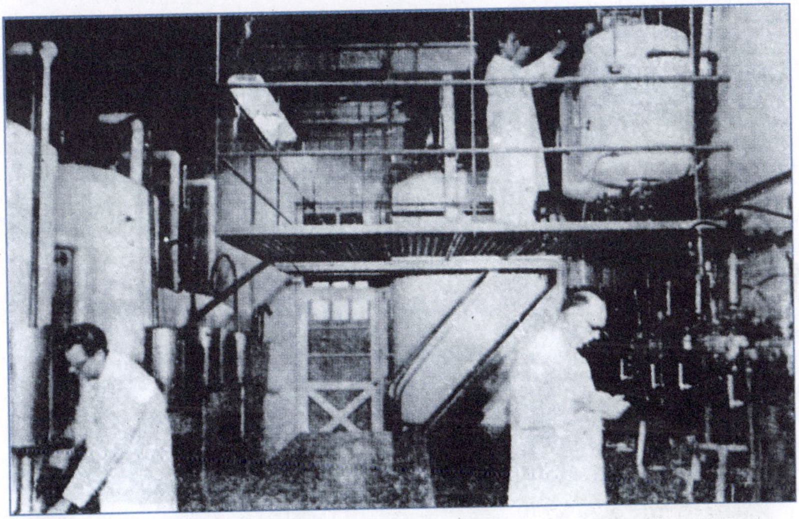

Figure 23.11. Fermentor room for growing various strains of rhizobia bacteria to be used in the preparation of legume inoculant. Photo courtesy of the Nitragin Co.

MUSHROOMS

Mushrooms, the fruiting bodies of various Basidiomycetes, are used as a food and as a flavoring agent in soups and sauces. The common mushroom of commerce, *Agaricus bisporus*, is grown on compost beds in mushroom houses or caves, although it also can be grown in submerged fermentation in its mycelial phase, but the flavor in the latter instance does not match that for compost-grown mushrooms.

For the growth of this mushroom on compost, the spores first are germinated on agar, and the resulting white mycelium then is transferred to sterile wheat, rye, or kaffir corn so that, on incubation, mycelial "spawn" is produced. This spawn then is mixed with a specially prepared and pasteurized compost and, after two to three weeks incubation to allow extensive mycelium formation (Figure 23.12), a thin layer of soil (1 to 1 1/2 inches) is placed over its surface (it is "cased") to induce production of the fruiting bodies (Figure 23.13).

Another possibly less well-known mushroom, the morel mushroom, (*Morchella hortensis*), can be grown in submerged fermentation in the mycelial form to provide a commercially acceptable product. This is accomplished by a three day fermentation, which produces spherical nodules of hyphae approximately 1/4 to 1 inch in diameter. The flavor of this product is typical for the morel mushroom but differs from that of *Agaricus bisporus*, and it has been proposed that the morel mushroom be used as a protein source or as a flavorful protein supplement.

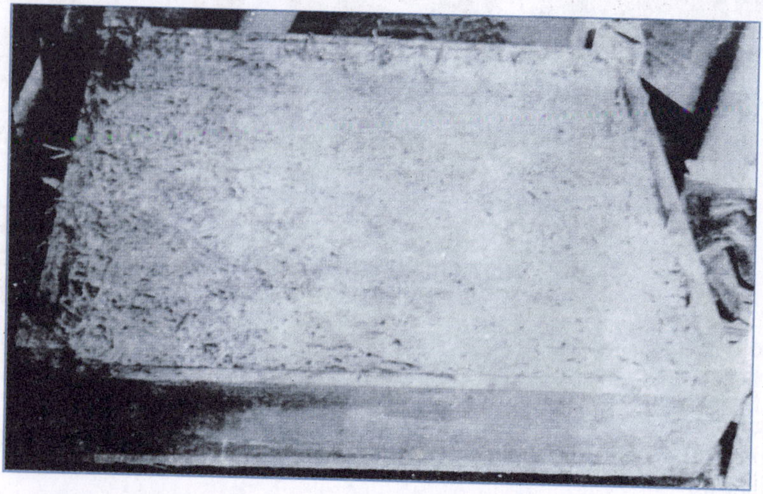

Figure 23.12. Mycelial growth of *Agaricus bisporus* ready for casing. Photo courtesy of the Mushroom Laboratory of the Pennsylvania State University.

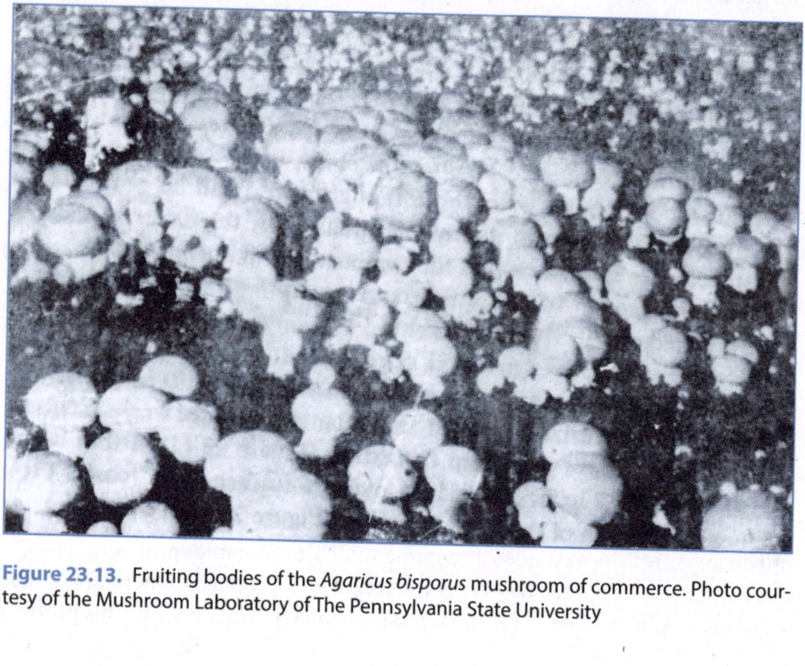

Figure 23.13. Fruiting bodies of the *Agaricus bisporus* mushroom of commerce. Photo courtesy of the Mushroom Laboratory of The Pennsylvania State University

References

Mushrooms

Litchfield, J. H. 1964. The mass culture of *Morchella* species in submerged culture and their potential uses as sources of protein. Pp. 327–337 in *Global impacts of applied microbiology* (ed. by M. P. Starr). John Wiley and Sons, Inc., New York.

Robinson, R. F., and R. S. Davidson. 1959. The large-scale growth of higher fungi. *Adv. Appl. Microbiol.*, **1**, 261–278.

Sebek, O. K. 1961. Synthesizing chemicals and biologicals by microorganisms. *Am. Perfumer Aromat.,* **76,** 27–35.

ALGAE

Algae are a potential source of human food and animal feed, providing good sources of protein, vitamins, fats, and carbohydrates. Also, algae present a certain appeal as a fermentation source of food or feed, because they use carbon dioxide and photosynthesis to obtain their carbon source for growth, and because certain of the algae also fix gaseous nitrogen from the air as their nitrogen source for growth. Thus, under these conditions, only inorganic salts need to be added to the medium. However, there also are less favourable fermentation aspects. The algae grow only slowly, and there is a problem in getting enough carbon dioxide and light to the individual algal cells. Finally, there is a requirement for some type of processing to improve digestibility of the cells. *Chlorella ellipsoidea* has received extensive study as a fermentation source of food and feed, and other algae of potential value are *Chlorella pyrenoidosa, Chlorella vulgaris, Scenedesmus*, and the blue-green nitrogen-fixing algae *Nostoc*.

Algae fermentations provide further distinct interest, because of the possibility for their use in closed ecological systems for space exploration. Thus, the algae would be employed to remove carbon dioxide from the atmosphere, replacing it with oxygen, and at the same time to serve as a source of food during extended space flights.

References

Algae

Krauss, R. W. 1962. Mass culture of algae for food and other organic compounds. *Am. J. Bot.,* **49**., 425–435.

Rose, A. H. 1962. Modern trends in industrial microbiology. *The School Sci. Rev.,* **152,** 16–17.

Chapter 24

Vitamins and Growth Stimulants

Various microbial fermentation products find commercial application for their use in animal and human nutrition. In addition, a group of compounds, the Gibberellins, are utilized to stimulate plant growth.

Antibiotics added to feed stimulate the growth of domestic animals and chickens, although the mechanism by which this occurs still remains obscure. When antibiotics are used in this manner, they need not receive the costly purification steps associated with veterinary and medical uses of the antibiotics and, in fact, crude dried concentrates of the fermentation broths often are adequate. Several vitamins are produced during the normal metabolism of microorganisms, but only riboflavin and B_{12} (cobamide) have found extensive commercial production. However, vitamin A, as the beta-carotene fermentation, has received extensive study, and this fermentation may well enjoy extensive industrial exploitation in the near future.

VITAMIN B_{12} (COBAMIDE)

For a period of years, intensive studies were conducted to determine the component of liver extract which was active in the treatment of pernicious anemia. Finally, Rickes *et al* (1948a) recovered a small amount of active material from liver, crystallized it as vitamin B_{12}, then showed that it was a cobalt complex (Rickes *et al*, 1948b). At the time of the latter studies, Stokstad *et al* (1948) demonstrated that something that occurred in cultures of the bacterium *Flavobacterium solare* was active in the animal-protein-factor assay in chicks and in the treatment of pernicious anemia in human patients, but these workers, because of the impurity of the preparations being studied, could not prove whether the microbial factor was, in fact, the same as the antipernicious anemia factor. This point was demonstrated, however, when Rickes *et al* (1948c) recovered active crystalline vitamin

B_{12} (Figure 24.1) from a *Streptomyces griseus* culture (which also produced the antibiotic grisein). Further studies by other workers then revealed that at least small amounts of cobamide were synthesized by many different types of microorganisms, but particularly bacteria and actinomycetes, and that the ability to synthesize large amounts of this vitamin was particularly prevalent among microorganisms from intestinal habitats. Also, at this time, it was realized that the synthesis of cobamide in nature probably was limited exclusively to microorganisms, although different microorganisms might produce different cobamides.

Thus, vitamin B_{12} is not a single compound, but a group of closely chemically related cobamides which demonstrate varying effects on animal growth. A somewhat similar group of cobamides, which also are produced by microorganisms, promote growth only in microorganisms; these cobamides are known as the pseudo-B_{12} group. The true B_{12} vitamins are essential for normal growth in man and most domestic animals and, in domestic animals, they are known to increase the utilization of vegetable proteins.

The cobamides all contain a cobalt porphyrin nucleus to which is attached ribose and phosphate. However, the various cobamides differ in the purine, benzimidazole, or other base, found in the nucleotidelike portion of the molecule, and in the chemical group attached to the cobalt atom. Vitamin B_{12}, as recovered from liver preparations, is known as cyanocobalamin or 5, 6-dimethyl- α- benzimidazolyl cobamide cyanide. A similar B_{12} is synthesized by microorganisms, and cyanide as a precursor can be added to the fermentation medium, although its toxicity precludes the addition of more than trace amounts.

The status of vitamin B_{12} in the human or animal body is as yet unclear. However, there is evidence that it exists as coenzymes with an adenine moiety attached to the cobalt atom.

The first commercial fermentation production of vitamin B_{12} was as a by-product of various *Streptomyces* antibiotic fermentations, particularly that for streptomycin, and as a by-product of the acetone-butanol fermentation. However, as regards its by-product status in the streptomycin fermentation, the mutation of *Streptomyces griseus* to higher antibiotic yield capacity decreased its vitamin B_{12} yields. The subsequent discovery of relatively high concentrations of this vitamin in sewage is sludge solids also allowed its recovery and commercialization from this source in at least one or two localities in the United States. Actually, most of the vitamin B_{12} in the sludge solids is synthesized by microorganisms during the activated sludge treatment of the sewage. The addition of cobalt salts during sewage processing, however, only slightly increases the vitamin B_{12} yields in comparison to the more marked responses obtained on addition of these salts to pure-culture microbial vitamin B_{12} fermentations.

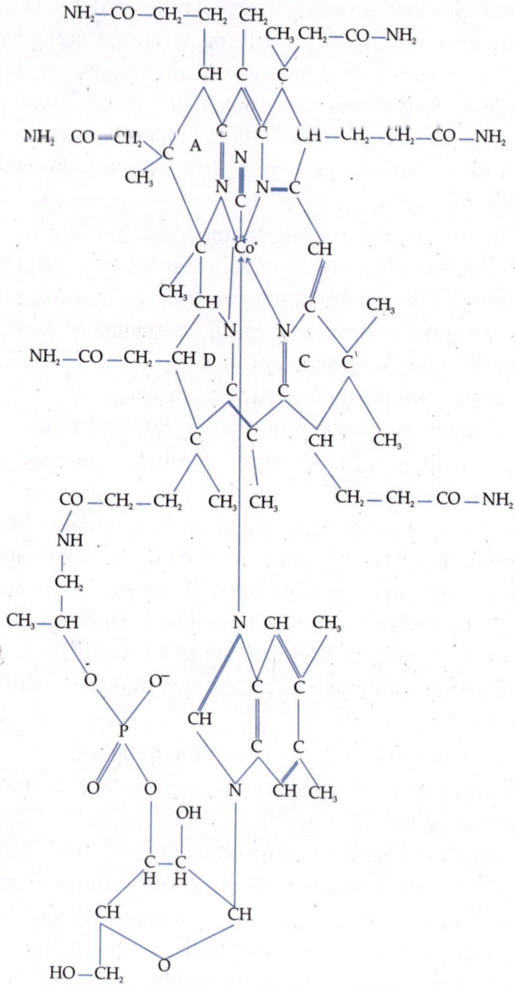

Figure 24.1 Vitamin B_{12}.

Vitamin B_{12} has also been produced commercially by a direct fermentation utilizing *Streptomyces* species such as *Streptomyces olivaceus* (Figure 24.2). This organism is grown with aeration at 27°C in a nutritionally rich crude medium with glucose as a major carbon source. Cobalt chloride ($CoCl_2 \cdot 6H_2O$) at approximately 2 to 10 ppm is added to this medium as a precursor;

the organism scavenges low levels of cobalt from the medium, but higher levels are toxic. The duration of the fermentation is about 3 to 4 days, or until mycelium lysis begins to occur. Thus, most of the vitamin B_{12} remains within the microbial cells until autolysis sets in, and therefore the recovery of the vitamin from the fermentation broth is simplified by harvesting before autolysis has become serious, that is, while the vitamin is still contained within the mycelium. At harvest, the solids and mycelium are filtered or centrifuged, to separate them from the fermentation broth, and then dried for use as B_{12}-enriched animal- or chicken-feed supplements. In alternate recovery procedures, the vitamin is released from the cells by procedures such as acidification, heat, alcohol treatment, and so forth. For example, the completed fermentation broth is acidified, sodium sulfite is added to protect the vitamin, and the culture plus broth is heated. The residual solids and spent mycelium then are separated by centrifugation or filtration, and the fluid portion is evaporated under vacuum. Actually, only relatively small amounts of the vitamin are further purified and crystallized for the treatment of pernicious anemia and for other medical uses.

Vitamin B_{12} has also been commercially produced by a fermentation utilizing *Bacillus megaterium*, and the fermentative recovery approaches for this fermentation are similar to those for the *Streptomyces* organisms. The bulk of the present-day production of this vitamin, however, is by aerated submerged bacterial fermentations that employ strains of *Propionibacterium* or *Pseudomonas* with a beet-molasses medium and cobalt addition. Specific details concerning these fermentations are not generally available.

References

Vitamin B_{12}

Mervyn, L., and E. L. Smith. 1964. The biochemistry of vitamin B_{12} fermentation. Pp. 151–201 in *Progress in industrial microbiology*, vol.5 (ed. by D. J. D. Hockenhull). Gordon and Breach Science Publishers, Inc., New York.

Perlman, D. 1959. Microbial synthesis of cobamides. *Adv. Appl. Microbiol.*, **1**, 87–122.

Prescott, S. C. and C. G. Dunn. 1959. *Industrial microbiology*. 3rd Ed., pp. 482–496. McGraw-Hill Book Co., Inc., New York.

Rickes, E. L., N. G. Brinck, F. R. Koniuszy, T. R. Wood, and K. Folkers. 1948a. Crystalline vitamin B_{12}. *Science*, **107**, 396–397.

Rickes, E. L. N. G. Brinck, F. R. Koniuszy, T. R. Wood, and K. Folkers. 1948b. Vitamin B_{12}, a cobalt complex. *Science*, **108**, 134.

Rickes, E. L., N. G. Brinck, F. R. Koniuszy, T. R. Wood, and K. Folkers. 1948c. Comparative data on vitamin B_{12} from liver and from a new source, *Streptomyces griseus*. *Science*, **108**. 634–635.

Stokstad, E. L. R., A. Page, Jr., J. Pierce, A. L. Franklin, T. H. Jukes, R. W. Heinle, M. Epstein, and A. D. Welch. 1948. Activity of microbial animal protein factor concentrates in pernicious anemia. *J. Lab. Clin. Med.*, **33**, 860–864.

RIBOFLAVIN

Riboflavin (Figure 24.3) is a vitamin essential for the growth and reproduction of both humans and animals and, thus, it often is employed as a feed additive for the nutrition of various domestic animals. It is produced commercially by microbial fermentation, although this source now encounters strong competition from that produced by chemical synthesis.

Various microorganisms can be employed for the fermentation production of riboflavin. Thus, riboflavin is a by-product of the acetonebutanol fermentation, as carried out by microorganisms such as *Clostridium butylicum*, *Clostridium acetobutylicum* and related species. However, it is produced commercially by direct fermentation utilizing the Ascomycetes, *Eremothecium ashbyii* and *Ashbya gossypii*. Various *Candida* species such as *Candida guilliermondia* and *Candida flareri* also produce riboflavin in good yield, but fermentations with these organisms as yet have not been employed commercially.

Ashbya gossypii and *Eremothecium ashbyii* both are plant pathogens causing diseases of cotton and other plants. This attribute makes it mandatory that cultures and fermentation residues be sterilized before discard or commercial usage. The two Ascomycetes are morphologically similar, although some differences do exist. However, from an industrial fermentation standpoint, the principal difference between these two organisms is the greater stability of the riboflavin-producing capacity of *Ashbya gossypii*, since this organism does not degenerate as readily as does *Eremothecium ashbyii* to forms lacking the ability to accumulate riboflavin.

The Ascomycete riboflavin fermentations utilize media containing a semipurified sugar, such as glucose, plus additional crude organic nutrients. In certain instances, however, the glucose may be totally replaced by a lipid such as corn oil, or a low level of corn oil may be added to the glucose to stimulate riboflavin yields. The medium is initially adjusted to pH 6 to 7.5 and the *Ashbya gossypii* fermentation is conducted at a temperature of 26 to

28°C for approximately 4 to 5 days. It is a submerged, aerated fermentation, but high-level aeration must be avoided, because excess air inhibits mycelial production and reduces the riboflavin yields. At harvest, the culture is evaporated and dried to serve as a feed supplement. Riboflavin fermentation by *Eremothecium ashbyii* closely resembles that for *Ashbya gossypii*.

Those riboflavin fermentations utilizing species of *Candida* are extremely sensitive to the presence of traces of iron and, as a result, iron or steel fermentation equipment cannot be used. In fact, it has been proposed that the fermentation equipment be lined with plastic. Cobalt, which at proper concentrations stimulates the Ascomycete fermentations, can also be employed in the *Candida* fermentation to partially counteract the iron toxicity. The *Candida* fermentation does have one advantage, however, in that it is carried out at relatively low pH values which inhibit bacterial growth and negate a requirement for sterilization of the fermentation medium.

Various studies have been directed toward attempting to define the mechanism by which the Ascomycetes are able to accumulate large amounts of riboflavin. While these studies as yet have not yielded definitive answers, they have brought forth several interesting observations on the fermentation and have allowed the advancement by Kapralek (1962) and Starka (1957) of at least a partial explanation. Thus, these workers demonstrated that the fermentation progresses through three phases. In the first phase, rapid growth occurs with little riboflavin production. The glucose is rapidly utilized and oxidized, and a pH decrease occurs because of an accumulation of pyruvic acid. By the end of this phase, the glucose is exhausted and growth ceases. In the second phase, sporulation occurs, and the pyruvate decreases in concentration. Ammonia accumulates, because of an increase in deaminase activity, so that the pH values become alkaline. There is rapid synthesis of cell-bound riboflavin, occurring mainly as flavin adenine dinucleotide (FAD) as well as some flavin mononucleotide (FMN) (See Figure 24.3). Thus, apparently, the cellular regulatory mechanisms for FAD synthesis break down at this point. This phase also is accompanied by a rapid increase in catalase activity and a disappearance of cytochromes. In the last of the three phases, autolysis occurs, releasing free riboflavin into the medium as well as some riboflavin in the nucleotide form. From these observations, it was concluded that at about the time of sporulation there is a shift from the initial cytochrome type of terminal respiration to a terminal respiration utilizing flavoproteins, and that this flavoprotein respiration is accompanied by an overproduction of the flavin prosthetic group.

Other workers have demonstrated that certain purines, but not pyrimidines, stimulate riboflavin production without simultaneously stimulating growth. This observation was clarified when it was shown that

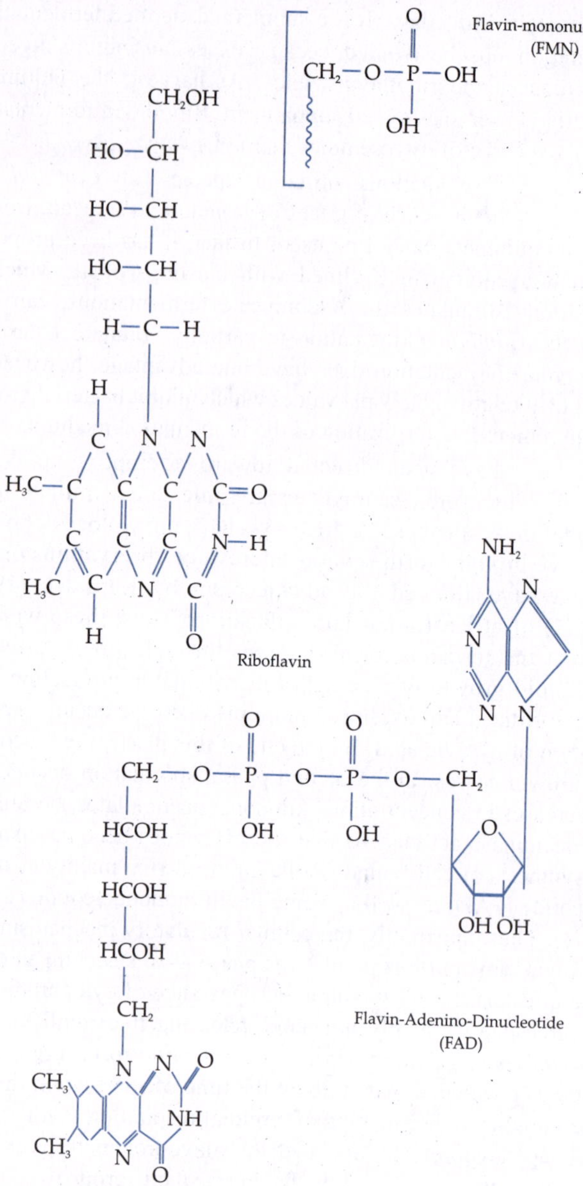

Figure 24.3 Riboflavin in the free state and as a component of the coenzymes FMN and FAD.

purines or purine precursors are used by the microorganism to construct the middle and right-hand rings of the riboflavin molecule (Figure 24.3).

References

Riboflavin

Goodwin, T. W. 1959. Production and biosynthesis of riboflavin in microorganisms. Pp. 137–177 in *Progress in industrial microbiology*, vol. I (ed. by D. J. D. Hockenhull). Interscience Publishers, Inc., New York.

Hickey, R. J. 1954. Production of riboflavin by fermentation. Pp. 157–190 in *Industrial fermentations*, vol. 2 (ed. by L. A. Underkofler and R. J. Hickey). Chemical Publishing Co., Inc., New York.

Kapralek, F. 1962. The physiology of riboflavin production of *Eremothecium ashbyii*. *J. Gen. Microbiol.*, **29**, 403–419.

Pridham, T. G. 1952. Microbial synthesis of riboflavin. *Econ. Botany*, **6**, 185–205.

Starka, J. 1957. Properties of *Eremothecium ashbyii* strain producing riboflavin. *J. Gen. Microbiol.*, **17**, VI.

VITAMIN A

β-Carotene (Figure 24.4), also known as provitamin A, occurs naturally as a component of various agricultural products, and particularly as a component of green plants. When ingested, β-carotene is converted in the animal body to vitamin A (Figure 24.4). Although β-carotene can be produced by microbial fermentation, the yields at the present time, nevertheless, are relatively low for good economic competition with chemically synthesized vitamin A.

β-Carotene is produced by various organisms, but particularly by members of the Choanephoraceae family of the Phycomycetes. Thus, *Phycomyces blakesleeanus*, *Choanephora cucurbitarum*, and *Blakeslea trispora* have received extensive study for their ability to produce β-carotene. The β-carotene fermentations for the latter two microorganisms are unusual in that they utilize the concept of heterothallism and, in this regard, Barnett, Lilly, and Krause (1956) discovered that increased yields of β-carotene result with *Choanphora cucurbitarum* if both the plus and minus marting types of the organism are grown together (Figure 24.5). Other workers then demonstrated a similar phenomenon for mating types of *Blakeslea trispora* (Hesseltine and Anderson, 1957). However, according to the report of Lilly, Barnett, and Krause (1960), this phenomenon does not hold true for all β-carotene producers, since mixed growth of the plus and minus mating types of *Phycomyces blakesleeanus* produce no more β-cartone than does the minus mating type alone.

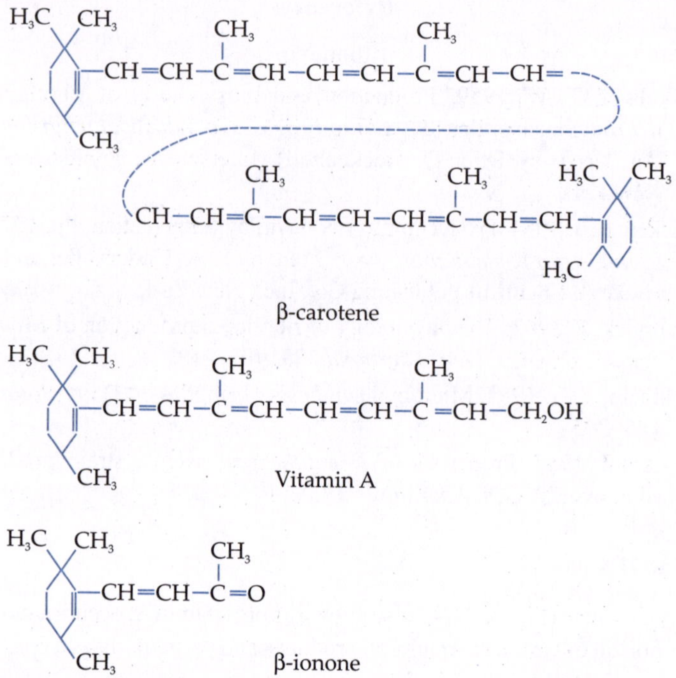

Figure 24.4 Chemical structures of β-carotene, vitamin A and β-ionone.

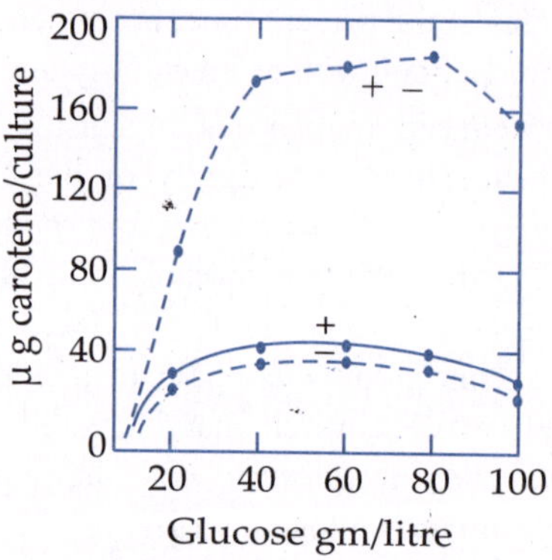

Figure 24.5 Maximum yields of carotene by +, −, And mixed + and − cultures of *Choanephora cucurbitarum* when the glucose concentration in the glutamic acid medjum varied between 20 and 100 g/Liter. (Chu and Lilly. 1960. *Mycologia*, **52**, 80-96).

The fermentation medium among various ingredients includes β-ionone, nonionic detergent, and vegetable oils, fats, fatty acids, waxes, or white grease. The β-ionone (Figure 24.4), although it would appear to be a possible precursor of β-carotene, apparently is not directly incorporated into the β-carotene, molecule. Instead, it is regarded as a "steering" factor associated with bringing about the presence and activity of the enzymes responsible for β-carotene formation. Inoculum of each mating type is grown separately, and approximately 5 percent of each is added to the fermentation medium, although it is not necessary that both mating types be added simultaneously. The β-ionone is aspetically added to the fermentation approximately 48 hours after inoculation.

References

Vitamin A

Barnett, H. V., V. G. Lilly, and R. F. Krause. 1956. Increased production of carotene by mixed + and – cultures of *Choanephora cucurbitarum*,. *Science*, **123**, 141.

Chu, F. S., and V. G. Lilly. 1960. Factors affecting the production of carotene by *Choanephora cucurbitarum. Mycologia*, **52**, 80–96.

Hesseltine, C. W., and R. F. Anderson. 1957. Microbiological production of carotenoids. 1. Zygospores and carotene produced by intra-specific and inter-specific crosses of Choanephoraceae in liquid medium. *Mycologia*, **49**, 449–452.

Lilly, V. G., H. L. Barnett, and R. F. Krause. 1960. The production of carotene by *Phycomyces blakesleeanus*. West Virginia University Agricultural Exp. Station Bull. 441T.

Margalith, P. 1964. Secondary factors in fermentation processes. *Adv. Appl. Microbiol.*, **6**, 81–84.

GIBBERELLINS

The gibberellins are plant hormones that elicit amazing results when applied to plants. Thus, these compounds promote growth by both cell enlargement and cell division, so that the observable effects resulting from application of even small amounts of gibberellins include lengthening of stems and internodes, acceleration of seed germination, breaking of dormancy, and hastening of flower formation and seed setting (Figure 24.6 and 24.7).

The gibberellins comprise a group of closely related compounds; three gibberellins and gibberellic acid (gibberellin X) promote plant growth, although the latter (Figure 24.8) is the most active form. So far as is known, the gibberellins are produced by only one microorganism, the fungus *Gibberella fujikuroi*, which is a pathogenic fungus for rice seedlings and is the conidial or perfect stage of *Fusarium moniliforme*. In recent years, however, it has been realized that green plants naturally contain small amounts of gibberellinlike compounds, but the natural source of these compounds is not known.

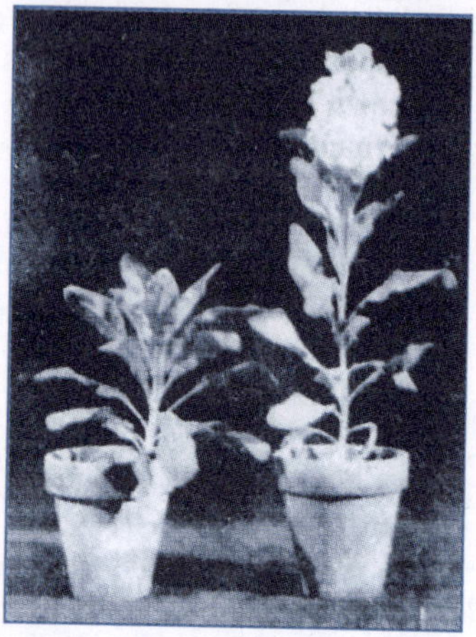

Figure 24.6 Early blooming of hyacinth brought on by gibberellic acid. Photo courtesy of the Michigan State University.

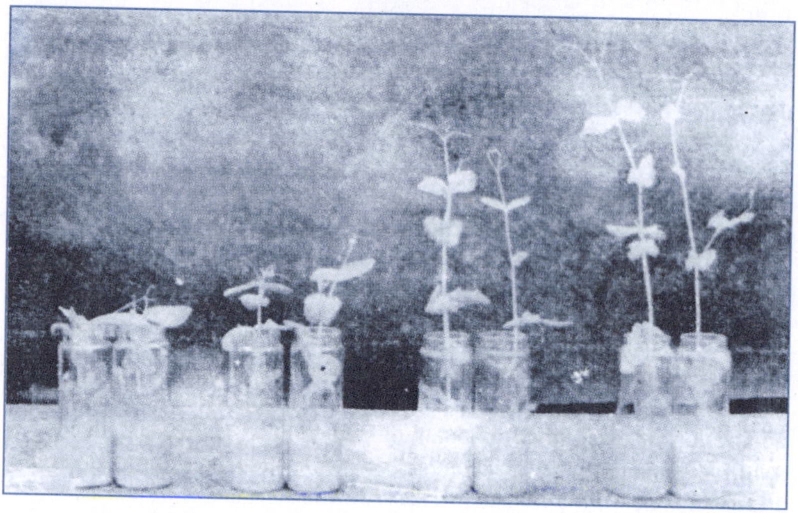

Figure 24.7 Effect of increasing concentrations of gibberellic acid (left to right) on the growth of peas. Photo courtesy of Abbott Laboratories.

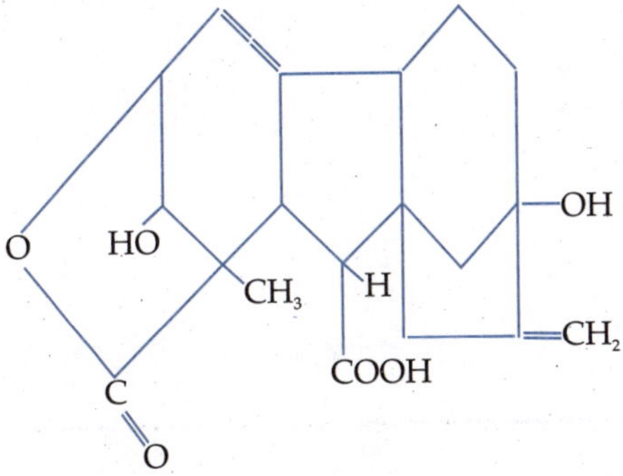

Figure 24.8 Presumed structure of gibberellic acid

Gibberellin production by *Gibberella fujikuroi* is conducted in aerated submerged fermentation culture at 25°C for a period of 2 to 3 days. A simple glucose-salts medium of slightly acidic pH is employed, and the most of the gibberellin production occurs after maximum growth of the fungus.

The gibberellins, and particularly gibberellic acid, would appear to be a great boon to agriculture. However, to date, the cost of the gibberellins has been great enough to preclude their extensive use for plant growth promotion, except for certain high-value plants such as flowers and other ornamentals.

References

Gibberellins

Brian, P. W. 1961. Gibberellins : a new group of plant hormones. *Sci. Progr.*, **49**, 1–16.

Brian, P. W., and J. F. Grove. 1957. Gibberellic acid. *Endeavour*, **16**, 161–171.

Darken, M. A., A. L. Jensen, and P. Shu. 1959. Production of gibberellic acid by fermentation. *Appl. Microbiol*, **7**, 301–303.

Stodola, F. H. 1958. Source book on gibberellin, 1828–1957. Agricultural Research Service 71-11. U.S. Dept. of Agriculture.

Stodola, F. H., K. B. Raper, D. I, Fennell, H. F. Conway, V. E. Sohns, G. T. Longford, and R. W. Jackson. 1955. The microbiological production of gibberellins A and X. *Arch. Biochem. Biophys.*, **54**, 240–245.

Wittwer, S. H., And M. J. Bukovac. 1958. The effects of gibberellin on economic plants. *Econ.*, **12**., 213–255.

Chapter 25

Enzymes as Fermentation Products

Microbial cells contain or produce a variety of enzymes and, as we have seen, these enzymes are the biological catalysts for the biochemical reactions leading to microbial growth and respiration, as well as to the formation of fermentation products. In certain instances, however, some of these enzymes may in themselves become fermentation products, so that one then is specifically interested in obtaining high yields per se of particular enzymes, instead of a high-level activity of the enzymes as they mediate fermentation processes of the cells.

Enzymes are either adaptive or constitutive. A constitutive enzyme is always produced in amounts usable by the cell regardless of whether the particular substrate of the enzyme is present in the growth medium. In contrast, microbial cells produce adaptive enzymes in usable amounts only in response to the presence of the particular enzyme substrate in the fermentation medium ; the microorganism produces an adaptive enzyme only if required to do so to bring about degradation or change in a particular nutrient substrate otherwise not available to the cell. Microorganisms, however, vary greatly from one to another in their ability to produce adaptive enzymes. Thus, various *Pseudomonas* species are known for their outstanding ability to produce adaptive enzymes in response to many different types of chemical compounds.

Enzymes also may be either exocellular or endocellular. An endocellular enzyme is produced within the cell or at the cytoplasmic membrane, and normally does not find its way into the fermentation medium surrounding the cell. Exocellular enzymes, which include most of the enzymes produced by microbial fermentation for commercial usage, are also produced by the microbial cell, but in addition are liberated to the fermentation medium so that the enzyme can hydrolytically attack and degrade polymeric substances

Table 25.1 Industrially produced enzymes and their applications

Name of Enzymes	Source	Applications	Notes	Commercial Importance
		Starch Liquifying Amylases		
Diastase	*Malt*	Digestive aid. Supplement to bread. Syrup	α-amylase activity, β-amylase activity	+++
Takadiastase	*A. oryzae*	Same as for diastase	Contains many other enzymes, protease, RNase	+++
Amylase	*B. subtilis*	Desizing textiles. Syrup. Alcohol fermentation industry. Glucose production	Crude preparation contains protease	+++
Acid-resistant amylase	*A. niger*	Digestive aid	Optimum pH 4-5	+
		Starch Saccharifying Amylases		
Amyloglucosidase	*Rhizopus niveus* *A. niger* *Endomycopsis fibuliger*	Glucose production		+++
Invertase	*S. cerevisiae*	Confectionaries, to prevent crystallization of sugar. Chocolate. High-test molasses		
Pectinase	*Sclerotina libertina* *Coniothyrium diplodiella* *A. oryzae* *A. niger* *A. flavus*	Increase yield and for clarifying juice. Removal of pectin. Coffee concentration	Scrase(Sankyo). Pectinol (Rohm and Hass Company) Takamin e Pectinase Clarase (Takamine Lab.). Filtragol (I. G. Farbenind)	+++
		Animal and Vegetable Proteases		
Trypsin	Animal pancreas	Medical uses. Meat tenderizers. Beer haze removal		+++
Pepsin	Animal pancreas	Digestive aid. Meat tenderizer		+++

Table 25.1 Industrially produced enzymes and their applications (continued)

Name of Enzymes	Source	Application	Notes	Commercial Importance
α-Chymotrypsin	Animal stomach	Medical uses		
Rennet	Calf stomach	Cheese manufacture		+++
Pancreas protease	Animal pancreas	Digestive aid. Cleaning. Leather-bating. Dehairing. Feed improvement		++
Papain	Papaya	Digestive aid. Medical uses. Beer haze removal. Meat tenderizer		+++
Bromelin. Ficin	Pineapple, fig	Same as for papain		++
		Microbial Proteases		
Protease	*A. oryzae*	Flavoring of sake. Haze removal in sake		+
Protease	*A. niger*	Feed, digestive aid	Acid resistant protease. Optimum pH 2-3	++
Protease	*B. subtilis*	Removal of galatin from film (recovery of silver). Fish solubles. Meat tenderizer	Optimum pH 7	+++
Protease	*Streptomyces griseus*	Same as above	Optimum pH 8	++
Varidase	*Streptococcus sp.*	Medical use	Lederle Lab.	++
Streptokinase	*Streptococcus sp.*		Profibrinolysin	++
		Other Commercial Enzymes		
Penicillinase	*B. subtilis*	Removal of penicillin	Takamine Lab.	+
	B. cereus		Schenley Lab.	
Glucose oxidase	*A. niger, Dee O, Dee G*	For removal of oxygen or glucose from various foods. Dried egg manufacture.	Takamine Lab.	++
	P. chrysogenum	For glucose determination	Negase Co.	

Table 25.1 Industrially produced enzymesC and their applications (continued)

Name of Enzymes	Source	Applications	Notes	Commercial Importance
Hyaluronidase	Animal, bacteria	Medical use		+
Lipase	Pancreas, Mold (Rhizopus)	Digestive aid, Flavouring of milk products		+
Cytochrome C	Yeast (Candida)	Medical use	Sankyo Co.	+
Catalase		Sterilization of milk		
Karatinase	Streptomyces fradiae	Removal of hair from hides	Merck Co.	+
		Nucleotic and Other New Enzymes		
5′-Phosphodiesterase	P. citrinum S. griseus, B. subtilis	Inosinic acid and guanylic acid mnufacture. (5′-nucleotides)	Yamasa Co. Takeda Co.	+++
Adenylic acid deaminase	A. oryzae	AMP $\rightarrow$ IMP	In Takadiastase	+
Microbial rennet	Mucor sp.	Cheese manufacture	Meito Sangyo Co.	+
Naringinase. Hesperidinase	A. niger	Removal of better taste from citrus juice	Rohm and Haas	+
Glucose isomerase	L. brevis	Glucose $\rightarrow$ Fructose	Optimum pH 6-7	
Laccase	Coriolus versicolor	Drying of lacquer		
Cellulase	Tricoderma koningi	Digestive aid	Optimum ph. 4–6	

Source. Arima. 1964. *Global impacts of applied microbiology*. Pp. 277-294.

too large or insoluble to pass through the microbial cell wall, or in some other manner inaccessible to the cell. Examples of exocellular enzymes are amylases attacking starch, and proteases, attacking protein.

Enzymes are proteins and, hence, they possess the physical and chemical characteristics of proteins. Thus, some enzymes are inherently unstable, their protein being easily denatured so that enzymatic activity is lost. Each enzyme has its own pH and temperature optimum for activity, although there may be more than one enzyme capable of attacking a specific substrate, but varying in these conditions of pH and temperature optima. Enzymes demonstrate specificity for the particular substrates that they attack, and this property is of competitive economic advantage for the commercial usage of enzymes since, because of this specificity, the side reactions often accompanying chemical reactions usually are not associated with enzymes. Enzymes act at relatively low temperatures, that is, temperatures below those which denature the enzyme protein, and not under the high-temperature, catalyst-associated conditions often required for chemical reactions. Since enzymes are easily denatured, an enzyme reaction can be stopped at an opportune moment simply by denaturing the enzyme, as for instance by the application of acid, heat, and so forth. The protein nature of enzymes also provides an additional bonus as regards their relative ease of recovery from fermentation culture broths. Thus, common protein precipitants, such as various alcohols or ammonium sulfate, can be used to accomplish precipitation. Microbial enzymes sometimes are marketed as stabilized culture filtrates, but more often they are prepared as protein precipitate, and diluted to an acceptable potency level with an inert material such as starch, salt, or flour. Except for specific applications, these enzyme preparations usually are not further purified.

Although the activities of microbial enzymes have been observed and even utilized for many centuries, it has been only in relatively recent times that the use of microbial enzymes has been commercialized. Thus, although ancient oriental civilizations are known to have employed crude fungal preparations to bring about starch hydrolysis for brewing, the first commercial usage of fungal enzymes occurred just before the 20th century, and that of bacterial enzymes at the time of **World War I.** Since this time, microbial enzyme fermentations have encountered little if any competition from the synthetic chemical industries, but microbial enzyme preparations have had to compete with crude enzyme preparations as obtained from plant and animal sources. Thus, the latter enzymes, such as those from the pancreas, stomach mucosa, malt, and papaya fruit, are mainly amylases or proteases finding use in the textile, leather, brewing, and other industries. Nevertheless, the enzymes from the plant and animal sources are somewhat difficult to recover from the source materials and, as a result, the cost involved has been great enough to allow commercial competition by microbial enzymes.

Commercial microbial enzyme production utilizes mainly various fungi, bacteria, and yeasts and, in fact, bacteria and fungi often produce similar enzymes, although the particular enzymes from these sources may vary somewhat in pH and temperature optima as well as in other characteristics. Also, within any one broad group of organisms, such as the bacteria or fungi, there is great variation between various genera as to their ability to produce a specific enzyme. This variability also extends to the species within a genus and even to strains within a species. In addition, the production of a particular enzyme varies with the particular medium employed and with various physical and chemical factors of the fermentation. Genetic stability of the microbial strains also plays an important role and, as a result, cultures must be preserved in such a manner as to maintain their enzyme-producing ability. Thus, microbial strains are carefully selected so that they possess high enzyme yield capacity and genetic stability under the particular conditions employed in the fermentation.

Microbial enzymes produced by fermentation include amylesss proteases, pectinases, invertase, catalase, penicillinase, glucose-oxidase, streptokinase-streptodornase, and others (Table 25.1). Moreover, cellulases, pentosanases, and hemicellulases possibly also may find future applications as industrial microbial enzymes. Additional enzymes are produced by microorganisms, some in relatively large amounts, and these too may find eventual commercial usage, if a demand should arise for the particular activities of these enzymes.

AMYLASES

Various bacteria and fungi produce α-amylases, although the enzymes from these two sources are not identical. These amylases are employed commercially for the preparation of sizing agents and removal of starch sizing from woven cloth, preparation of starch sizing pastes for use in paper coatings, liquefaction of heavy starch pastes which form during heating steps in the manufacture of corn and chocolate syrups production of bread, and removal of food spots in the dry-cleaning industry where the amylase functions in conjunction with protease enzymes. In addition, these amylases also can be employed as a replacement for malt for starch hydrolysis in the brewing industry.

Fungal Amylase

Fungal amylase, as employed in the "Amylo"process to hydrolyze starch for yeast-alcohol production, is not separated from the fungal mycelium.

Thus, to prepare the mash for the yeast, the grain is first soaked in water and then heated to solubilize its starch. The resulting mash is acidified, inoculated with a *Mucor* or *Rhizopus* fungal species, and incubated approximately one day before further inoculation with the yeast. However, in a modification of this process, the yeast is added simultaneously with the fungus to bring on quicker alcohol formation.

Fungal amylase production (in which the enzyme is separated from the mycelium and the mycelium is discarded) utilizes strains of *Aspergillus oryzae* for stationary culture with wheat bran, and strains of *Aspergillus niger* for submerged aerated-agitated culture. As regards these alternative processes, the wheat-bran stationary culture has been employed extensively for the production of fungal amylase. For this process, the wheat bran, spread in relatively thin layers in trays (or even in rotary drum fermentors), is moistened with water or dilute acid, sterilized, and inoculated with spores of a fungus such as *Aspergillus oryzae*. After growth, the fungus plus bran can be dried at 50°C or less and then ground to serve as an amylase preparation. However, more often the amylase is extracted by water from the wheat-bran culture, precipitated from the aqueous solution by the addition of alcohol, and dried at 55°C or less. The submerged fermentations for amylase production have recently become economically feasible and, although strains of both *Aspergillus niger* and *Aspergillus oryzae* have been studied extensively for their possible use in submerged fermentation, *Aspergillus niger* growing in a starch-salt medium has now been commercialized.

Fungal amylase concentrates prepared as above must compete successfully on an economic basis with the acid hydrolysis of starch, and with amylase preparations from other sources such as pancreatin, malt, and bacteria. In this respect, it has been reported that, in at least one instance, fungal amylase provided a slightly better alcohol yield for a yeast fermentation and better economics than did a similar process in which malt was employed for saccharification.

Bacterial Amylases

Various bacteria elaborate amylases, but only those from *Bacillus subtilis* and *Bacillus diastaticus* have been produced on a commercial basis. Bacterial amylase is employed commercially under those conditions in which fungal amylase, or amylases from other sources, hydrolyze starch less well. For instance, bacterial amylase has an optimum temperature for activity at approximately 55°C, and the enzyme is relatively heat resistant. As a result, the bacterial enzyme finds particular application in situations in which starch hydrolysis must be conducted at higher temperatures.

Strains of *Bacillus subtilis* are specially selected for amylase with high starch liquefying and dextrinizing activity and, consequently, this amylase produces relatively less fermentable sugars when acting on starch. High yields of bacterial amylase are obtained when *Bacillus subtilis* is grown in stationary culture. The amylase is constitutive and, surprisingly, a medium is employed which contains a high level of crude protein ; a high carbohydrate level in the medium stimulates protease production and depresses amylase production. Nevertheless, some of the insoluble protein of the medium may first be partially hydrolyzed by boiling in dilute acid or by enzymatic treatment. The pH of the medium is near neutrality, and the fermentation proceeds for approximately 6 days (ranging from 3 to 7 days) at an incubation temperature of 25 to 30°C. *Bacillus subtilis* in this stationary liquid culture produces a heavy surface-pellicle growth, which apparently is associated with high amylase yield, and fresh sterile air is circulated over the pellicle to improve aeration. At harvest, the culture is filtered or centrifuged, the recovered aqueous portion is concentrated by evaporation to yield an amylase concentrate, and salt and an antiseptic are added. As an alternate recovery procedure, the amylase can be precipitated from aqueous solution by the addition of cold acetone, ethanol, isopropanol, or ammonium sulfate. In addition to their amylase content, these preparations also demonstrate some protease activity which is produced by *Bacillus subtilis* concurrently with the amylase.

Bacillus subtilis amylase can also be produced in highly aerated submerged culture by employing a special highly starchy medium. However, the ability to produce amylase is a somewhat unstable characteristic of this organism, and culture degeneration, which is difficult to detect, may occur during the fermentation. This culture degeneration, however, is not as serious a problem with the stationary, pellicle-forming *Bacillus subtilis* fermentation.

PROTEOLYTIC ENZYMES

Proteolytic enzymes are produced by various bacteria, such as species of *Bacillus*, *Pseudomonas*, *Clostridium*, *Proteus*, and *Serratia*, and by fungi such as *Aspergillus niger*, *Aspergillus oryzae*, *Aspergillus flavus*, and *Penicillium roquefortii*. However, the enzymes associated with these microorganisms are actually mixtures of proteinases and peptidases, with the proteinases usually being excreted to the fermentation medium during growth, while the peptidases often are liberated only on autolysis of the cells. At present, the proteinases are of more commercial interest than are the peptidases.

Among the commercial applications of proteolytic enzymes is the bating of hides in the leather industry. Here, the enzymes bring about changes in the hides to provide a finer grain and texture, greater pliability, and better general quality. Proteolytic enzymes also are employed in the textile industry to remove proteinaceous sizing, and in the silk industry to liberate the silk fibres from the naturally occurring proteinaceous material in which they are imbedded. In addition, these enzymes are employed in the tenderizing of meat, and they also are the active ingredient in spot-remover preparations for removing food spots in the dry-cleaning industry. The fungal proteases present a wider pH activity range than do animal or bacterial proteases, and to a certain extent this results in a wider range of uses for the fungal proteases.

Fungal Protease

Various fungi produce protease enzyme in good yield, and the commercial production of fungal protease has utilized *Aspergillus flavus*, *Aspergillus wentii*, *Aspergillus oryzae*, *Mucor delemar*, and *Amylomyces rouxii*. The fungus is usually grown on wheat bran, although other media are sometimes employed, under fermentation conditions similar to those for amylase production. At sporulation, the various fungal proteolytic enzymes are present in the medium, and the proteases are recovered by procedures similar to those for mold amylases. Submerged fermentation procedures for fungal protease production have been studied, and the indications are that such fermentations may become commercially feasible.

Bacterial Protease

Bacterial protease production again utilizes strains of *Bacillus subtilis*, and the fermentation conditions are similar to those for amylase production by this organism. However, the *Bacillus subtilis* strains are specially selected for high protease activity and not for amylase activity. As stated previously, a high carbohydrate content medium is utilized to stimulate protease activity and depress amylase production, although the final product does contain some amylase activity. The fermentation is incubated 3 to 5 days at 37°C in pans containing a shallow layer of fermentation medium, and the harvest procedure is similar to that for bacterial amylase, except that concentration of the broth is carried out at reduced pressure and at temperatures of less than 40°C in order to protect the enzyme from denaturation.

PECTINASES

Pectinase enzymes are utilized to eliminate pectin and pectinlike protective colloids in fruit juices (thus facilitating clarification of the juice) and as a means of preventing gelling of the juices during the concentration steps of processing. Pectinases are produced by various bacteria and fungi, although commercial microbial pectinase production probably utilizes species of *Penicillium* or *Aspergillus*. Pectinase production by these fungi is stimulated by the presence in the fermentation medium of pectin or pectin-containing compounds. Since the pectinase, in part, is retained in the cells and, in part, in excret to the medium, the enzyme is recovered from both sources. Thus, at harvest, the mycelium is dried and ground, and its pectinase is excreted with water. It is then precipitated from this aqueous solution and from the culture broth by procedures similar to those employed for amylases. The commercial enzyme preparation contains at least two types of pectinase, differing from each other by the extent to which they degrade pectin, as well as a few other nonpectolytic enzymes, and the ratios of these enzymes in the commercial product depend on the particular fungal strain employed.

INVERTASE

Invertase, also known as sucrose or saccharase, is an enzyme that hydrolyzes sucrose to yield glucose and fructose, although the enzyme also acts on some tri- and tetra-saccharides. It is widely distributed in nature, occurring in animal and plant tissues, and it is prevalent among various bacteria, yeasts, and fungi. Certain yeasts contain considerable quantities of this enzyme, but the enzyme as produced by yeast differs from that which occurs in fungi. Thus, yeasts produce a fructosidase-type invertase, while the fungal enzyme is a glucosidase. Nevertheless, both types of enzymes provide similar hydrolysis products from sucrose, the difference in the enzymes being in the products occurring on hydrolysis of the tri-and tetra-saccharides.

Invertase is employed commercially to prepare invert sugar from sucrose. The inversion of the sucrose increases its sugar solubility so that sugar crystallization is diminished and, thus, the use of this enzyme prevents sugar crystallization during the preparation of food products, such as certain candies and ice creams. The invert sugar formed by the enzyme is somewhat hygroscopic, a property that also helps to maintain the moisture content of the product. Invertase, in addition, is employed to enzymatically yield invert sugars for use as plasticizing agents in the paper industry.

Invertase is produced commercially from bakers' or brewers yeast, or a direct fermentation is employed utilizing special strains of *Saccharomyces cerevisiae*. In the latter fermentation, enzyme yield responds to the presence of sucrose in the fermentation medium. Invertase is an endoenzyme, liberated to the fermentation medium only on autolysis of the cells. Therefore, the enzyme is recovered from the yeast either by mechanical disruption of the cell wall, or by autolysis induced by chloroform, ethyl acetate, or toluene. The enzyme then is precipitated from aqueous solution by alcohol addition.

OTHER ENZYMES

Catalase, an enzyme decomposing hydrogen peroxide to water and oxygen, is produced by a fungal aerated-submerged fermentation. This enzyme finds use in peroxide bleaching and in the peroxide sterilization of milk for cheese making. Penicillinase, which is employed to inactivate penicillin, is produced by an aerated-submerged fermentation of *Bacillus cereus* or *Bacillus subtilis*, and the enzyme is precipitated and marketed as a dry enzyme concentrate. Glucose-oxidase is produced in association with catalase by *Aspergillus niger* in submerged-aerated fermentation. This enzyme is commercially employed to remove glucose from egg white and whole eggs before drying; the enzymatic hydrolysis of the glucose prevents browning and deterioration of the dried egg. A mixture of streptokinase and streptodornase, as produced by a hemolytic *Streptococcus* grown in aerated-submerged culture, is employed to clean debris from wounds and burns. Finally, a recent process (Sardinis, 1967) employs *Endothia parasitica* for the commercial production of a rennetlike enzyme used in the curdling of milk for cheese manufacture.

Cellulases, as well as the related pentosanases and hemicellulases, occur in various microorganisms, although probably no microbial process for their production has as yet been commercialized. The formation of cellulase appears to be largely adaptive in fungi, but constitutive in those bacteria having the ability to produce the enzyme. The development of a microbial process, such as with the fungus *Myrothecium verrucaria*, to produce cellulose or related enzymes should find commercial acceptance, with the enzymes being employed for the conversion of wood, wood by-products, and various cellulosic agricultural by-products to fermentable substrates. Enzymes of this type also could be utilized to increase the digestability of brewers' grains and other cellulosic industrial and agricultural by-products for use in chicken and certain animal feeds.

References

Arima, K. 1964. Microbial enzyme production. Pp. 277–294 in *Global impacts of applied microbiology* (ed. by M. P. Starr). John Wiley and Sons, Inc., New York.

Hoogerheide, J. C. 1954 Microbial enzymes other than fungal amylases. Pp. 122-154 in *Industrial fermentations*, vol. 2(ed. by L. A. Underkofler and R. J. Hickey). Chemical Publishing Co., Inc., New York.

Prescott, S. C. and C. G. Dunn. 1959. Saccharifying agents : methods of production and uses. Pp. 836–885 in *Industrial microbiology*, 3rd Ed. McGraw-Hill Book Co., Inc., New York.

Sardinis, J. L. 1967. U.S. 3,275,453.

Sizler, I. W. 1964. Enzymes and their applications. *Adv. Appl. Microbiol.*, **6**, 207–226.

Underkofler, L. A. 1954. Fungal amylolytic enzymes. Pp. 97–121 in *Industrial fermentations*, vol. 2 (ed. by L. A. Underkofler and R. J. Hickey). Chemical Publishing Co., Inc., New York.

Underkofler, L. A., R. R. Barton, and S. S. Rennert. 1958. Production of microbial enzymes and their applications. *Appl. Microbiol.*, **6**, 212-221.

Windish, W. W., and N. S. Mhatre. 1965. Microbial amylases. *Adv. Appl. Microbiol.*, **7**, 273–304.

CHAPTER 26

Organic Acids

Various microorganisms possess the ability to convert carbohydrate to high yields of organic acids. This property is demonstrated by various bacteria, as for example, species of *Clostridium* produce acetic and butyric acids. *Lactobacillus* and *Streptococcus* species produce lactic acid, *Acetobacter* species produce acetic, gluconic, and ketogluconic acids, and *Pseudomonas* species produce 2-ketogluconic and α- ketoglutaric acids. Fungal acids produced commercially, or at least studied extensively, include citric, fumaric, gluconic, itaconic, kojic, and gibberellic acids. Those fermentations yielding gluconic and gibberellic acids are described in Chapters 21 and 24, respectively.

Citric, fumaric, and itaconic acids either are intermediate components of the tricarboxylic acid cycle, or they are compounds closely related to members of this cycle. However, the high-percentage conversions of carbohydrate observed in the formation of these acids by fungal fermentation require that the acid accumulation proceed via routes other than or in addition to the tricarboxylic acid cycle, since the tricarboxylic acid cycle per se cannot function properly if high levels of some intermediate are continuously withdrawn from the cycle. Thus, special mechanisms must be postulated to explain the accumulation of these acids and, in most instances, the actual mechanism by which the accumulation occurs still is only poorly understood. Nevertheless, in several instances it is known that the organic acid accumulation is associated with an apparent nutritional deficiency which is imposed by the fermentation conditions, and that this nutritional deficiency is the factor that limits the amount of substrate carbon utilized for growth so that the substrate carbon is shunted to organic acid formation rather than to growth. As we shall see, this nutritional deficiency often appears to be associated with the levels of particular trace metals in the medium in such a manner that more than minimal amounts of these metals hinder organic acid accumulation, although the presence of at least trace amounts nevertheless, may be required for growth and organic acid accumulation.

Among the industrially important organic acid-forming fungi, any one genus or species may have the ability to accumulate organic acids in addition to the acid of interest, and there also may be great variability among strains of a particular species as to whether they can or cannot accumulate a particular organic acid. As a result of these considerations, careful strain selection and adjustment of the media and fermentation conditions usually are necessary to obtain a fungal strain and develop a fermentation that will yield high concentrations of a particular organic acid. Another point to be considered, however, is that a fungal strain chosen for its ability to accumulate an organic acid in its growth medium may or may not be tolerant to the resulting high acidity of the medium. Thus, the accumulation of certain organic acids may require that the acid be continuously neutralized as it is produced in the fermentation medium, while, as will be noted shortly, for certain other organic acids the high acidity of the fermentation medium may be beneficial or even required to bring on acid accumulation.

CITRIC ACID

Citric acid (Figure 26.1) occurs naturally as a component of many fruits and, in fact, commercial citric acid for many years has been recovered from fruit-processing by-products. This acid also is produced by a fungal fermentation, and in the United States most of the commercial citric acid now is obtained in this manner. To date, there is no chemical synthesis competitive with the fungal fermentation although, for some purposes, other organic acids may be used in place of citric acid.

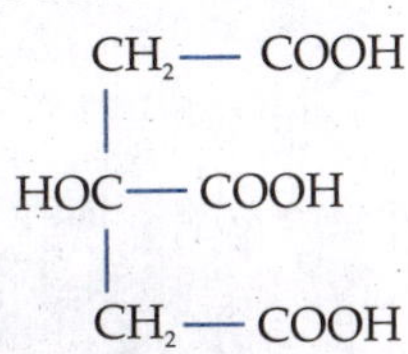

Figure 26.1 Citric acid.

Commercial citric acid finds many uses. It is employed as an acidulant in the food and pharmaceutical industries, and it finds extensive use in the production of carbonated beverages. In addition, it is employed commercially as a chelating and sequestering agent, and citrate and citrate esters are used as plasticizers.

Citric acid accumulates during the controlled fermentative growth of particular species of *Penicillium* and *Aspergillus*. Thus, various *Penicillium*-like fungi first were studied for citric acid accumulation, but the discovery during **World War I** that *Aspergillus niger* (Figures 26.2 and 26.3) could be induced to accumulate large amounts of citric acid while growing on a carbohydrate medium has made this organism the principal fungus for commercial citric acid production. *Aspergillus niger*, however, seems to be more a group of closely related fungi than a well-defined species, with great variation being observed from one strain to another in regard to morphology and physiology. Strains of *Aspergillus niger*, therefore, are carefully selected for the positive characteristics of citric acid yield, amount of sporulation, strain stability, and so forth, and for the negative characteristics of lack of ability to degrade the citric acid product, and of lack of concurrent formation of other acids such as oxalic, gluconic, malic, and 5-ketogluconic. Once a strain has been selected, it is carefully watched during stock-culture maintenance for culture degeneration. Various procedures of stock culture maintenance have been employed but, overall, the cultures are best stored in the form of dry spores.

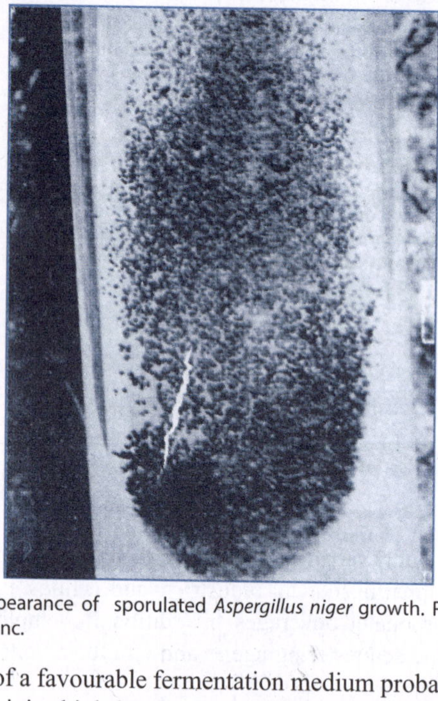

Figure 26.2 Gross appearance of sporulated *Aspergillus niger* growth. Photo courtesy of Charles Pfizer and Co., Inc.

The selection of a favourable fermentation medium probably is the most critical factor in obtaining high-level accumulations of citric acid by *Aspergillus niger*. Thus, a nutrient deficiency in the form of trace metals or phosphate is required, although the particular required deficiencies vary with the particular *Aspergillus niger* strains employed. The medium should be slightly deficient in phosphate, or in one or more of the metals manganese, iron, zinc, and probably coppper. Of these, manganese appears to be particularly important. The effects of these metals, however, are interrelated so that the proper level of one metal may depend on the concentrations of other metals present in the medium. Also, it has been found that methanol, added to the medium at a slightly toxic level, is not metabolized but increases the tolerance of the fungus to zinc, iron, and manganese. A beet-molasses medium containing in the range of 10 to 20 percent sugar often is employed in this fermentation, and ammonium nitrate, magnesium sulfate and KH_2PO_4 are usually added to the medium. Hydrochloric acid then is used to adjust the medium to a low pH value. The beet molasses, however, contains too great a quantity of trace metals, and this excess is reduced during a pretreatment of the molasses by complexing the metals with ferrocyanide or ferricyanide, although it is also possible to utilize a cation-exchange resin to adjust the metal concentration of beet molasses. Thus, as regards the latter procedure, invert molasses pretreated with a cation-exchange resin has been used in submerged-aerated citric acid fermentations with *Aspergillus niger*.

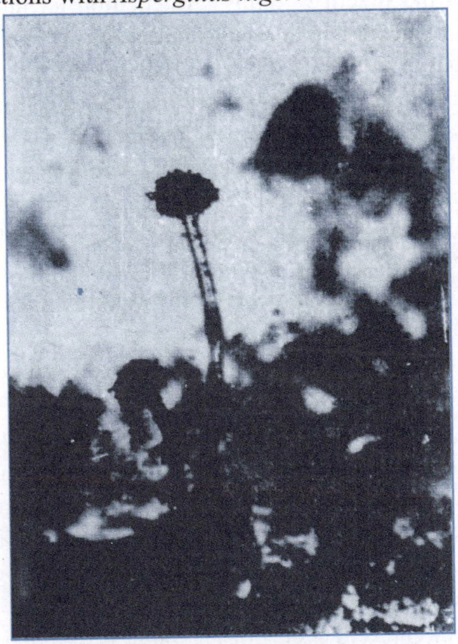

Figure 26.3 *Aspergillus niger* conidiophres as photographed at 130 fold magnification.

The effect of trace metals on the citric acid *Aspergillus niger* fermentation also applies to the growing of spores to be used as inoculum for the fermentation. Thus, trace amounts of manganese salts in the agar medium, unless balanced against proper concentrations of zinc or iron salts, can reduce citric acid yields in the succeeding fermentation in which these spores are used.

Citric acid fermentations presently are conducted on an industrial scale both by the submerged-aerated technique and by a procedure utilizing stationary pans or trays containing a shallow layer of medium. The latter is the older of the two methods, but it is still practiced, because the submerged-aerated fermentation has not as yet equalled the high-level conversions of sugar to citric acid provided by the stationary fermentation. Both fermentations utilize somewhat similar pretreated molasses media, and the fermentations are conducted at approximately 28 to 30°C, with proper aeration being of importance.

Very little actually is known generally about the commercial stationary-tray fermentation, because the principal industrial concern producing citric acid by this procedure has maintained secrecy concerning its process and has not obtained patents that might reveal process details. However, it is known that, in the practice of this fermentation technique for citric acid, the medium is inoculated by blowing spores across the surface of a shallow layer of medium (1 to 2.5 cm in depth, but sometimes up to 8 cm) so that they float, and that air is blown gently over the resulting mycelial mat, or the air is changed at intervals to provide additional aeration. As might be expected with this method of aeration, contamination by other fungal species at times becomes a problem. The trays are harvested after approximately 7 to 10 days of incubation, with the citric acid yields being reported to be on the order of 60 to 80 g (or greater) of anhydrous citric acid per 100 g of added sugar. Replacement culture can be employed for both the stationary-tray fermentation and the submerged-aerated fermentation, but experience has been that citric acid yields based on sugar utilized are greater when the mycelium is not reused.

The citric acid is difficult to recover from the harvested fermentation broth, and the recovery is further complicated by the presence of unfermented sugars, other acid fermentation products, and inorganic impurities. The usual procedure, therefore, is to precipitate the citric acid as calcium citrate from hot neutral aqueous solution, followed by the addition of sulfuric acid to remove the calcium as calcium sulfate.

The tricarboxylic acid cycle does not appear to function properly during citric acid accumulation by *Aspergillus niger*. Thus, it has been observed that, during the accumulation of this acid, the fungus demonstrates decreased activity of the condensing enzyme and almost no activity for the isocitric dehydrogenase and aconitase enzymes. In light of these observations, various theories have been advanced to explain just how citric acid is able to accumulate during this fermentation. For instance, one of the main theories proposes that glucose is first split to yield two 3-carbon fragments, followed by the decarboxylation of one of the fragments to yield a 2-carbon compound, and the carboxylation of the other fragment to yield a 4-carbon compound. The 2-carbon and 4-carbon compounds then would be combined to yield citric acid. Obviously, much study is yet required to explain the high conversion of carbohydrate to citric acid in this fermentation.

FUMARIC ACID

The fungal production of fumaric acid (Figure 26.4) is an example of a microbial fermentation with good yields but little demand for the fermentation product, although at least small amounts of this acid have been produced on an industrial scale by a fungal fermentation. The picture for this fermentation is not hopeless, however, because if the fermentation costs could be reduced, there might be some demand for fumaric acid in the manufacture of resins and, possibly, wetting agents. Also, fumaric acid can be converted to maleic acid by heating in acid solution, and the demand for maleic acid is increasing for the manufacture of alkyd resins, unsaturated polyester coating compounds, rosin adducts, and plasticizers.

Most microorganisms produce small amounts of fumaric acid as a fleeting intermediate of the tricarboxylic acid cycle, but very few microorganisms accumulate this acid as an end product of metabolism. This property is primarily associated with various members of the *Mucorales*, and particularly among species of the genus *Rhizopus* such as *Rhizopus nigricans* (Figure 26.5). Strain selection is of great importance for this fermentation, since some strains of *Rhizopus* do not produce fumaric acid, while others produce fumaric acid or a mixture of fumaric and acids. Also, certain species

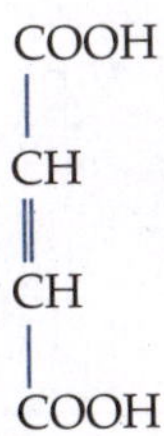

Figure 26.4 Fumaric acid.

of *Rhizopus*, including *Rhizopus nigricans*, lack invertase activity and, therefore, cannot utilize sucrose. Thus, with the latter organisms, molasses cannot be used as a carbon substrate unless its sucrose is first inverted with mineral acid or invertase.

The fumaric acid fermentation with *Rhizopus nigricans* is highly aerobic; in fact, a deficiency of oxygen during the fermentation allows accumulation of ethanol. The fermentation is conducted as 28 to 33°C by surface or submerged techniques, and with or without the use of replacement culture. The medium contains a hexose, salts, and ammonia or urea, but a proper ratio of carbon to nitrogen compounds in the medium is important, since this ratio controls not only the yields of fumaric acid but also the formation of fermentation acids other than fumaric acid. The levels of trace metals in the fermentation medium also play a role, and of these trace metals, zinc is particularly critical and should be slightly limiting, since an excess allows the formation of additional acids. However, the exact level of zinc to be used in the medium depends on the levels of other trace metals. In analogy to the citric and fermentation, the addition of methanôl to the medium is beneficial to fumaric acid formation, but in the latter instance, the mechanism may possibly be different in that at least some of the methanol appears to be fixed into the fumaric acid molecule.

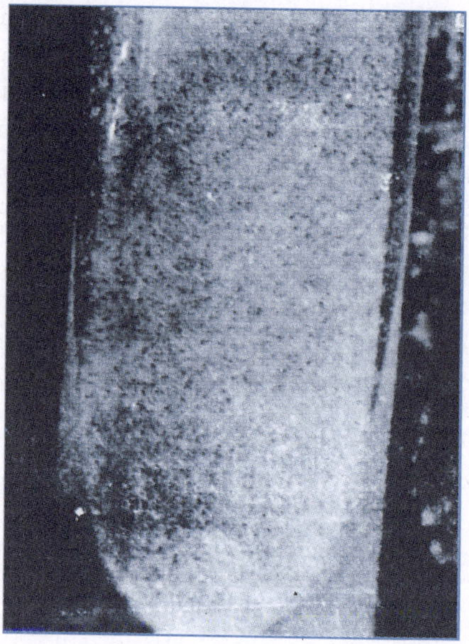

Figure 26.5 Gross appearance of sporulated *Rhizopus nigricans* growth. Photo courtesy of Charles Pfizer and Co., Inc.

Fumaric acid is only poorly soluble in water, with saturation occurring at approximately 0.7g per 100 ml. As a result, fumaric acid crystallizes in the medium to form gels that cause thickening of the medium and coating of the mycelium. Under the latter conditions the fermentation slows or comes to a stop. *Rhizopus nigricans* also cannot withstand a high acidity of its medium for either growth or fumaric acid production. Therefore, to neutralize the acidity and to prevent crystallization of fumaric acid, an intermittent addition of sodium or potassium carbonate is employed to maintain a pH value of between 5 and 6. Calcium carbonate cannot be used for this purpose, because calcium fumarate also crystallizes from the medium and forms gells.

The fumaric acid is harvested from the fermentation medium by acidifying so that the acid crystallizes. It is then recrystallized from hot water.

The biosynthetic mechanism for fumaric acid formation in this fermentation remains obscure. Apparently, the fumaric acid does not arise as a direct result of an accumulation of fumaric acid formed via the tricarboxylic acid cycle. There is some evidence, however, for a mechanism by which two 2-carbon fragments condense to yield fumaric acid, but other mechanisms also apparently are operative to yield the acid.

ITACONIC ACID

Itaconic acid (Figure 26.6) is used in the resin and detergent industries. It is produced by an *Aspergillus terreus* fermentation, but chemical processes for its production also are available which employ either the pyrrolysis of citric or cis-aconitic acids, or the heating of calcium aconitate (a by-product of the sugar refining of cane molasses) in acid solution.

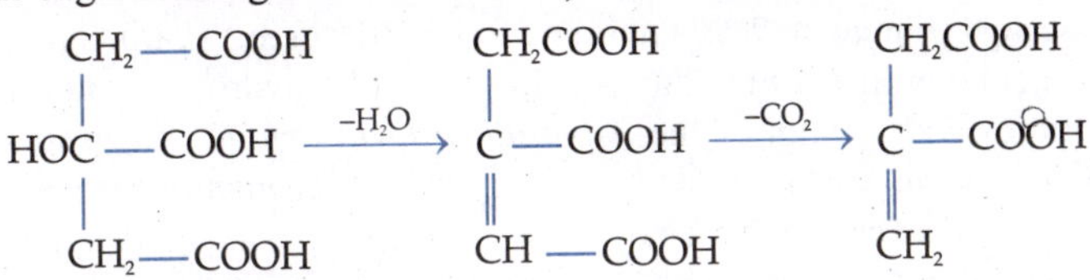

Citric acid Cis-aconitic acid Itaconic acid

Figure 26.6 Itaconic acid in relation to citric and cis-aconitic acids of the TCA cycle.

The fermentation-derived itaconic acid results either through stationary or through submerged fermentation, but commercial production is by the latter procedure. The fermentation is highly aerated at an incubation temperature of 30 to 35°C, and the molasses-salts medium is maintained during the fermentation at a pH value below 2.2. The reason for this adjustment is that at pH values greater than 2.6, *Aspergillus terreus* utilizes or degrades the itaconic acid, while no itaconic acid is produced at pH 6. Obviously, fermentor liners must be fabricated of acid-resistant material. As in the fumaric acnd citric acid fermentations, the accumulation of itaconic acid is sensitive to the levels of trace metals in the fermentation medium.

Some workers have reported that a relatively low inoculum level should be employed, and that the mycelial inoculum should be in the form of small pellets. In fact, it has been stated that the numbers of pellets added as inoculum per volume of medium should be determined and duplicated for each production run. This inoculum procedure is said to provide less mycelial growth and greater yields of itaconic acid. In contrast to these reports, however, other reports state that an inoculum level of 5 to 10 percent is optimum.

Approximately 85 percent of the acid produced during the fermentation can be accounted for as itaconic acid, with the residual acidity being attributed mainly to succinic and itatartaric acids or to itatartaric lactone. At harvest, the mycelium is separated from the broth, and the broth is evaporated to allow crystallization of the itaconic acid. The crystals then are washed in cold water and can be recrystallized from hot water.

As may be seen in Figure 26.6, itaconic acid is closely related to cis-aconitic acid of the tricarboxylic acid cycle. *Aspergillus terreus* possesses the enzymes of the tricarboxylic acid cycle, and it is assumed, therefore, that the itaconic acid arises from cis-aconitic acid during the operation of the cycle.

KOJIC ACID

Kojic acid (Figure 26.7) is a pyrone compound lacking a carboxyl group. Thus, its acidic properties are attributed to its enolic hydroxyl group. Kojic acid is produced by fungi of the *Aspergillus flavus-oryzae* and *Aspergillus tamarii* groups in surface culture. Submerged fermentations also are a possibility, but as yet they have not been investigated to any extent, because no commercial use has yet been found for this acid.

High yields of kojic acid occur during growth on a medium containing ammonium nitrate, salts, and glucose, sucrose, or xylose. However, low-level additions of ethylene chlorohydrin provide yet further increased yields. Iron must be carefully excluded from the medium to prevent its interaction with kojic acid to form a deep-red color. The latter reaction, nevertheless, is of interest because kojic acid was first observed as a fermentation product of *Aspergillus oryzae* by the color that developed when ferric chloride was added to a culture of the organism. Kojic acid is recovered by crystallization on evaporation of the culture liquor.

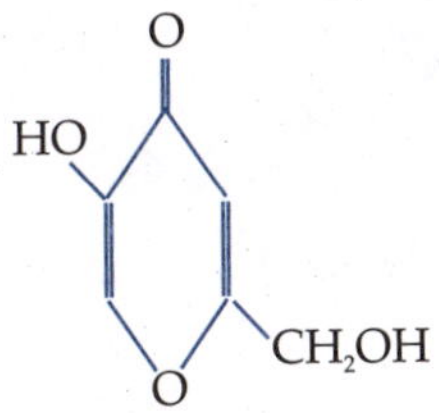

Fig. 26.7 Kojic acid.

BACTERIAL GLUCONIC AND α-KETOGLUTARIC ACID FERMENTATIONS

Various species of *Acetobacter* oxidize glucose to gluconic acid, galactose to galactonic acid, and so forth. However, the *Acetobacter* gluconic acid fermentation does not successfully compete with the fungal fermentation, because of the tendency of the *Acetobacter* species to further oxidize the gluconic acid to various ketogluconic acids.

Many *Acetobacter* strains oxidize glucose to 5-ketogluconic acid (Figure 26.8), and specially selected strains oxidize calcium gluconate to 5-ketogluconic acid. Thus, *Acetobacter suboxydans* oxidizes glucose to gluconic acid (neutralized by calcium carbonate), but then after most of the glucose is gone and cell multiplication has ceased, it oxidizes the gluconic acid to 5-ketogluconate. During the latter part of the fermentation, the calcium 5-ketogluconate precipitates from the medium so that at harvest it is separated by filtration. It is then dissolved in dilute acid for further purification and precipitation. 5-Ketogluconic acid is utilized as an intermediate in the chemical production of D-tartaric acid, although the economics of fermentation-produced D-tartaric acid, (via 5-ketogluconic acid) are poor in comparison to the direct recovery of tartaric acid as a by-product of the wine industry and the chemical-oxidation production of D-tartaric acid from starch.

The 5-ketogluconic acid in the *Acetobacter suboxydans* fermentation usually accompanied by small amounts of 2-ketogluconate, and specially selected strains of *Acetobacter suboxydans* have been found which will yield mainly the 2-ketogluconate. However, a fermentation utilizing *Pseudomonas fluorescens* would appear to have more promise for the production of 2-ketogluconate from glucose.

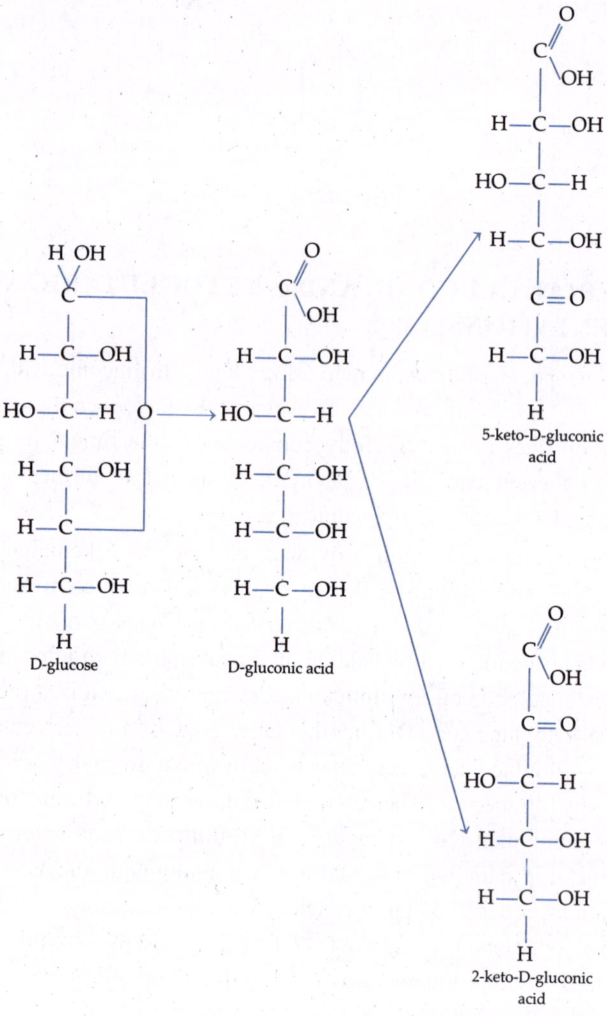

Figure 26.8 Oxidation of glucose to ketogluconic acids

Many common soil-derived species of *Pseudomonas* oxidize glucose to gluconic to 2-ketogluconic acids, and the fermentative production of 2-ketogluconic acid by strains of *Pseudomonas fluorescens* has received considerable study. This organism's submerged fermentation has a high oxygen requirement, since limited aeration tends to yield carbon dioxide and

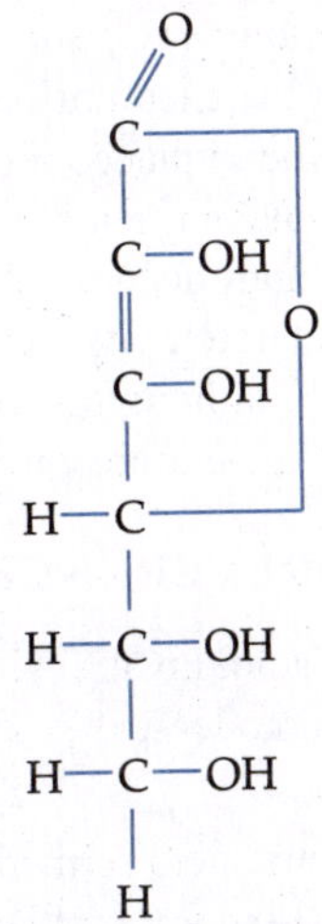

Figure. 26.9 D-Araboascorbic acid.

water instead of 2-ketogluconate. The fermentation medium utilizes urea as a nitrogen source and calcium carbonate to neutralize the 2-ketogluconic acid. At harvest of the culture broth, the acid is recovered as the calcium salt on evaporation of the filtered

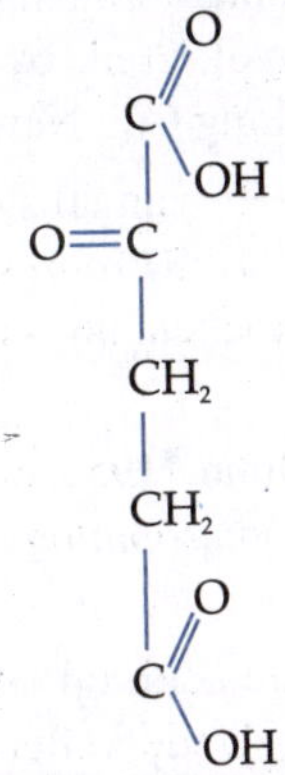

Figure. 26.10 α-Ketoglutaric acid.

broth at relatively low temperatures. 2-Ketogluconate can be used commercially as an intermediate in the preparation of D-araboascorbic acid (Figure 26.9), which provides vitamin C antioxidant sparing action for the preservation of fruits and other foods. However, 2-ketogluconate fermentations probably have not been commercialized, because the D-araboascorbic acid must compete with L-ascorbic acid, which is relatively inexpensive.

Certain strains of *Pseudomonas fluorescens* produce 2-ketogluconate which, after the nitrogen of the medium has become limiting and growth has stopped, disappears to be replaced in good yield by α-ketoglutaric acid (Figure 26.10). Additional fermentative control is applied by having the aeration rate after maximum accumulation of the 2-ketogluconate has occurred. Calcium α-ketoglutarate may precipitate during the fermentation and can be recovered as such, although recovery of the α-ketoglutaric acid usually consists in acidifying the culture and extracting with ethyl acetate.

REFERENCES

Foster, J. W. 1954. Fumaric acid. Pp. 470–487 in *Industrial fermentations*, vol. I (ed. by L. A. Underkofler and R. J. Hickey). Chemical Publishing Co., New York

Johnson, M. J. 1954. The citric acid fermentation. Pp. 420–445 in *Industrial fermentations*, vol I (ed. by L. A. Underkofler and R. J. Hickey). Chemical Publishing Co., New York.

Lockwood, L. B. 1954. Itaconic acid. Pp. 488–497 in *Industrial fermentations*, vol. I (ed. by L. A. Underkofler and R. J. Hickey). Chemical Publishing Co., New York.

Lockwood, L. B. 1954. Ketonic fermentation processes. Pp. 1–23 in *Industrial fermentations*, vol. 2(ed. by L. A. Underkofler and R. J. Hickey). Chemical Publishing Co., New York.

Perlman, D., And C. J. Sih. 1960. Fungal synthesis of citric, fumaric and itaconic acids. Pp. 167–194 in *Progress in industrial microbiology*, vol. 2(ed. by D. J. D. Hockenhull). Interscience Publishers, Inc., New York.

Prescott, S. C., and C. G. Dunn. 1959. The citric acid fermentation. Pp. 533–575 in *Industrial microbiology*, 3rd Ed. McGraw-Hill Book Co., Inc., New York.

Schopmeyer, H. H. 1954. Lactic acid. Pp. 391–419 in *Industrial fermentations,* vol. I (ed. by L. A. Underkofler and R. J. Hickey). Chemical Publishing Co., New York.

Underkofler, L. A. 1954. Gluconic acid. Pp. 446–469 in *Industrial fermentations*, vol. I (ed. by L. A. Underkofler and R. J. Hickey). Chemical Publishing Co., New York.

PART IV
THE FUTURE

Chapter 27

Outlook for Industrial Microbiology

It is difficult to say just what place in our society the future holds for industrial microbiology. Many different factors are involved, and it is the interaction of these factors which will controls its future.

It is apparent that many different industrial fermentations are presently available for commercial usage, but that relatively few are actually practiced. Some of these fermentations were practiced in the past but, because of changes in the competitive positions of the fermentation products, they are no longer able to compete on the open market. This state of affairs was brought on by increased costs of substrate materials and labor and equipment, by competition from chemical synthesis routes, and by the discovery of other compounds or products more suitable for the particular applications over which the fermentation products had held rein.

Another group of available industrial fermentation processes which are not practiced at present include those for which a fermentation process has been developed, but for which a public demand has not been created. Included in this group are fermentation-derived products that are not quite as good as or do not perform quite as efficiently for specific uses as do other compounds already in commercial usage. Also included are fermentation products which, because of high production costs, including low yields and recoveries, have not been in a position to compete on the open market.

A third group of fermentations is concerned with a vast array of microbial metabolic by-products for which workable fermentation processes, other than small-scale laboratory studies, have not yet been developed. These metabolic by-products are often unusual compounds not yet producible by chemical synthesis, but frequently no commercial usage can be found for them. Thus, Raistrick (1950) has described many unusual and often chemically reactive compounds produced by fungi, but these compounds have not been studied in enough detail or considered thoroughly enough from the commercial standpoint for their present commercial exploitation. Of course, the development of fermentation processes for the production of these compounds also is deterred because of a poor patent position. Without a defined demonstration of utility (which of course strengthens the case for the granting of a patent), the economic drive for process development is lacking. These various groups of presently unused industrial fermentation processes all could find commercial exploitation in the future if changes should occur in the economic and demand pictures for their respective fermentation products.

But what about those industrial fermentation processes presently being practiced? What will be their future status in the open market? It has already been observed that chemical synthesis routes to products similar to those produced by fermentation have made deep inroads into the fermentation market. A notable example, of course, is that of petroleum-derived chemicals. These petrochemicals will probably become a yet greater threat to industrial fermentations, particularly as the chemical synthesis technology advances and the costs of fermentation substrates increases. Thus, the production of the simpler chemical molecules will probably be relegated to the chemical synthesis industries. However, microbial processes for producing the more complex organic molecules, the molecules for which biologically active isomers are required, and the molecules requiring microbial enzymatic transformation steps should retain their competitive position on the market. This can also be said for biologically active microbial products such as various enzyme preparations.

Certain fermentation products have enjoyed, in the past, and still do enjoy an unusual economic position. In particular, beverage alcohol has had no problem in competing with petrochemical alcohol, while fermentation-derived industrial alcohol has not been in such a fortunate position. These two types of alcohol are in actuality the same compound, the difference being that government regulations protect the fermentation production of beverage alcohol. The question may be raised, however, as to whether government protection will continue. For the most part, this is not a bothersome question, because the flavor, aroma, and other complex characteristics of the various beverage alcohol products are difficult if not impossible to reproduce by purely chemical means, so that fermentations of this type should continue to be able to compete on their own merit. Nevertheless, the question might be raised as to whether other industrial fermentation processes should be protected by government regulations against the competitive inroads by chemical synthesis processes. This question can be answered by stating that there probably is little need for this coddling of the fermentation industry. There are enough possibilities, both explored and unexplored, for economically sound industrial fermentations that such regulations should not be required.

Government regulations of fermentation processes and products presently play a large role in another area of the fermentation industry, that of the safety of pharmacological compounds used in medical practice. Obviously, such regulations are of benefit to the public as well as to the fermentation industry. This is true, however, only so long as these regulations are wisely defined and administered. Tremendous strides have already been made in discovering and developing processes for fermentation-derived products for the treatment of disease, and it is hoped that government regulation of these products in the future will be such that the economic reward accruing to those who search for new products of this type will be great enough to entice them to continue their search.

Government regulation in the form of patent grants is a boon to the industrial fermentation industries. The cost of research is so great that the gamble is considered worthwhile only if it is known that strong patent protection for the product or process can be obtained. Thus, the future statement and workings of our patent laws will have a profound effect on industrial microbiology. In this regard, however, there are distinct indications of impending changes in the patent laws, although most of these changes may take place in countries other than the United States. There have been discussions concerning the possibility that, at least in portions of Western Europe, a single patent might be granted that would provide protection in several countries to the inventor – a multination patent. There is also the possibility that countries such as Italy may change their outlook on the issuing of pharmaceutical patents. The question of patent protection in the underdeveloped nations, obviously, is unanswered at the present time. The patent laws of these nations are bound to change, particularly as developments occur in the availability of fermentation substrates, requirements for fermentation products, and economic climates for fermentation industries. Although not presently included in the protection provided by patent grants, it is likely that courts in the United States and in other countries will deem it necessary to provide greater protection than is presently available for company secrets, microbial cultures, and so forth, since these are vital factors in the ability of a fermentation process or product to maintain a competitive position in the market.

Those industrial fermentation processes that are presently practiced will require continued research and development. In particular, many of these fermentations will require increased yield capacity if they are to maintain their economic positions. An important aspect of the yield capacities for these fermentations involves continuous research on strain selection, both from natural sources, and through induced changes such as by mutation or hybridization in strains already at hand. Alternatively, other organisms (even organisms from quite different genera or families) with the capacity to produce a particular fermentation product should be evaluated as a substitute for the organism normally utilized as the fermentation agent.

To obtain and evaluate organisms for these processes, as well as to obtain organisms for new and different fermentation processes, will require the development of better and more efficient primary and secondary screening techniques, including those techniques for the detection and assay of fermentation products. The latter also includes the ability to detect the presence in fermentation broths of new fermentation by-products, whether or not these compounds have ever been previously observed from any source. Some of these techniques should allow the screening of groups of microorganisms from soil and marine environments which, as yet, have not been investigated to any extent, or which, although existing in these environments, have rarely or possibly never been cultured successfully in the laboratory. For instance, a group of microorganisms (Casida, 1965) which occurs in soil in large numbers, but which is difficult to grow in the laboratory by conventional techniques, has as yet not been evaluated for its possible ability to produce fermentation products of value. Also, another potential group of industrial organisms, the nonspore-forming obligate anaerobes, is known to be present in soil, but little is known of their numbers and types in this environment. Thus, the vast numbers of possible microorganisms and strains of these organisms existing in natural microbial sources, compounded with the mutational and metabolic control possibilities for each individual strain, should allow virtually unlimited source material for investigation.

The mutational and other genetic approaches to obtaining industrially important microbial strains offer fascinating possibilities. Included among these approaches are the use of mutagenic agents, hybridization of fungi, and various transfers of genetic material in bacteria. In a sense, the fermentation industry is waiting for the microbial geneticist to determine for it the finite points of the genetic make-up of the cell, and to develop better means for its manipulation. With this knowledge at hand, greater use could be made of genetic blocks to unmask useful but minor metabolic sequences of the cell, and of genetic transfers to introduce new genetic material into cells. New mutagenic agents are continuously being discovered that enhance the frequency of specific mutation types. We hope that new mutagenic agents also will be found that will broaden, through mutation, the total phenotypic spectrum of individual microorganisms so that new commercially valuable strains of microorganisms with undreamed-of synthetic capabilities will result.

Greater use also should be made of nongenetic manipulations of the regulatory mechanisms of the cell. Specific enzyme poisons and various substrate and product inhibitions of specific metabolic pathways should be employed in the order to bring into play minor but valuable metabolic sequences from the industrial standpoint.

A somewhat similar approach would be to make use of the faulty metabolism of aging microbial cultures; that is, cultures which have been incubated for considerable periods of time. This is the approach employed so successfully by Raistrick (1950) to discover chemical products of microbial metabolism not previously observed. However, Raistrick's approach was laborious in that he often had to employ difficult and involved chemical fractionation procedures to detect and characterize these products. In contrast, however, modern-day procedures will detect and often characterize products in one or a few perations and the use of these procedures should markedly simplify the detection and characterization of products such as those studied by Raistrick.

The application of new screening techniques, as well as of these presently available, should engender success in the search for alternate products present in fermentation broths of commonly practiced industrial fermentations, products which, thus far, have been overlooked. These fermentations were developed with one product in mind, because that product could be easily identified and possessed commercial value. However, other potentially valuable products also may be present in these broths. For example, the presence of 6-aminopenicillanic acid in penicillin fermentation broths was overlooked for many years, although this compound at the present time has considerable economic value for the production of new penicillins. It is difficult to predict what other compounds might be present in various fermentation broths without first performing a thorough search for such compounds, assuming of course the availability of the methods for their detection. Thus, it is entirely possible that the culture broths of some fermentations may contain compounds with pharmacodynamic action if we could but devise methods for the detection of these compounds.

The possibilities for the existence of valuable by-products in fermentation broths are multiplied when mutation and other regulatory controls of the metabolism of the organism are employed since, even though these metabolic controls are directed towards increasing the yield of a specific and known product of economic value, the alterations in unconsidered metabolic pathways may well yield other valuable products during the prime fermentation which remain only to be detected. In fact, it is always possible that such alternate products may be of more economic value than the primary fermentation product, so that the fermentation could be redesigned to make such a product the primary product of the fermentation.

It is obvious from the foregoing discussion that vast screening programs may be required to attain these ends. But screening programs are becoming increasingly more expensive in labor, time, and materials. Obviously, the better designed a screening program is, the more quickly will it yield the desired organisms and with the least cost. Nevertheless, even the best of designed screening programs are still expensive, and methods for decreasing screening costs obviously will need to be worked out. One approach to reducing screening costs, now being employed to a limited extent, is to have the screening carried out in nations that have low labor and overhead costs. While this solution may be attractive at present, it certainly is not a long-term answer.

Spent fermentation medium should be studied not only for its potential content of valuable by-products, but also to find better uses for it than to be sewered to become a problem of waste disposal. The same applies to spent microbial cells at the termination of a fermentation. The spent media and cells still contain a lot in the way of fermentation nutrients and, if properly handled, could well be used to supply at least some of the nutrients for fresh fermentation media. This is analogous to the slopping-back procedure employed in the acetone-butanol fermentation. The use of spent microbial cells may require that the cells first by lysed or broken up in some manner, thus liberating their store of potential fermentation nutrients. Obviously, such reuse of spent medium and microbial cells would contribute greatly to the economic position of a fermentation, since this procedure would help hold down the high cost of fresh fermentation nutrients. Spent media and cells also could find further use a animal feeds or feed supplements. In addition, with an improvement in their patability and acceptability, they might find use as food for man.

To date, most industrial fermentation processes have been developed to comply with the existing designs of fermentation equipment. This equipment may or may not be ideal for individual fermentations and, in fact, there are fermentations (for instance, those utilizing hydrocarbons as substrates) which probably would provide greater yields in a shorter period of time if the fermentation tanks and auxiliary equipment were redesigned specifically for these fermentations. Thus, at least for some fermentations, the fermentation equipment should be designed for the fermentation instead of vice versa.

The design of fermentation tanks and auxiliary equipment should tanks several factors into account. There may well be a greater future use of continuous fermentations, multistep fermentations, and even fermentations employing mixed cultures or unusual microorganisms. Thus, specific equipment will need to be designed to provide a high level of efficiency for such fermentations. Special fermentation tanks also will be needed for highly oxygen-sensitive anaerobic microorganisms, for fermentations employing gaseous substrates, and for other fermentations employing unusual substrates or microorganisms having unusual or sensitive growth requirements. Fermentation tanks should also be designed to provide better aeration and agitation with less power input and, in addition, the design should consider means for more adequate foam control and prevention of contamination. More refined electronic controls for the monitoring and control of pH, temperature, nutrient addition, and so forth, and for the programming of these variables in a defined manner, should be made an integral part of the fermentation equipment. Computers should more frequently be associated with production fermentors, especially in order to make immediate decisions between alternative steps to be taken if contamination or the biological variability of the fermentation microorganism should gain the upper hand in the fermentation. It is assumed, of course, that these refinements or changes in the design of fermentation equipment will not only provide fermentations with higher yields in a shorter period of time, but also will greatly reduce the total expense associated with the fermentation.

As has been pointed, out, the expense of media sterilization is great enough that certain industrial fermentations employ unsterile media so as to maintain economic feasibility for the process. Also, it has been noted that the media employed in some industrial fermentations are difficult to sterilize because of their crude organic substrate components, and that the heat requirement for sterilization of these media components can mean that other components of the media become overcooked. Thus, new, more efficient, and cheaper means of media sterilization are needed. Gaseous sterilization, as with ethylene oxide, is a possibility, but this procedure is probably far from any semblance of economic feasibility for large-scale fermentation processes.

The availability of cheap organic compounds as fermentation medium carbon sources today is a critical problem of fermentation economics, and it will become more serious as time progresses. In fact, it is possible that carbohydrate and protein fermentation nutrient sources in the temperate areas of the world in the future will become so expensive that they cannot be employed as fermentation nutrients. Because of the rise in population density, these nutrients will have to be channeled for use as human food and animal feed. However, carbohydrate sources for fermentation media are presently available in high quantity and low price in the tropics, and it is likely that, in the near future, various fermentation (including those yielding microbial cells as food and feed as well as those yielding fuel alcohol) will be practiced more extensively in this part of the world. Other fermentations also may gain prominence as some of the underdeveloped nations in these areas achieve a higher technological level.

Obviously, new sources of fermentation nutrients, particularly carbon nutrients, will have to become available. Hydrocarbons as fermentation substrates have already been discussed, and it is probable that hydrocarbons will be employed much more extensively as the carbon substrate for the fermentative production of chemical compounds as well as for the production of microbial cells for food and feed. Also, hydrocarbons may find extensive utilization as substrates for microbial conversions, such that in a one- or two-step transformation a reactive chemical group or groups becomes incorporated into the hydrocarbon molecule to make it acceptable for various commercial uses and as a starting point foi further chemical alterations or syntheses. Cellulosic agricultural by-products present a possible source of carbohydrate fermentation nutrient, but for most fermentations the cellulose will need to be hydrolyzed by some means. Acid hydrolysis is possible, as is the use of microorganisms (or their enzymes) which have strong cellulolytic activity. Spent fermentation media and the exhausted cells from harvested fermentations, as previously stated, also are possible sources of fermentation nutrients. Another possible source rich in available nutrients is domestic sewage. For most fermentation processes, the sewage waters would need to be sterilized before they could be used, but the expense of sterilization, as contrasted to the expense of a source or readily available fermentation nutrients, might be minimal. A similar source of fermentation nutrients exists in the high BOD wastes from food-processing plants.

The potential for industrial microbiology applications to agriculture and food production is vast, and certainly has been only nominally explored. Various fermentation products already find extensive use in agriculture (for instance, the use of antibiotics in the prevention of plant and animal disease, as an animal-growth stimulant when incorporated into feeds, and as an aid in food preservation.) Vitamins, gibberellins, auxins, and related substances also should find continued and possibly expanded use as plant- and animal-growth stimulants. However, microorganisms may well find other extensive applications in agriculture. Thus, batches of microorganisms grown in fermentors could be incorporated into the soil to fight soil-borne plant diseases although, admittedly, more information on the ecology of soil microorganisms will be required to increase the feasibility of this application. Microorganisms also could be added to soil to release plant nutrients that are bound in soil in form unavailable to growing plants. Non-symbiotic nitrogen fixation in soil has received considerable study in the past, but without resulting in the discovery of any decisive means for increasing the content of the fixed nitrogen of the soil. Russian investigators on many occasions have reported increased crop yields on incorporation of *Azotobacter* strains into soil, but this may have been more a growth-stimulation phenomenon for the plants than due to the actual nitrogen fixation by the organisms. Therefore, the possibilities for adding nitrogen-fixing strains of *Azotobacter* or *Clostridium* species to soil, or for incorporating various chemicals into soil to adjust the soil ecology in favor of the nitrogen-fixing microorganisms, are still areas for exploration. *Rhizobium* inoculant has been and still is employed extensively for the inoculation of legume seed. A somewhat similar symbiotic association, that of the mycorrhizal fungi with the roots of trees and other plants (Figure 27.1), should receive extensive study for possible commercial exploitation. Although the exact reasons why the mycorrhizal fungi stimulate plant growth are not yet clear, these fungi obviously are beneficial to the plant, and possibly could be grown in large volumes in fermentors for incorporation into soil with seeds or seedlings of the proper plant species.

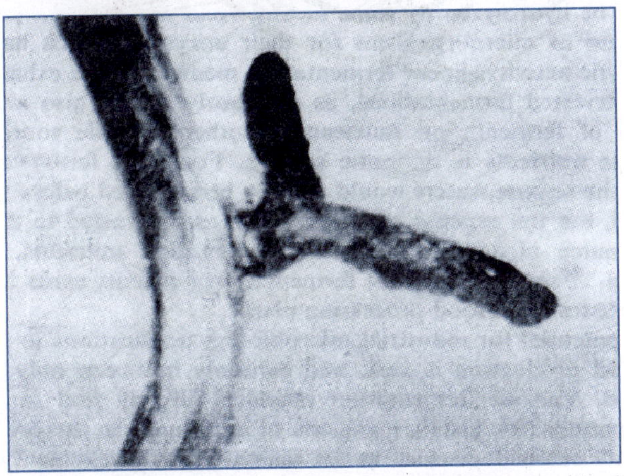

Figure 27.1 *Mycorrhizae of Cenococcum* graniforme projecting from a Douglas-fir root. Courtesy of J. M. Trappe.

Microorganisms such as *Bacillus thuringiensis* which destroy insects have present agricultural applications, and other microorganisms with this capability doubtlessly will be evaluated and find use in agriculture. Microorganisms that destroy lower animal forms also may well find application in agriculture, for instance, the nematode-trapping fungi that entrap and kill these tiny wormlike parasites of the roots of growing plants

(Figure 27.2). A word of warning is in order, however. The above and other similar uses of microorganisms in agriculture can cause limited to extensive alterations in the ecological balance of the microorganisms that occur in soil, on plants, and in the intestinal tracts of animals, birds, and so forth, so that a better understanding of microbial ecology again would be of distinct value. This also is true for those situations in which antibiotics and nonmicrobially produced chemicals such as herbicides, fungicides, bactericides, and insecticides are incorporated into the soil, onto plants, and into other natural environments.

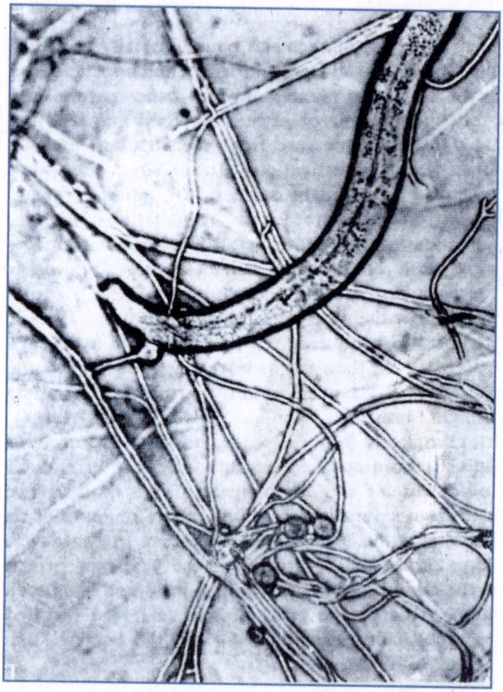

Figure 27.2 Nematode trapped by the predaceous fungus *Dactylella drechsler*. The nematode has become trapped by the adhesive knobs on the fungal hyphae and wil serve as nutrient for the fungus. Other nematode trapping fungi employ doughnutshaped protuberances from the hyphae which impinge nematodes unlucky enough to crawl through the opening. Courtesy of D. Pramer.

The production of microbial cells for food and feed probably will come under increased pressure from the population explosion in all parts of the world. Investigations already are underway to evaluate *Torula* yeast, as produced by sulfite-waste liquor fermentations, and *Candida* yeast, from hydrocarbon fermentations, for this purpose. Cellulosic agricultural by-products are potential carbohydrate sources for growing yeasts of this type, but these substrates will require preliminary acid hydrolysis of the cellulose, or the use of cellulolytic microorganisms or their enzymes for the hydrolysis. Present fermentation procedures for producing yeast protein from hydrocarbons utilize liquid hydrocarbons ; the yeast removes most of the paraffinic portion of the hydrocarbon, leaving behind the aromatic fraction and some of the more highly branched paraffins. This aromatic fraction is difficult to separate completely from the cells at harvest – a procedure, however, which must be accomplished because of the potential carcinogenic activity of certain of the components of the residual hydrocarbon. The protein from several yeasts is low in one or more of the essential amino acids, and this has caused hesitation in the development of fermentation processes for growing these yeasts as protein sources. However, the critical amino acids can be produced by specific bacterial fermentations, so that the yeast protein could be fortified with the deficient amino acid(s) as obtained from the bacterial fermentation sources (Bunker, 1964).

Microorganisms other than yeasts are also known to produce protein in good yields. Various bacteria produce considerable protein during growth, including some that do so during growth on hydrocarbons, and these organisms may well be useful as a protein source if their cells can be made palatable and acceptable as a food or feed. Studies are already underway (C. and E. News, 1966) to utilize methane and other small molecular weight gaseous hydrocarbons as the carbon substrate, so that no residual hydrocarbon will be associated with the bacterial protein. Algae and, possibly, photosynthetic bacteria are particularly attractive sources of protein, because their photosynthetic capabilities practically negate the requirement for substrate organic carbon nutrient. Again, however, palatability, digestibility, and acceptability of these organisms as food or feed must be evaluated.

The fat-producing yeast *Rhodotorula gracilis* is a particularly intriguing source for food and feed. This organism undergoes normal cellular growth during its logarithmic growth phase in a medium containing adequate nitrogen. However, at the onset of nitrogen starvation, this organism accumulates large amounts of lipid within its cells. It has been pointed out, however (Bunker, 1964), that the protein-lipid ratio occurring in this organism can be varied at will by the way in which its nitrogen nutrition is handled, while at the same time allowing it to produce other products, such as B vitamins, ergosterol, and pro-vitamin A.

The discovery and development of microbially mediated means for producing new foods and flavoring agents for human consumption, and of better methods for the production of similar presently available foods and flavoring agents, are distinct possibilities. For instance, the mushroom of commerce, the *Agaricus* mushroom, presently is grown in a commercially acceptable form only on compost beds, and it would be hoped that submerged, aerated fermentations to yield this organism in an acceptable form will be accomplished in the near future. The somewhat exotic foods such as soy sauce, various cheeses, and fermented milks have been microbially produced for centuries. Monosodium glutamate is presently produced by fermentation, and the nucleotide flavoring agents are under study. There is no reason to believe that similar or even other types of foods and flavouring agents will not soon be discovered and developed as products of microbial action.

The rumen of the cow is known to be a vital component of the metabolism of this highly productive animal. The rumen allows the functioning of an anaerobic balanced ecology designed for the natural fermentative breakdown of cellulose and for the conversion and degradation of other natural compounds. Since the rumen exists within the living animal, the temperature and certain other incubation conditions are constant, so that the rumen actually in an ideal fermentation vat. This raises the possibility that the rumen of the living animal, or even an artificially established rumen in the laboratory, could be employed to produce defined chemicals of commercial value simultaneously with its normal metabolic function. Obviously, the microbial ecology of the rumen would have to be well understood, and the specific chemical fermentation products would have to be nontoxic to the animal and not absorbed by it. The latter, of course, would not be pertinent of the artificial rumen were employed.

Many good antibiotics have been discovered in recent years, and new antibiotics are still being discovered. New uses for antibiotics may well be found so that additional impetus will be applied to the search for organisms producing new antibiotics, and for ways of chemically modifying those antibiotics that presently are of little commercial value because of toxicity or other problems. Antibiotics are needed which are active against common viruses, against L-form bacterial states (which apparently are induced in the body by continuous antibiotic therapy), and against various carcinomas. Already there is some evidence that antibiotics are effective for these treatments, and that there is sufficient difference in the toxicity level for the disease agent as contrasted to the healthy tissue. The build-up of antibiotic resistance in certain pathogenic microorganisms, such as *Staphylococcus*, has caused alarm in the past, and the search will continue for new antibiotics to use in instances in which this has occurred. Chemical or microbiological modifications of the structures of existing antibiotics have already yielded a certain amount of success, for instance, in the use of microbial enzymes to remove the side chain (**R** group) of penicillin to yield 6-aminopenicillanic acid so that new penicillins can be synthesized. There is no reason why success should not be achieved in the modification of other antibiotic structures in order to reduce toxicity, broaden the microbial inhibition spectrum range, or introduce specific activities into the antibiotic molecules. Antibiotics previously discarded because of high toxicity, or for other reasons, may soon find pharmacological, agricultural, deterioration prevention, and other uses for their biological activity. Antibiotics such as tetracycline are presently being employed for the preservation of fish and poultry. It is possible that a similar application of antibiotics for the preservation of meat and other foods will gain acceptance, and it is also possible that, if the particular economic situation will allow it, antibiotics will be used for protection against microbial deterioration of many other forms of natural and man-made materials.

Microbial enzymes enjoy extensive present-day usage, and there is no reason why this usage should not be expanded. It is hoped that enzymes from microbial sources will gradually replace those obtained from the tissues of higher plants and animals. In favor of this is the high rate of production of microbial enzymes, the relatively lower production and purification costs, and the possibility that enzymes of commercial value may be found which are unique to microorganisms. Enzymes from microbial sources may well find further medical uses, particularly if a means can be found to safely utilize pure crystalline enzymes for intravenous injections. Enzymes also may find further use in the improvement of food quality, especially if they can be utilized to remove undesirable substances or components of foods (Arima, 1964).

Microbial enzymes, either cell-free or retained within the organisms that produce them, will find greater application in the mediation of specific steps of chemical syntheses and of transformations difficult by purely chemical means. This is already being accomplished in the modification of specific sites on steroid molecules ; such transformations should also be feasible on antibiotics and other complex molecules. Thus, in specific instances, it should be possible to change the molecular configuration of a complex molecule such that specific chemical properties are either added, retained, or deleted from the molecule.

Increased knowledge of the treatment of municipal and industrial wastes doubtlessly will provide means for treating these wastes in a manner such that the effluent waters, which contain oxidized inorganic salts promoting aquatic weed and algal growth, and toxic and obnoxious inorganic or organic materials that survive present procedures of waste treatment, do not find their way into natural bodies of water. The modifications in waste-water treatment procedures required for obtaining these ends at least to some extent will necessitate a better understanding of the natural microbial ecology that occurs during the various treatment steps of the processing of the waste waters.

Industrial and municipal wastes undergoing treatment are a gigantic and continuous reservoir of highly nutritive materials for microbial growth and, as such, it is possible that by-products can be recovered from the treated waste waters. Vitamin B_{12} occurs naturally in these waters and, in certain instances, it presently is being recovered commercially. It should also be possible to direct the microbial activities of waste-water treatment microorganisms such that other products of commercial value can be recovered, either from the waters or from the settled sludge. Another possibility, although obviously more remote, is the utilization of waste-water treatment facilities as a giant microbial fuel cell for the production of electricity. We shall discuss this later on in this chapter.

Microbial deterioration has always been a problem, and it will continue to be so. Much study will be required to find means for preventing the deterioration of paper, fabrics, food and feed, wood, metals, concrete, and so forth. Also, means for preventing the fouling of submerged objects in marine environments will require extensive study.

The fact that microorganisms can be employed as scavengers is only beginning to be realized. Thus, microorganisms should find use in the scavenging of phosphate and other ions from waste waters, and from phosphate and other mining waters. In addition, they should find use in scavenging heavy and rare metals from mining process waters, sea water, and waters resulting from nonmining-related industrial processes. There also is some evidence that microorganisms can be employed to scavenge radioactive materials from water, food, soil, and so forth.

Fermentation processes employing unique microorganisms, or unique means for making use of the activities of microorganisms, may well be commonplace in the year to come. Thus, fermentative agents for producing commercially valuable products could include protozoa, lichens [with either a fungal or *Streptomyces* species component (Lazo and Klein, 1965)], microbial spheroplasts or protoplasts, stable bacterial L-forms (or unstable L-forms purposely maintained in this state), and animal or plant cells maintained as reproducing tissue cultures. As a specific example, the tissue-culture approach might yield alkaloids, hormones, and other biologically active compounds.

Chemosynthetic or photosynthetic autotrophs also could serve as fermentation microorganisms, particularly if mutated to expose components of their complete biosynthetic metabolisms. Unless introduced during mutation, a carbohydrate nutritive requirement would not be involved, hence these microorganisms would by-pass this costly ingredient of fermentation media make-up. Separate from or complimentary to this use of these organisms is the ability of some of them to oxidize inorganic ions ; perhaps, more application will be found for the ability of the thiobacilli to oxidize hydrogen sulfide, mineral sulfides and sulfur to sulfuric acid.

Microorganisms may be useful as agents to partially degrade highly viscous petroleum so as to reduce its viscosity. This would allow the oil to be more easily pumped through long pipelines. This property of microorganisms also could be employed to release oil from underground reservoirs ; the reduced viscosity would allow the petroleum to become detached from the sand and rock to which it is bound so that it could flow underground toward the location of oil wells. This would require that the organisms be introduced into the ground along with the waters used in secondary oil recovery. Microorganisms also might be employed for the releasing and removal of the contaminating metals, sulfides, and so forth which occur in crude oil fractions. Another potential microbial application as regards hydrocarbons relates to the fact that hydrocarbons are completely reduced compounds and, as such, they contain considerable quantities of hydrogen in their molecules. Therefore, microorganisms might be employed to release this hydrogen as gaseous hydrogen for use in chemical catalytic reductions.

Microbial spores as fermentative agents for mediating chemical transformations of various compounds probably will find greater exploitation. These spore fermentations would be analogous to the present use of spores in methyl ketone fermentations and steroid transformations. The nonspore-forming, highly oxygen-sensitive anaerobe has never really been investigated for its fermentation potential. Thus, it is not known just what products of commercial value these organisms might produce, if means could be found for their growth under mass culture conditions. Microbial dextrans and other polymers are known to be synthesized in high yield by microorganisms ; more and better uses should be found for these polymers. Poly-β-hydroxybutyrate is a specific example of a polymer produced in large amounts by many organisms. This compound could serve as a basal material for chemical modification, or it could be partially or totally hydrolyzed. Nucleic acids and their partial degradation products are already being recovered from cultures of microorganisms and these compounds should find increased applications in medicine, as food-flavoring agents, and in other ways.

The advent of space travel has generated several microbial problems that need solving. Leaving and returning spacecraft require some means for decontamination. Sampling devices and auxiliary equipment are needed for detecting and, possibly, identifying the microbial life on other planets. Algal and other balanced ecosystems for space travel are under study, as a means for supplying oxygen and removing carbon dioxide from the air, and as a means for decomposing and utilizing human wastes. Biochemical fuel cells also might be employed for utilizing human wastes and, at the same time, for producing electricity for space travel.

Microbial fuel cells, or as they are more often known, biochemical fuel cells, are of various types, but at least one type could be described as a unit made up of electropositive and electronegative half-cells joined by a potassium chloride agar bridge with each half-cell containing an electrolyte and an electrode. Reducing conditions are maintained in the electronegative cell by microbial activity on a nutrient substrate, and the electropositive side

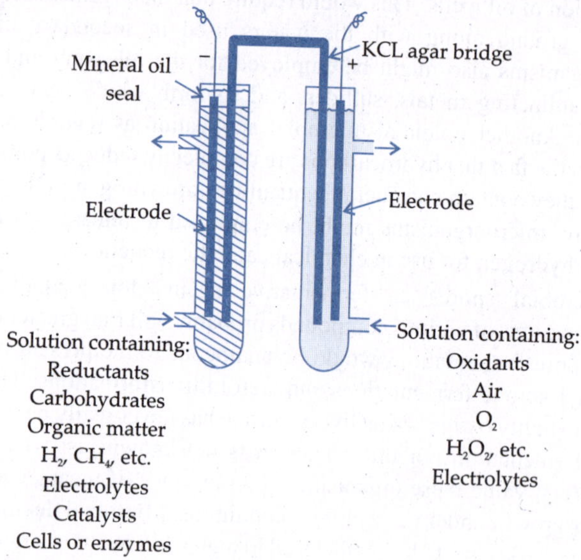

Figure 27.3 Biochemical fuel cell (Sisler, 1964, *Global impacts of applied microbiology*, p. 346).

is maintained by oxidizing conditions such as by air, oxygen, hydrogen peroxide, and so forth (Figure 27.3). Apparently, the microorganisms can tolerate a high electric charge, but other problems remain to be solved for these fuel cells (Sisler, 1964). For instance, they rapidly discharge under load, because the media are not sufficiently poised for accumulation of a sustained charge. Also, unfavorable reaction kinetics are encountered which lead to a sluggish electromotive response. It is theoretically possible that, if the problem of these fuel cells could be solved, electricity could be generated for municipalities. Thus, the activated sludge system or other microbial processes employed by municipal sewage-treatment plants could be used as the electronegative half-cell.

It should now be obvious that industrial microbiology presents many possibilities for the future, and many directions in which to go. Industrial microbiology does not stagnate. The thinking of man may stagnate at times, but usually someone manages to make the critical observation or discovery, design the proper equipment, and evaluate the market so that financial rewards accrue. Advances in the understanding and practice of the industrial applications of microorganisms will occur in university, government, and industrial laboratories, and it is only through working together and understanding each other's goals and purposes that the apparently purely theoretical discoveries made in these laboratories will have industrial significance. By the same token, research carried out in industrial microbiology laboratories would do well to include more of the basic or theoretical approaches that may seem to have little if any potential for economic return in the foreseeable future. Thus, what appears at first glance to be a purely theoretical discovery may, when considered from the proper viewpoint, be the key to a profitable industrial fermentation process.

REFERENCES

Anonymous. 1966. Bacteria metabolize methane. *Chem. and Eng.* news, *June* 20, pp. 20–21.

Arima, K. 1964. Microbial enzyme production. Pp. 277–294 in *Global impacts of applied microbiology* (ed. by M. P. Starr). John Wiley and Sons, Inc., New York.

Bunker, H. J. 1964. Microbial food. Pp. 234–240 in *Global impacts of applied microbiology* (ed. by M. P. Starr). John Wiley and Sons. Inc., New York.

Casida, L. E., Jr. 1965. Abundant microorganism in soil *Appl. Microbiol.*, **13**, 327–334.

Lazo, W. R., and R. M. Klein. 1965. Some physical factors involved in actinolichen formation. *Mycologia*, **57**, 804–808.

Raistrick, H. 1950. The chemistry of fungi. A region of biosynthesis. *Eripains-inos*: *Suomen Kemistilehti*, **10A**. 221–246.

Sisler, F. D. 1964. Electrical energy from microbiological fuel cells. Pp. 344-353 in *Global impacts of applied microbiology* (ed. by M. P. Starr). John Wiley and Sons, Inc., New York.

Starr, M. P., ed. 1964. *Global impacts of applied microbiology*. John Wiley and Sons, New York. 572 pp.

APPENDIX

Reagents and Buffers

CASEIN SOLUTION (2%)

Ingredients	Grams
Casein	2.0
Borate buffer (0.1 M)	80 mL

Adjust the pH 7.6 and completely dissolved by heating on a steam bath for 15 min. Cool this solution, adjust the pH to 7.6 and make the volume up to 100 mL by the borate buffer.

GRAM-STAINING REAGENTS

(A) Safranin (counterstain) Solution

Ingredients	Grams
Safranin	2.5 g
Ethyl alcohol (95%)	100 mL

For a working solution, dilute stock solution 1/10 (10 mL of stock safranin to 90 mL of distilled water).

(B) Crystal Violet

	Ingredients	Grams
(*a*)	Crystal violet (85%)	2.0 g
	Ethyl alcohol (95%)	20.0 mL
(*b*)	Ammonium oxalate	0.8 g
	Distilled water	80.0 mL

Add solution (*a*) to solution (*b*). Let stand for a day, and then filter. If the crystal violet is too concentrated, solution (*a*) may be diluted as much as 10 times.

(C) Decolorizer

95% Acetone of Ethyl alcohol

(D) Gram's Iodine Solution (mordant)

Ingredients	Grams
Iodine crystals	1.0 g
Potassium iodide	2.0 g
Distilled water	300.0 mL

Store in an amber bottle; discard when the colour begins to fade.

GUM ARABIC (10%)

Ingredients	Grams
Gum Arabic	10.0 g
Make the Volume up to 100 mL with distilled water	

METHYLENE BLUE SOLUTION (1 : 250,000)

The Methylene blue concentration used in 1 part of dye in 3,00,000 parts of milk. Presently tablet forms are available. One tablet dissolved in 200 mL of hot, distilled water produces the stock dye solution for addition to the milk. Although this solution is stable when it is refrigerated and protected from light, it is safer to prepare the solution weekly.

PHENOPTHALEIN (1%)

Ingredients	Concentration
Phenolphthalein	0.1
Ethyl alcohol	89–91
Methanol	4–6
Deionized water	4–6

SODIUM PHOSPHATE BUFFER (pH 7)

Solutions	Ingredients	Grams/Lit
Stock solution A	Monobasic sodium phosphate, monohydrate (2 M)	276.0
Stock solution B	Dibasic sodium phosphate (2 M)	284.0
Final pH: 7.0 ± 0.2 at 25°C		

Mixing an 39.0 (mL) of A and 61.0 (mL) of B as diluting to a total volume of 200 mL, a 1 M phosphate buffer of the required pH at room temperature.

NaOH (N/10)

Ingredients	Grams
NaOH	0.4
Distilled water	100 mL

NEWMANN'S STAIN

Ingredients	Grams
Methylene blue chloride	0.6 g
Ethyl alcohol (95%)	52 mL
Tetrachlorethane	44 mL
Glacial acetic acid	4 mL

TCA SOLUTION (10%)

Ingredients	Grams
Trichloroacetic acid	10.0
Anhydrous sodium acetate	10.0
Glacial acetic acid	2 mL
Make volume up to 100 mL	

SOLUBLE STARCH (1%)

Ingredients	Grams
Soluble starch	1.0
Heated water	100.0

SULFURIC ACID (2N)

Ingredients	mL
Sulfuric acid	55.0 mL
Distilled water	45.0 mL
Make final up to 1000 mL	

Index